THE COSMOLOGICAL DOCTORS OF CLASSICAL GREECE

Why did some doctors in Classical Greece feel compelled to study the universe as a whole? How could cosmological principles be employed in clinical practice? This book explores the works of the cosmological doctors, such as *On Breaths, On Flesh,* and *On Regimen,* and argues that they form part of a much broader reorganization of medical knowledge in the fifth and fourth centuries BCE. These healers used cosmological principles as a supplement to, rather than a replacement of, more traditional approaches to health and disease, creating theories about the cosmos whose obscurities can best be understood as the products of medical thinking. Through fresh readings of many ancient sources, the book revises customary views of the intersections between medicine and cosmology in Classical Greece and advances our understanding of one of the most remarkable periods in the history of ancient thought.

DAVID H. CAMDEN holds the Alexander Smith Cochran Chair in Greek Language and Literature at St. Paul's School in Concord, NH. He obtained his doctorate in Classical Philology at Harvard University.

THE COSMOLOGICAL DOCTORS OF CLASSICAL GREECE

First Principles in Early Greek Medicine

DAVID H. CAMDEN

St Paul's School

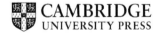

CAMBRIDGE
UNIVERSITY PRESS

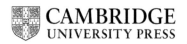

Shaftesbury Road, Cambridge CB2 8EA, United Kingdom

One Liberty Plaza, 20th Floor, New York, NY 10006, USA

477 Williamstown Road, Port Melbourne, VIC 3207, Australia

314–321, 3rd Floor, Plot 3, Splendor Forum, Jasola District Centre,
New Delhi – 110025, India

103 Penang Road, #05–06/07, Visioncrest Commercial, Singapore 238467

Cambridge University Press is part of Cambridge University Press & Assessment,
a department of the University of Cambridge.

We share the University's mission to contribute to society through the pursuit of
education, learning and research at the highest international levels of excellence.

www.cambridge.org
Information on this title: www.cambridge.org/9781009202992

DOI: 10.1017/9781009203012

First published 2023

A catalogue record for this publication is available from the British Library.

Library of Congress Cataloging-in-Publication Data
NAMES: Camden, David H., 1982– author.
TITLE: The cosmological doctors of classical Greece : first principles in early Greek
medicine / David H. Camden.
DESCRIPTION: Cambridge ; New York, NY : Cambridge University Press, 2023. |
Includes bibliographical references and indexes.
IDENTIFIERS: LCCN 2022058753 | ISBN 9781009202992 (hardback) |
ISBN 9781009203005 (paperback) | ISBN 9781009203012 (ebook)
SUBJECTS: LCSH: Medicine, Greek and Roman. | Cosmology, Ancient.
CLASSIFICATION: LCCR138 .C36 2023 | DDC 610.938–dc23/eng/20230302
LC record available at https://lccn.loc.gov/2022058753

ISBN 978-1-009-20299-2 Hardback

For Liz

Contents

Acknowledgments

I owe a great deal of thanks to many people, without whose support I would never have completed this project. Special thanks are due to Frances Fisher, who first introduced me to the study of the ancient world, and who is the indisputable *arche* for my interest in antiquity; my dissertation adviser and long-time mentor, Mark Schiefsky, to whom I owe much of my thinking about what early Greek medicine is all about; countless friends and teachers from Harvard, Emory, and St. Paul's School, too many to name here; my parents, Betty and Rodney Camden, and my brother, James; my sons, Benjamin and Henry Camden, whose energy, joy, and curiosity make me strive every day to do better; and most importantly, my best friend and wife, Elizabeth Engelhardt. This book is dedicated to her.

Citations and Abbreviations

With the exception of Galen, abbreviations of Greek authors and their works are taken from Liddell, Scott, and Jones, hereafter LSJ. Abbreviations for Latin authors are taken from Lewis and Short. Titles of Galen's works are abbreviated in accordance with the appendix to Nutton (2020). Works in the Hippocratic Corpus are first cited by their paragraph and section number, then by their volume and page number in Littré, hereafter L. The paragraph and section numbers are taken from the most recent editions, with preference given to the *Corpus Medicorum Graecorum*, Budé, and Loeb editions, in that order. All Greek texts are based on these same editions, although I have occasionally found it preferable to adopt my own readings, the most significant of which are explained in the footnotes. Where applicable, the works of Galen are cited according to their volume and page number in Kühn, hereafter K. The following abbreviations have also been used:

AbhMainz	*Abhandlungen der geistes- und sozialwissenschaftlichen Klasse der Akademie der Wissenschaften und der Literatur, Mainz*
AMT	Thompson, R. C. 1923. *Assyrian Medical Texts from the Originals in the British Museum.* Oxford University Press
BAM	Köcher, F. 1963–2007. *Babylonisch-assyrische Medizin in Texten und Untersuchungen.* De Gruyter
BNJ	*Brill's New Jacoby*
BNP	*Brill's New Pauly*
CP	*Classical Philology*
CQ	*The Classical Quarterly*
DK	Diels, H., and Kranz, W. 1952. *Die Fragmente der Vorsokratiker.* Sixth edition. Weidmann
HSCP	*Harvard Studies in Classical Philology*
IG	*Inscriptiones Graecae*

IStrat.	Sahin, M. C. (ed.). 1981–90. *Die Inschriften von Stratonikeia.* Habelt
JHS	*Journal of Hellenic Studies*
K–A	Kassel, R., and Austin, C. 1983–2001. *Poetae comici Graeci.* De Gruyter
OF	Bernabé, A. 2004–5. *Orphicorum et Orphicis similium testimonia et fragmenta*, vols. 1–2. Saur
RE	*Paulys Realencyclopädie der classischen Altertumswissenschaft*
REG	*Revue des Études Grecques*
SpTU	*Spätbabylonische Texte aus Uruk*
STT	Gurney, O., and Finkelstein, J. J. (eds.). 1957–64. *The Sultantepe Tablets.* British Institute of Archaeology at Ankara

Unless otherwise noted, all translations are my own.

Introduction

I.1 The "Cosmological Doctors"

On the broadest possible application of the term, we all engage in "cosmology" whenever we step back from the world of everyday experience to talk about what is real, permanent, and universal. When Pericles tells the Athenian assembly that their power may one day diminish, "for all things naturally depreciate" (πάντα γὰρ πέφυκε καὶ ἐλασσοῦσθαι, Th. 2.64.3), or when the Athenians inform the Melians that they will not relent, for the stronger rule the weaker "on all occasions by a natural necessity" (διὰ παντὸς ὑπὸ φύσεως ἀναγκαίας, Th. 5.105.2), these speakers offer "cosmological" explanations in the sense that they account for specific actions or events by appealing to the operation of universal laws. In these two examples, the fall of the Athenian empire and the invasion of Melos are historically defined events, confined to a specific point in time, but they are governed by principles that hold true διὰ παντός (at all times and in all places). The principles underlying these events are "cosmological" in the sense that they present the world as a cosmos, a natural order that is both consistent and universal. The cosmologist observes the orderly progression of nature – the rising and setting of the sun, the waxing and waning of the moon, the changes in the seasons, the rotation of the heavens – and extrapolates from these a more general assumption that all things form part of a natural order, which governs both the world around us and, by implication, our own interactions with that world.

The following study concerns a group of physicians I will call, for lack of a better term, "cosmological doctors." These doctors all lived in the Greek-speaking world during the fifth and fourth centuries BCE. What defines them as "cosmologists" is their attempt to base the art of healing on the first principles of all things in general. The precise nature of their first principles varied greatly depending on the author. Some of these doctors focused on the material elements from which all things are composed. Others emphasized the fundamental "powers" (δυνάμεις) that govern all things. Many isolated the general patterns that can be found in all corners of the universe, drawing analogies between the macrocosm of the universe and the microcosm of the human body. What unites these thinkers is not the identity of their first principles but their emphasis on the *universality* of such principles. These doctors isolated principles that govern all things in general, and they applied those principles to the everyday practice of treating and preventing disease.[1]

For most students of Greek literature, the best-known example of a "cosmological doctor" is the physician Eryximachus. His speech in Plato's *Symposium* defines *eros* ("love") as a universal power, present "in the bodies of all animals, in the things that grow in the earth, and in practically all that is" (ὡς ἔπος εἰπεῖν ἐν πᾶσι τοῖς οὖσι, 186a). In support of this thesis, Eryximachus constructs what amounts to an argument by induction. He compares the role of *eros* in six crafts (medicine, gymnastics, agriculture, music, astronomy, and divination) in order to show that this principle "extends over everything, both human and divine" (186b) and "has a great, a strong, nay an absolute power" (188d). The Hippocratic treatise *On Breaths* describes *pneuma* ("breath, wind") in similar terms. *Pneuma* is "the greatest potentate in the universe and over the universe" (μέγιστος ἐν τοῖσι πᾶσι τῶν πάντων δυνάστης, 3.2, 6.94 L.), and it is also the "starting point and source" (ἀρχὴ καὶ πηγή, 1.4, 6.92 L.) of all diseases in the sick. *On Regimen* asserts that all animals, including humans, are composed of fire and water. Fire has the "power" (δύναμις) to move all things, water the power to nourish all things, and these two substances are "sufficient in themselves, both for each other and for everything else" (αὐτάρκεά ἐστι τοῖσί τε ἄλλοισι πᾶσι καὶ ἀλλήλοισιν, 3.1, 6.472 L.). Another text, *On Flesh*, presents anatomy in a framework of anthropogony. It begins by dividing the cosmos into the hot, the cold, and the wet, and it then explains how each part of the body, with the aid of the "fatty" (τὸ λιπαρόν) and the "glutinous" (τὸ κολλῶδες), arose from these three substances. Then there is the *Anonymus Londiniensis*, a first-century papyrus that summarizes earlier medical theories, which mentions several Greek doctors with an interest in cosmology. To cite just one example, Philistion of Locri is said to have held that humans are composed of four "forms" (ἰδέαι): fire, air, water, and earth. To each of these forms he

---

[1] Of course, it is impossible to know whether all the figures I call "cosmological doctors" were *personally* engaged in the treatment of patients. For the sake of this study, I will use the terms "doctor" and "physician" very loosely to refer to anyone who presents the treatment and prevention of disease as their primary field of interest.

assigned a "power" (δύναμις). To fire he assigned the hot, to air the cold, to water the wet, and to earth the dry (XX.25–37).[2]

This list could be expanded with other known cosmological doctors: figures such as Petron of Aegina, the unnamed opponents of *On Ancient Medicine*, and Polybus of Cos (the presumptive author of the treatise *On the Nature of the Human Being*). Together, they suggest that the Classical period was a time when many Greek doctors were interested in cosmology. It was a time when medical writers were attempting to base the art of healing on a limited number of principles, generalized to the highest possible degree, while asserting that the same "powers" (δυνάμεις) that govern the universe in its entirety are also the "starting point" (ἀρχή) of all changes in the body. As the author of *On Ancient Medicine* succinctly notes, many doctors in this period were attempting to speak or write about medicine "after laying down a foundation for their account" (ὑπόθεσιν αὐτοὶ ἑωυτοῖσιν ὑποθέμενοι τῷ λόγῳ, 1.1, 1.570 L.). They were "narrowing down the starting point of the cause [τὴν ἀρχὴν τῆς αἰτίης] of diseases and death for human beings," and making that starting point "the same for all," setting up "one or two" principles like "the hot, the cold, the wet, the dry – or whatever else they please" (1.1, 1.570 L.).

One of the goals of this study is to understand how these cosmological doctors came to be. What led them to adopt such universalizing theories, and what can their theories tell us about the priorities of Greek doctors in the fifth and fourth centuries BCE? These questions are not easy to answer, primarily because the intermixture of medicine with cosmology cannot be attributed to any single, centralized authority. There was no "school" of cosmological medicine, no one thinker to whom all of these doctors were responding. Nowadays, most would agree that an important role was played by the "inquiry into nature" (περὶ φύσεως ἱστορία), the tradition of cosmological speculation that is commonly said to have begun with Thales, Anaximander, and Anaximenes of Miletus in the sixth century BCE. It is now generally agreed that this tradition lent authority and inspiration to the cosmological doctors. The precise nature of its contribution, however, has never been clearly defined.[3]

---

[2] Such, at least, is the doxographical report. My own reservations about this report can be found in Chapter 1.

[3] The phrase "inquiry into nature" comes from Plato (*Phd.* 96a; cf. *Ly.* 214a–b, *Prt.* 315c, *Phlb.* 59a, *Ti.* 47a), although echoes of this expression can be found in other texts from the Classical period (e.g., Heraclit. DK 22 B123, Emp. DK 31 B110.5, Philol. DK 44 B1, B6, Archyt. DK 47 B1, Critias DK 88 B19.2, E. fr. 910 K, *Dialex.* 8.1, and X. *Mem.* 1.1.11, 1.1.14). On the cosmological scope of these inquiries, see Long (1999) and Laks (2006: 6–12), both of whom argue that a common goal of these

I.2 Medicine and Philosophy?

In previous treatments of the cosmological doctors, scholars have tended to begin with the framework of medicine's interactions with "philosophy." Under this rubric, the cosmological doctors are presented as either aspiring participants in the "inquiry into nature" or as passive recipients of philosophy's spreading influence. In the third volume of his *Paideia: The Ideals of Greek Culture*, Jaeger (1944: 4–16) exemplifies this approach when he describes a three-stage process of mutual influence between medicine and philosophy: first, philosophy influenced medicine, then medicine philosophy, and finally philosophy and medicine fell in danger of being confused. "It was entirely natural," Jaeger concludes, "that, when the great concepts of natural philosophy were taken over into medicine, its cosmological ideas should enter along with them and disturb men's minds." Jaeger's characterization of cosmology as something that "entered into" medicine can be found in numerous accounts of the cosmological doctors. It has its roots in a modern tendency to distinguish "medicine" from "philosophy," to separate "empirical" doctors, the supposed forerunners of positive science, from their more ambitious, "philosophical" colleagues. As one commentator writes in reference to *On Flesh*, "it is difficult to see that π. σαρκῶν is typically a 'medical' treatise, in spite of its self-description in its first sentence. It is certainly not concerned practically with medicine."[4] Another says of *On Regimen* and *On Flesh* that they were written by "a new type of doctor, a very attractive type, because he tries to achieve *avant la lettre* a kind of symbiosis between positive science and philosophical thought."[5] Many historians have described the cosmological doctors as sophists, "health experts" – anything but real doctors.[6] They were "under the influence of philosophy," following its lead "to so great a degree as to interfere with and destroy the positive scientific outlook."[7] In other words, the cosmological doctors were not just nonmedical; they were *antithetical* to medicine. Jones captures this sentiment when he writes that "During the

---

investigations was to provide a comprehensive account of "the totality of things" (τὰ πάντα). Sometimes, these inquiries were also associated with the word *kosmos*, the "order" that structures the world in which we live (cf. E. fr. 910 K, X. *Mem.* 1.1.11, Pl. *Grg.* 508a, *Ti.* 27a, and *Phlb.* 29e), although there is disagreement over the precise point at which the word *kosmos* came to mean not just "order" but a "world-order" (for which see Horky 2019). In this study, the phrase "inquiry into nature" will function as a shorthand for all cosmological speculations *except* those produced by the cosmological doctors. It should be stressed, however, that my use of such terminology is primarily a matter of convenience. No sense of unity, differentiation, or self-awareness should be presupposed in my employment of this phrase.

[4] Peck (1936: 62).   [5] Bourgey (1953: 124).   [6] For the term "health expert," see pp. 206–207.
[7] Miller (1949: 314).

fifth century B.C. philosophy made a determined effort to bring medicine within the sphere of its influence. . . . Medicine was here face to face with a deadly enemy."[8]

More recently, scholars have moved away from this narrative of a single, true "medicine" struggling against its enemies. Instead, it has been pointed out that "medicine" and "philosophy" were fluid concepts in the Classical period, and that any boundary between these two disciplines was liable to be crossed by doctors and philosophers alike.[9] In some cases, we see this overlap between "medicine" and "philosophy" explicitly mentioned in Classical Greek literature. In the *Phaedo*, Plato cites investigations into human physiology as an integral part of the "inquiry into nature" (96a–c). Elsewhere, he refers to Egyptians who study "everything concerning the cosmos down to divination and the art of healing that aims at health" (*Ti.* 24b–c). Aristotle twice notes that investigations "concerning nature" should conclude with the first principles of health and disease, while the best doctors tend to begin their inquiries with first principles derived from philosophy (*Sens.* 436a17–b1, *Resp.* 480b21–30). In *On Ancient Medicine*, the author complains about certain doctors and "sophists" who speculate about the fundamental constitution of human beings (20.1, 1.620 L.). Such speculations, he asserts, are not relevant to medicine but rather "tend towards philosophy, just like Empedocles or others who have written, concerning nature, what a human being is from the beginning, how it originally came to be, and from what it was compounded." By arguing for a clear demarcation between medicine and "philosophy," the author of *On Ancient Medicine* reinforces the idea that, at the time of his writing, such a demarcation did not yet exist. Anyone could give a speech, participate in a debate, or disseminate a text about "nature" (φύσις). The intended audience of such a contribution included both medical practitioners and educated laymen, who were in turn expected to develop their own opinions on whatever was being discussed.

---

[8] Jones (1923b: xlv). For further designations of philosophy as an "enemy" of medicine, see Jones (1923a: xxiv, 1946: 23–25), Longrigg (1963: 150–155, 2001: 29–33), Ducatillon (1977: 89), and Thivel (1981: 145, 254). Jouanna (1999: 259) picks up on this language of opposition when he writes that "the debate over medicine and philosophy is at the very heart of the Hippocratic Collection as a whole" and that "the essential problem of method that was debated had to do with the relation of medicine to philosophy." Note also Vegetti's (1976: 11) description of *On Regimen* as a work "of non-Hippocratic inspiration" and Mansfeld's (1980a: 347) assertion that "a consistently cosmological brand of medicine is to be found only in marginal treatises of the *Corpus*" – both attempts to separate the cosmological doctors from more "professional" experts in health and disease.

[9] Thivel (1983: 221), Orelli (1998), Craik (1998: 2–3, 2015: xviii, 2018: 218–219), Lloyd (2002), Agge (2004: 13), Nutton (2004: 44), van der Eijk (2005a: 8–14, 2018: 304–307), and Laks and Most (2016b: 298–299). An early expression of this point can already be found in Heidel (1914: 153).

This "fluid-boundary" explanation for the cosmological doctors stresses the sheer openness of intellectual discourse in the Classical period. It explains why Greek doctors were *permitted* to speculate about the cosmos, but it does little to clarify the precise origins, motivations, and methods of the doctors who sought out the first principles of all things. Even if we say that the Classical period saw no clear demarcation between "medicine" and "philosophy," we do little to challenge the modern assumption that "philosophy" is still the most appropriate label for defining cosmological thinking. To cite one recent example, Bartoš (2015) provides one of the most sensible analyses of a cosmological doctor to have appeared in modern scholarship. However, even he separates the "medical" and "philo-sophical" interests of his subject, observing that the author of *On Regimen*'s "elemental theory may seem obsolete from the dietetic and medical point of view ... but regarding the tradition of philosophical inquiries into nature, it is an appropriate device for explaining natural processes" (98–99). For most historians of ancient thought, "philosophy" remains the preferred category for approaching the systems of the cosmological doctors. The upshot, of course, is that when these doctors are said to combine medicine with "philosophy," it is still generally supposed that they are either undermining the former for the sake of the latter or else creating an amalgam in which the "philosophical" elements can easily be separated from the "medical."

For my part, I prefer to avoid any reference to the cosmological doctors as practicing a "philosophical" brand of medicine. I do not object to this term on the ground that these physicians should not qualify as "philo-sophers." Instead, I wish to stress that an equation between "cosmology" and "philosophy" oversimplifies what it means to investigate first prin-ciples. On the one hand, many participants in the inquiry into nature were devoted cosmologists, by which I mean their primary objective was to understand and describe the universe as a whole. However, cosmology can also be a framework for organizing and explaining *other* sciences, a mode of high-level thinking that elucidates phenomena by referring to the funda-mental nature of all things. A doctor might take some principle from his clinical experience (e.g., hot compresses draw fluids from the body), compare that principle with other, nonclinical phenomena (e.g., the sun draws water from the sea), and further generalize it so that it applies not merely to the body but to the universe as a whole (e.g., heat attracts all fluids). If the doctor then applies this new principle to other, related aspects of clinical decision-making, we would say that he is thinking in "cosmological" terms. That does not mean, however, that the doctor has necessarily departed from a specifically "medical" mode of thought.

By equating cosmology with "philosophy" and by assuming that cosmological speculations are the exclusive purview of "philosophers," we run the risk of ignoring what the doctors themselves might have brought to the table. Furthermore, if we assume that cosmology was simply imported into medicine, we are forced to choose between several unsatisfactory explanations for how the cosmological doctors came to be. It has often been asserted, for example, that the introduction of cosmology into medicine was *unavoidable* given the influence of the inquiry into nature. According to Festugière (1948: xix), "It was inevitable that the physicians of Ionia, in their investigation of the cause of the evils which afflict human nature, would have recourse to the theories elaborated by their compatriots concerning universal Nature." Similarly, Lonie (1981: 56) writes that "Greek speculative medicine could hardly avoid being governed, to a very large extent indeed, by the concepts and the categories of pre-Socratic philosophy," implying that this movement was so transformative that Greek doctors could not help but be swept along with it. Some have attributed the entire phenomenon of cosmological medicine to the influence of one or more participants in the inquiry into nature. In these studies, one commonly finds references to supposed "schools" of cosmological medicine, whether they are Empedocles's "Sicilian school" or even the "Eleatic school" of Parmenides and his followers.[10] It has also been popular to attribute the beginning of cosmological medicine to Alcmaeon of Croton, a shadowy figure who is sometimes presumed to have invented the definition of health as the balance between pairs of opposing powers.[11] One problem with such great-man narratives, of course, is that the works of the cosmological doctors contain widely disparate opinions about the nature of

---

[10] On the "Sicilian school" of medicine, sometimes also labeled the "Italian" or "West Greek" school to incorporate the Pythagoreans of southern Italy, see Wellmann (1901), Burnet (1930: 200–202), Diller (1938), Bidez and Leboucq (1944), Jones (1946: 10–13), Vegetti (1976: 43–45), Gourevitch (1989), Longrigg (1993: 104–148, 2001: 35–36), Michler (2003), Barton (2005), Sisko (2006), and Primavesi (2009). For the supposed "Eleatic" origin of tracing all diseases back to a single cause, see Littré (1839, vol. 1: 559), followed by Kühn (1956: 33n1); note also Thivel (1981, 1992), who attempts to distinguish a "West Greek" (i.e., Eleatic, Pythagorean, Empedoclean) group of doctors from those who adopted an "Ionian" outlook. On the assignment of the cosmological doctors to the "Cnidian school" of medicine, a debunked categorization once advocated by scholars such as Ilberg (1894), Gomperz (1901: 285–288), and Rey (1946: 420–444), see the bibliographical survey of Thivel (1981: 58–63, 86n233, 154–155).

[11] See Jones (1923a: xi, 1946: 3–6), Wellmann (1929, 1930: 301–302), Kahn (1960: 190), Kudlien (1970: 4–5), Mudry (1982: 60), Longrigg (1993: 48), Jouanna (1999: 262), and Cruse (2004: 34). The one testimony that reports Alcmaeon's definition of health (quoted on p. 36) never actually says that he was the first person to hold this view.

the universe. If these doctors were simply followers of this or that cosmologist, we would expect their systems to have many more details in common. At the very least, we would expect them to engage in similar *forms* of cosmological thinking, but whereas some of these doctors focused on the material elements from which all things are composed, others simply speculated about the fundamental forces that have more "power" than anything else.

Some have suggested that the works of the cosmological doctors were influenced by Zoroastrianism or the Ayurvedic healers of ancient India.[12] These suggestions, like other attempts to emphasize the influence of outside thinkers, are worthy of investigation when limited to particular details, but when they are used to explain entire systems, or even, in some instances, the entire phenomenon of cosmological medicine, they feed into a more general tendency to view cosmological medicine as somehow aberrant and therefore only explicable by pointing to some external origin. Götze (1923: 79) justifies the supposed Zoroastrian origin of *On Sevens* (another work by a cosmological doctor) by observing that this text is "an erratic block in Hellas." West (1971: 385–388), by contrast, stresses that *On Sevens* is "far from being an erratic block," being "put together from parts that very obviously belong in a known tradition of speculation."[13] West further adds that "In approaching the question of non-Greek material ... we should not think in terms of any direct influence upon the work before us, but at most of the absorption of such material into a certain current of Greek thought at an earlier period." Like other Greek thinkers from the Classical period, the cosmological doctors speculated about the universe in ways that have certain echoes in other cultures. That does not mean, however, that the entire phenomenon of cosmological medicine can be explained by simply pointing to these parallels. Even if we presume the transference of some ideas from one culture to the next, we would still need to explain the conditions that made these ideas attractive to Greek-speaking healers of the fifth and fourth centuries BCE.

Other attempts to explain the cosmological doctors have simply listed all the benefits that come from cosmology: it is comprehensive, precise, persuasive, easy to teach, distinguishes one doctor from another, and so

---

[12] For example, Götze (1923), Ilberg (1925: 6), van der Eijk (2004), Craik (2015: xxxi), and Matsui and Cornelli (2017: 30n19).

[13] On this point, see already Wellmann (1933) and Kranz (1938), both of whom stress the many parallels between *On Sevens* and other Greek descriptions of the cosmos. Compare also Duchesne-Guillemin (1956).

on. Building off of statements from *On Ancient Medicine*, Schiefsky (2005) endorses all of these points while further suggesting that the cosmological doctors could have been responding to outside criticisms that the "art" of medicine does not actually exist, which spurred them to give medicine the "starting point" (ἀρχή) and "method" (ὁδός) that would make it qualify as a genuine "craft" (τέχνη). As we will see, such concern for medicine's status and methods was certainly a contributing factor to the rise of the cosmological doctors. However, a more precise explanation is needed to account for why these doctors would have taken their "starting points" all the way to cosmological principles. As for the idea that cosmology distinguishes one doctor from another, this explanation has been especially popular in modern scholarship, fostered by a heightened interest in the medical marketplace and in the physician's basic need to persuade.[14] I find it difficult, however, to understand how a full-blown cosmology is more persuasive than, say, a detailed theory of human physiology, especially since cosmological principles were notoriously susceptible to differing interpretations and were therefore viewed with suspicion by many people in the Classical period. Cosmologists were parodied in comedy, accused of impiety, and ridiculed for speculating about matters that were invisible, irrelevant, and ultimately irresolvable. If the cosmological doctors were simply looking for more students, more patients, or a higher place in society, why would they select such a controversial framework as "the things on high and under the earth" for presenting their views on disease? It is of course possible, even likely, that the cosmological doctors were interested in propping up both their own reputations and the reputation of their art. Before we factor in such social pressures, however, we need to understand why these doctors considered cosmological principles a viable option in the first place.[15]

The greatest shortcoming in all of these explanations is that they can be made with little knowledge of early Greek medical thought. In fact, they all treat medicine as a blank slate upon which new systems could be imposed. Medicine, of course, was not a blank slate. Greek doctors had their own traditional views on the etiology of disease, and they engaged in elaborate programs of medical inquiry in which they categorized phenomena in terms of commonalities and differences,

---

[14] For a discussion that emphasizes this explanation, see Chang (2008).
[15] A fuller rebuttal of this explanation will be offered in Chapter 4, where we will further see that many cosmological doctors actually sought to limit the extent to which they speculated about "the things on high" – an observation that does not lend itself well to the claim that these doctors engaged in cosmology primarily because they wanted to impress their patients.

universals and particulars at the same time that they speculated about the universe as a whole. To the best of my knowledge, no one has ever investigated how these preexisting theories and methods of inquiry may have contributed to the rise of cosmological doctors. In our haste to drive a wedge between medicine and "philosophy," we have awkwardly separated the cosmological doctors from the rest of the medical tradition.

I.3   The Scope of This Study

In this study, I will examine the cosmological doctors from a medical point of view. In particular, I will argue that if we want to understand how this phenomenon came to be, we need to consider the changing priorities of medical thinking in the fifth and fourth centuries BCE. By taking this approach, I do not intend to minimize or otherwise downplay the influence of the inquiry into nature on the cosmological doctors. Without a preexisting tradition of cosmological speculation, it is highly unlikely that this development would have ever taken shape. What I am stressing in this study is not that we should completely separate the cosmological doctors from other thinkers who inquired into the nature of all things. Rather, I intend to show that a simple gesture toward the inquiry into nature is insufficient for explaining how these doctors came to be.[16] In recent years, the monolithic edifice of "Presocratic philosophy" has given way to more specialized inquiries into the motivations and methods of individual thinkers. As a result, we are better able to understand how cosmological speculations were not simply a back-and-forth dialectic between self-identified "philosophers" but a multivalent mode of thinking that found reflection in many corners of Greek culture, a phenomenon that involved some fierce intellectual exchanges, to be sure, but that also needs to be placed within a broader range of social, religious, and cultural contexts. This study is a further step in the direction of complicating the old streamlined understanding of the inquiry into nature. It is not an investigation of medicine and philosophy but an exploration of what the cosmos meant to Greek doctors in the fifth and fourth centuries BCE. Along the way, I will of course have many opportunities to draw connections between the cosmological doctors and other thinkers who speculated

---

[16] On the need to take care when discussing lines of influence between the inquiry into nature and Greek medical texts, see Heidel (1914: 152–154), Jouanna (1992), Orelli (1998), Laks (1998, 2008: 260–262), and Schiefsky (2005: 2–3, 46–55).

about the universe as a whole. As I hope to show over the course of this study, however, we will ultimately arrive at more interesting conclusions if we ask why the cosmological doctors thought they *needed* to describe the first principles of all things before we consider their reliance on the theories of other thinkers.

My analysis will be divided into six chapters and a conclusion. First, I will examine three secondhand reports: (1) the testimonies on Petron and Philistion in the *Anonymus Londiniensis*, (2) the speech of Eryximachus in Plato's *Symposium*, and (3) *On Ancient Medicine*. I will then examine the four most important works by cosmological doctors to have survived from the Classical period: *On the Nature of the Human Being, On Breaths, On Flesh*, and *On Regimen*. For the sake of avoiding unnecessary distractions, I have chosen to omit any discussion of *On Sevens*. Nearly all the original Greek of this text has been lost, surviving only in a corrupt Latin translation.[17] In addition, there is significant disagreement about when *On Sevens* was written. Whereas some have dated the cosmological portion of this text as early as the sixth century BCE, Mansfeld (1971) has argued that it was actually composed half a millennium later, in the first century CE. To do this work justice would require a separate study in itself.[18] For a similar reason, I have also chosen to omit extended investigations into thinkers who have traditionally been grouped under the heading of "Presocratics." Figures such as Empedocles, Anaxagoras, Diogenes, Democritus, Hippon, and Philolaus had much to say about the human

---

[17] Of the fifty-two chapters in *On Sevens*, only nine survive in the original Greek, plus a few fragments from another seven. Some portions of the text are also preserved in the Arabic translation of a pseudo-Galenic commentary. For an edition of this commentary (with German translation), see Bergsträsser (1914). On the Latin translation, preserved in two ninth-century manuscripts, see Agge (2004: 19–23).

[18] Mansfeld's late date has attracted many challenges (e.g., Lebedev 2014: 92–93), but also some notable endorsements (e.g., Huffman 1993: 217). Compare also Thivel (1981: 227n221). Doubts over Mansfeld's dating have increased in recent years, with Craik (2015: 128) observing that "There is nothing to rule out a date in the fifth century BC." West (1971) dates the cosmological portion of *On Sevens* to the Classical period and provides what is still an essential discussion of the text. Further complicating the analysis of *On Sevens* are two modern claims about its process of composition. First, it has been asserted that *On Sevens* originated as two separate works composed by two different authors, one of whom wrote about the microcosm–macrocosm relationship (chapters 1–11), while the other discussed various aspects of fevers (chapters 13–53). Second, it has been claimed that certain passages *within* these two parts were added or changed in later periods. On these and other issues with the text, see the general overview of de la Villa Polo (2003: 453–471). By omitting a full analysis of *On Sevens*, I do not intend to endorse any of the above-mentioned conclusions about the composition and/or dating of this text. Instead, I simply believe that the many problems surrounding this work cannot be adequately addressed within the limits of this study. I will occasionally refer to *On Sevens*, but a separate chapter devoted to this text would have unreasonably extended what has already become a lengthy project.

body. Some of them even wrote separate works on the topic. However, my goal in this study is not to understand the place of anatomy, physiology, pathology, and therapeutics within the broader narratives of the inquiry into nature. Instead, my goal, as stated earlier, is to explore why some doctors for whom those topics were *paramount* felt compelled to also study the universe as whole. It would of course be interesting to come back to the inquiry into nature after arriving at a clearer picture of the cosmological doctors. It has been proposed that some figures such as Empedocles and Diogenes were practicing physicians, and it would therefore be interesting to compare their systems with the works presented in this study. It would also be interesting to think more generally about the intersections between cosmology and biology in the Classical period,[19] to explore the role of cosmology among medical writers of the Hellenistic and Roman periods,[20] and to compare the Greek phenomenon of cosmological medicine with the healing traditions of China, India, and other ancient civilizations. These are all worthwhile topics, for which I hope the present study will offer some support, but to take full account of such issues would have necessitated a very different book.

In Chapter 1, I will start by clearing away some common misconceptions about the cosmological doctors. Most importantly, I will point out that an interest in cosmological principles does not preclude more traditional explanations of health and disease. Petron, Philistion, and Eryximachus all combine their first principles with lower-level discussions of the humors, *pneuma*, and the "powers" of food and drink. Instead of replacing humors with cosmic principles, these doctors constructed multitiered narratives of pathogenesis, placing humors and cosmic principles at different points in the causal chain.[21] I will also point out that we can better understand some of the

---

[19] On this topic, see Jouanna (1999: 262–268), Zatta (2019), and the recent collection of essays in Salles (2021).

[20] Galen, of course, is the best-known example of a cosmological doctor from the Roman period. Also worthy of consideration would be the fragments of Asclepiades's *On Elements*, the "Pneumatic" school of medicine, and even the so-called commonalities of the Methodists.

[21] In this study, I will use the word "humor" as a shorthand for any bodily fluid that plays a determining role in either producing disease or maintaining health. There was no universally accepted term for "humor" in the Classical period, although the most common vocabulary refers to these bodily fluids as either "juices" or "moisture" (e.g., χυμός, χυλός, ἰκμάς, τὸ ὑγρόν). The precise identity of these fluids varied greatly from one author to the next. Depending on the author, a list of "humors" might include blood, bile, and phlegm, or alternatively flavor-juices like the sweet, the pungent, the acid, and the bitter, other fluids such as brine, water, or "serum" (ἰχώρ), or various combinations thereof. Greek authors postulated different numbers of humors, ranging from one to "myriad" (cf. *VM* 14.4, 1.602 L., *Nat. Hom.* 2, 6.34–36 L.). Some of these authors attached inherent flavors to the humors (referring, e.g., to "bitter bile" and "salty phlegm"), some associated them with various combinations of the hot, the cold, the wet, and the dry (although there was disagreement

more obscure aspects of these doctors' systems (e.g., Eryximachus's reference to a "healthy" and a "diseased" *eros* that exist within the body and are nourished by different things) by considering preexisting, widely attested beliefs about human physiology. After establishing this connection between more traditional theories of pathogenesis and the speculations of the cosmological doctors, I will then demonstrate that the polemical *On Ancient Medicine* is an unreliable witness to what the cosmological doctors were doing. Whereas the author of this text claims that the prioritizing of such principles as the hot and the cold is incompatible with the attribution of diseases to the humors, I will show that the cosmological doctors were in fact more than comfortable with combining first principles with more traditional beliefs about the body.

After making this observation, I will then turn in Chapter 2 to consider the relationship between cosmological principles and clinical decision-making. If the cosmological doctors still attributed diseases to substances like the humors, how did they incorporate cosmological principles into their systems of treatment? My investigation of this question will center around *On the Nature of the Human Being*, whose author I identify as Polybus of Cos. In this text, Polybus claims that the humors, like everything else, are composed of four primary substances: the hot, the cold, the dry, and the wet.[22] Polybus further claims that changes in these four qualities are

about which qualities should be attached to which humor, or even whether such qualities can be said to be inherent in the humors themselves), and we also commonly see the humors divided into subtypes (e.g., "white phlegm," "yellow bile," "black bile," etc.), which can be considered either subordinate to the humor after which they are named or even parallel with it. Some medical writers even claimed that one humor could change into another (e.g., *Anon. Lond.* XI.43–XII.8, *VM* 24, 1.634–636 L.). The familiar four-humor theory of blood, phlegm, yellow bile, and black bile is only fully developed in a single text from this period, *On the Nature of the Human Being*. Its widespread acceptance in later periods was due to the influence of Galen. Despite this variety of beliefs about the humors, it is remarkable that *some* version of humoral pathology can be found in virtually every text in the Hippocratic Corpus, suggesting that the attribution of diseases to bodily fluids was simply taken for granted by many, perhaps even all, of the authors in this collection. When I refer to more "traditional" explanations of health and disease, I am therefore referring to such lower-level beliefs about bodily fluids playing a role in pathogenesis rather than to any specific schematization of these fluids.

[22] As we will see in this study, Greek thinkers often refer to "the hot," "the cold," "the dry," and "the wet" as material substances that can combine, separate, interact with one another, and even undergo qualitative change. In Greek, these substances are usually denoted by combining the definite article with a neuter adjective (τὸ θερμόν, τὸ ψυχρόν, τὸ ξηρόν, τὸ ὑγρόν), which may have encouraged their treatment as material entities. Although the powers of heating, cooling, drying, and moistening were presumed to be inherent in these substances, it was often supposed that such qualities would not necessarily be perceptible, especially when they form part of a larger mixture. In Chapter 5, we will see the author of *On Flesh* constructing parts of the human body from various combinations of the hot, the cold, and the wet. In Chapter 6, we will find the author of *On Regimen* claiming that fire

responsible for the ebbing and flowing of four humors in the body, and that diseases can be prevented by treating "opposites with opposites"; that is, by counteracting the hot with the cold, the cold with the hot, the dry with the wet, and the wet with the dry. After establishing this theoretical framework, Polybus then appends a series of chapters that primarily focus on the topic of humoral flux. "Flux" is the idea that a single humor, after gathering in one part of the body, can create a wide range of effects by flowing to different parts. In this chapter, I will argue that Polybus's thinking about cosmological principles is closely tied to his interest in humoral flux. Both concepts are motivated by an interest in tracing diseases to their "source" (ἀρχή), and both ultimately establish a two-pronged approach to treatment, wherein doctors are expected to target both the proximate cause of a disease (i.e., a concentrated humor) and its remote cause (i.e., the factor(s) that initially caused that humor to separate out). Within this causal framework, the treatment of "opposites with opposites" is only applied to a disease's remote cause. The proximate cause, meanwhile, is still treated by identifying and then purging harmful humors from the body. In the final section of this chapter, I will observe that Polybus's emphasis on tracing diseases to their "source" is also tied to a more general interest in commonality and difference. Polybus is deeply interested in the many variables that can change from one case to the next, believing that treatments should be adjusted to the age, sex, habits, and physical constitution of the patient, the geographical location, the season of the year, and the fashion of the disease. However, such an interest in individual differences does not preclude a coexisting interest in cosmological principles. Instead, Polybus presents his cosmological principles as a solution to the problem of individual variation, identifying the shared "nature" (φύσις) of human beings as a high-level commonality that transcends individual differences.

---

contains the hot and the dry and water the cold and the wet, but also adding that fire simultaneously contains a certain amount of the wet, while water simultaneously contains a certain amount of the dry. Since these substances were viewed as material entities, Greek thinkers were generally comfortable with claiming that a single object might contain both members of a polarity at the same time. As Lloyd (1966: 81n1) observes, "The Greeks tended to consider 'hot' and 'cold' not as relative positions on a single temperature scale, so much as separate and distinct substances." Lloyd further observes that the words normally translated as "wet" and "dry" do not simply refer to the presence or absence of water; these adjectives also distinguish substances that are "solid" (= ξηρός) from those that are not (= ὑγρός, a term that encompasses both fluids and gases).

In Chapter 3, I will apply these lessons from *On the Nature of the Human Being* to the supposedly "radical" thesis of *On Breaths*. I will argue that the author's attribution of all diseases to *pneuma* is not as revolutionary as it initially appears. By relying on widely attested views about what *pneuma* tends to do within the body, this author is in fact remarkably conservative when constructing his own theories of pathogenesis. After making this point, I will then turn to the more important question of why this author felt compelled to identify a single cause of all diseases. On the one hand, we can point to the same interest in remote and proximate causes that we see in *On the Nature of the Human Being*. So many diseases are caused by *pneuma*, which naturally flows through the vessels and is the primary agent of bodily change, that the best way to ward off an illness is to remove anything that introduces noxious *pneuma* into the body. In this way, the author resembles Polybus in his application of cosmological principles to the *remote* cause of a disease, while the proximate cause does not deviate from more familiar narratives of pathogenesis. We should therefore resist the modern tendency to place *On Breaths* outside the "mainstream" of the Hippocratic Corpus; this author's views are not as radical as they often are portrayed. Of course, the otherwise practical consideration of remote and proximate causes does not explain why the author of *On Breaths* emphasizes the *universality* of his principle, and it also does not justify his more general assertion that *pneuma* is the most powerful force in the universe as a whole. On these points, the author seems to be driven by a separate "cosmological impulse," the belief that high-level commonalities, whatever their applicability, are inherently desirable and directly relevant to the medical art.

Chapter 4 addresses the central question of this study: how did cosmological medicine come to be? In this chapter, I will argue that the cosmological doctors arose as the result of a much wider realignment in Classical Greek medicine. As some doctors grew increasingly concerned about the many variables that can change from one case to the next, they rejected older forms of diagnostic handbooks in favor of new methods for organizing medical knowledge. We see this anxiety over individual differences not only in the works of the cosmological doctors but also in texts such as *On Regimen in Acute Diseases*, *Prognostic*, *Airs Waters Places*, and the seven books of *Epidemics*. In all of these texts, medical inquiry is defined, quite generally, as a search for commonalities. Doctors in this period were gathering together multiple accounts, noting the similarities and differences between those accounts, and isolating high-level generalizations that can unite and govern them all. Although the cosmological doctors took their search for commonalities farther than some of their contemporaries might have been willing to follow, they nevertheless responded to the same pressures that transformed nearly all the medical literature that survives from this period. Various social factors may have further encouraged some doctors to be more enthusiastic about their generalizations than others, but the very urge to generalize came from a research program that explicitly defined medical inquiry as the search for what is "common," a program that was itself driven by a central problem in clinical decision-making: the need to attain "precision" (ἀκρίβεια) when no two patients are exactly alike.

After providing this explanation for how the cosmological doctors came to be, I will turn to consider the details of their systems. In Chapter 5, I will propose solutions to some longstanding problems surrounding the anthropogony of *On Flesh*. First, I will show how the author's three main principles of the hot, the cold, and the wet reflect widely attested beliefs about the effects of heat and cold on bodily fluids. After that, I will argue that the author's two supplementary principles of the "fatty" and the "glutinous" are derived from a traditional dichotomy between bile and phlegm. The upshot of these observations is that the author of *On Flesh* uses the microcosm of the body as a tool for understanding the macrocosm of the universe. For this author, the natural world is primarily a reflection of the body (not the other way around), and it is specifically *medical* knowledge that gives him insight into the cosmos. Just as Eryximachus claims to have acquired his awareness of the universal power of *eros* "from medicine, our art" (ἐκ τῆς ἰατρικῆς, τῆς ἡμετέρας τέχνης, 186a), so the other cosmological doctors viewed medicine as a privileged starting point for contemplating the universe as a whole.[23]

In Chapter 6, I will conclude this study of the cosmological doctors with a wide-ranging consideration of *On Regimen*. This text is the longest and by far the most complex work by a cosmological doctor to have survived from the Classical period. Over the course of this chapter, I will show that *On Regimen* is a highly regular, unified, and richly detailed text. My most significant contribution will regard the author's views about divinity. As we will see, this author seems to consider the heavens to be the source of all souls within the universe. Anything that engenders either intelligence or movement is merely an emanation of this cosmic soul, and it represents

---

[23] For the microcosm–macrocosm analogy in the Hippocratic Corpus, see Olerud (1951), Joly (1960: 37–52), Magdelaine (1997), Le Blay (2005), Holmes (2010: 99–101), Bartoš (2015: 129–138), and Schluderer (2018). Democritus is usually credited with being the first person to explicitly state that "a human being is a small cosmos" (ἄνθρωπος μικρὸς κόσμος, DK 68 B34), although the underlying assumption that produced this analogy is attested already among the Milesians.

a unitary god from which all other divinities branch off. A brief consideration of this author's affinities with other thinkers will reinforce this interpretation. It will also illustrate how this understudied text can provide an invaluable lens for broadening our understanding of early Greek cosmology. As a medical writer, the author of *On Regimen* responded to pressures very different from what we see among other cosmologists. Nevertheless, he seems to have been deeply engaged with contemporary thinking about the cosmos, and therefore should serve as a helpful reminder that the Hippocratic Corpus is a critical resource for any student of Greek thought.

CHAPTER I

Three Secondhand Reports

1.1 *Anonymus Londiniensis*

The *Anonymus Londiniensis* is a Greek papyrus most commonly dated to the first century CE. It is divided into two parts, of which the first, sometimes called the *Menoneia*, draws on a Peripatetic source (perhaps the work of Menon, a collaborator of Aristotle) from the late fourth century BCE. This Peripatetic source was a collection of opinions on the etiology of disease. It was compiled under the direction of Aristotle, who saw the gathering and comparison of such opinions – a practice now known as "doxography" – as an important first step for the development of original theories. In addition to the work on medicine, Aristotle encouraged similar collections of opinions on mathematics, astronomy, and theology by Eudemus, as well as Theophrastus's *On Sensation* and the same author's widely influential *Opinions on Natural Philosophy*. Except for *On Sensation*, none of these collections have survived in their original form. Through intermediaries such as the *Anonymus Londiniensis*, however, we can access much of their content, providing invaluable insight into the early history of Greek thought.[1]

For our purposes, two entries in the *Anonymus Londiniensis* are of special interest. These are the entries for Petron of Aegina and Philistion of Locri, both of whom lived in the Classical period, sometime between 500 and 300 BCE.[2] Petron is datable from the report that Ariston was his student.[3] Galen mentions this Ariston alongside Euryphon, Phaon, and Philistion as

---

[1] In the *Anonymus Londiniensis*, there are entries for over twenty medical writers, seven of whom were unknown before the discovery of the papyrus. On the history of this papyrus and its relationship with Aristotle, see Manetti (1990, 1999a). For a modern edition, see Manetti (2011).

[2] On Petron (who is also called "Petronas" in some sources), see Deichgräber (1937), Touwaide (2007), and Manetti (2008b). On Philistion, see Wellmann (1901), Diller (1938), Nutton (2007a), Manetti (2008c), and Squillace (2017). The *Anonymus Londiniensis* also describes a third cosmological doctor, Polybus of Cos, whom we will discuss in Chapter 2.

[3] Anon. Paris. *De morbis acutis et chroniis* 10 (72.3–12 Garofalo).

a potential author of the treatise *On Regimen*, noting that all of these medical writers are "ancient" (παλαιοί) and that they are all either older than Hippocrates or contemporary with him.[4] Philistion, for his part, can be dated by his alleged connections with Eudoxus, Chrysippus, and Dionysius II of Syracuse. He is said to have taught medicine to both Eudoxus (ca. 390–340 BCE) and Chrysippus (*fl.* mid- to late fourth century BCE), while the Platonic *Second Letter* refers to Philistion's service in the court of Dionysius II, who ruled from 367 to 357 BCE.[5] On the strength of these testimonies, Manetti (2008c) suggests a *floruit* of 370–340 BCE for Philistion, although it is conceivable that he was active for several decades before this range.[6] Petron is at least one generation older than Philistion, which would place his birth at some unspecified point in the fifth century BCE.[7]

Beyond these biographical reports, very little is known about either Petron or Philistion outside the *Anonymus Londiniensis*. Petron is said to have administered the following treatment to fever patients: first, he covered them with blankets in order to encourage both heat and thirst; then, he administered a cold drink to purge the peccant humors through sweating and vomiting; and finally, he restored the patient's strength with roast meat and dark wine – a bold treatment that drew the attention of Erasistratus, Celsus, and Galen.[8] Philistion, meanwhile, is said to have described a machine for reducing dislocations (Orib. 4.344) and to have held a variety of opinions on anatomy and physiology. Among these opinions are the belief that respiration cools the body's innate heat and that drinks pass to the lungs – both

---

[4] Gal. *HVA* 15.455–456 K. See also Gal. *Alim. Fac.* 6.473 K., *Hipp. Aph.* 18a.8–9 K., and *Ind.* 26.

[5] D. L. 8.86, 8.89, Pl. [*Epist.*] 2, 314d–e. Like Ariston, Philistion is included in Galen's lists of "ancient" physicians; see Gal. *Alim. Fac.* 6.473 K., *MM* 10.27–28 K., and *HVA* 15.455–456 K. For a possible relationship between Philistion and Plato, see Pl. [*Epist.*] 2, 314d–e, where Plato is said to have invited Philistion to Athens, and Epicr. fr. 10 K–A, where a Sicilian doctor (unnamed but often assumed to be Philistion) is said to be present in Plato's Academy. There is also a modern tradition of detecting the influence of Philistion in Plato's *Timaeus*. In general, however, these discussions have not pointed out much that is uniquely "Philistionic," and they often invoke a supposed "Sicilian school" of medicine that modern historians are now finding increasingly difficult to accept (see note 48 in this chapter).

[6] Squillace (2017: 7) places him "between the end of the fifth century and the first half of the fourth century."

[7] Compare Jacques (2008), who dates Petron's "student" Ariston to 450–400 BCE, and Manetti (2008b), who dates Petron to 500–400 BCE.

[8] Gal. *HVA* 15.435–437 K., 15.451 K., [*Opt. Sect.*] 1.144 K., Cels. 3.9.2, and schol. T *ad Il.* 11.624. If neither sweating nor vomiting worked, Petron is said to have purged the patient's bowels with a saltwater drink. See also *Comp. Med. Gen.* 13.642 K., where Galen notes that he consulted Petron's works while trying to find the origin of a drug.

common assumptions in early Greek thought.[9] According to Rufus of
Ephesus, Philistion gave the name "eagles" (ἀετοί) to the temporal
vessels (*Onom.* 200–201), perhaps referring to their resemblance to
outspread wings.[10] To later generations, Philistion was especially famous as an authority on dietetics, which may explain his identification
as a potential author of the treatise *On Regimen*.[11] According to Pliny,
he recommended foodstuffs such as parsnips, cabbage, and basil for
a variety of diseases, including strangury, dropsy, tetanus, pleurisy,
epilepsy, jaundice, phrenitis, and cholera.[12] He is also said to have
drawn fine distinctions between different varieties of bread, noting
their powers to affect the body in accordance with their ingredients
and modes of preparation.[13] The specific powers that Philistion attributed to bread include the encouragement of either good or bad
humors and the production or repression of *pneuma*. He also appears
to have been very interested in digestion, noting how different varieties of bread are easier or more difficult to digest, are more or less
nourishing, and either relax or constrict the bowels.[14]

---

[9] Gal. *Ut. Resp.* 4.471 K., Plu. *Quaest. conv.* 699b–d, *De stoic. repugn.* 1047c–d, and Gell. *NA* 17.11.6.
On the use of respiration to cool the body's innate heat, compare *Anon. Lond.* XVIII.24–28
(Philolaus of Croton), *Cord.* 3, 9.82 L., 5, 9.84 L., *Hebd.* 8, and Pl. *Ti.* 70c–d. See also *P. Ebers*
855d with Bardinet (1995: 96). On the passage of drinks to the lungs, compare *Acut.* 15, 2.254–256 L.,
Morb. I 28, 6.196–198 L., *Int.* 23, 7.224 L., *Cord.* 2, 9.80–82 L., *Oss.* 1.2, 9.168 L., 13.2, 9.184–186 L.,
Alc. fr. 347a.1 Lobel–Page, Eup. fr. 158 K–A, E. fr. 983 K., and Pl. *Ti.* 70c, 91a, and note the
arguments against this view at *Morb. IV* 56, 7.604–608 L., Arist. *PA* 664b3–665a25, Erasistr. fr. 114
Garofalo and Macr. *Sat.* 7.15.1–24. For Philistion's general interest in anatomy and physiology, see
also Gal. *MM* 10.110–111 K. and *De anat.* 2.900–901 K.

[10] The term "ἀετός" was in fact applied to architectural gables for precisely this reason (LSJ s.v. ἀετός
IV). When the temporal artery becomes visible in patients with temporal arteritis, it displays
a distinctive "v" shape.

[11] For Philistion's status as an authority on dietetics, see Ath. 12.12 and Gal. [*Suc.*] 19.721 K.

[12] Plin. *HN* 20.xv.31 (parsnips), 20.xxxiv.86 (cabbage), and 20.xlviii.122 (basil). Although I have given
the traditional translations for these disease names, most of which are more or less transliterated
from the Greek, the reader should be aware that these ailments do not easily map onto modern
nosologies. It is especially important to be aware of this fact when ancient and modern terms overlap:
what the Greeks called "cholera," for example, is not to be confused with the disease that currently
bears this name. In general, Greek disease names tend to be associated with observable symptoms,
such as difficult urination (= strangury), fluid retention (= dropsy), yellowish skin (= *ikteros*, usually
translated as "jaundice"), violent shaking (= epilepsy or "the sacred disease"), paralysis and/or loss of
sensation (= apoplexy), a "fiery" fever (= *kausos*, usually translated as "ardent fever"), a twisting in the
intestines (= ileus), and so on.

[13] Ath. 3.83 (quoted on pp. 57–58).

[14] At Gal. *Adv. Typ. Scr.* 7.488 K., the reference to those who divide the year into seven seasons needing
someone like Philistion to mock them probably refers to the Augustan-era writer of mimes rather
than our doctor. Similarly, *pace* Smith (1867: 295), the reference to a Philistion at M. Aurel. 6.47
probably does not refer to Philistion of Locri but rather to the mimographer or else to a recently
deceased slave of the emperor; compare Hadot (1998: 276). It is unclear what we should make of the
two references to "Philistion's brother" at Cael. Aur. *Tard.* 3.8.147 and 5.1.22.

It is notable that none of these reports about Petron and Philistion say anything about their interests in cosmology.[15] Outside the *Anonymus Londiniensis*, the closest hint at their cosmological theories comes in a single passage from Galen. In this passage, Galen includes Philistion in a list of authorities who claimed that "the bodily parts of all animals are governed by the hot, the cold, the dry, and the wet, the one pair being active and the other passive, and that among these the hot has most power in connection with all functions, but especially with the genesis of the humors" (*Nat. Fac.* 2.110–111 K., trans. Brock, modified). It is possible that Galen cites Philistion in this passage because he actually wrote something to this effect. The testimony is extremely vague, however, and it groups Philistion with such a wide range of authorities (Hippocrates, Diocles, Praxagoras, Plato, Aristotle, Theophrastus) that its usefulness for reconstructing the views of Philistion is limited to say the least.[16]

It was not until Diels's publication of the *Anonymus Londiniensis* in 1893 that the cosmological interests of Petron and Philistion first came to the attention of modern scholars.[17] In this text, the author divides all medical writers into two camps, with one camp supposedly claiming that digestive "residues" (περιττώματα) are the primary cause of disease, while the other claims that "elements" (στοιχεῖα) are responsible for human illness.[18] The first camp includes Euryphon, Herodicus, Hippocrates, Dexippus, and at least twelve other medical writers. The second includes Plato and Philolaus, as well as four doctors: Polybus, Menecrates, Petron, and Philistion. To judge from these reports, "residues" denote any substance, either liquid or vapor, that arises from nutriment left to stagnate in the belly.[19]

---

[15] One source even identifies Philistion as a potential founder of the Empiricist sect (Gal. *Subf. Emp.* 1), although this report probably arose through confusion of his name with that of Philinus of Cos.

[16] On the limited usefulness of this passage, see van der Eijk (2001: 51–53). For similar passages that include Philistion among a list of physicians who all hold the same view, see Gal. *MM* 10.27–28 K., 10.110–111 K., and *Nom. Med.* 18.29–19.5 Meyerhof-Schacht. In these passages, Philistion is included among physicians who (1) distinguished the ways in which diseases resemble and differ from one another, (2) claimed that there are many types of disease and that each of these types requires a different treatment, (3) believed that nothing can be known or discovered about disease types without first knowing about the nature of human beings, and (4) said that fire (πῦρ) prevails in the body in cases of fever (πυρετός). Galen cites too many authorities alongside Philistion for us to reconstruct what the latter actually wrote about these topics. The division of diseases into various types, however, recalls Philistion's interest in drawing fine distinctions between different classes of foodstuffs.

[17] Compare, for example, the entries on Petron and Philistion in Smith (1867: 215, 295) with the entries in *RE* and *BNP* (cited in note 2 of this chapter).

[18] In *On Sensation*, Theophrastus similarly begins his doxography by dividing all thinkers into two camps, one of whom attributes sensation to similarity, the other to contrast.

[19] Such, at least, is the most common use of this term in the *Anonymus Londiniensis*. Note, however, Manetti (1992: 457–458, 1999a: 111–114) for an extension of its meaning. The specific term "residues" (περιττώματα) is Aristotelian in origin, although the notion that diseases arise from improper

"Elements," meanwhile, are the fundamental building blocks of human beings, identified as either bodily compounds (blood, phlegm, bile, and *pneuma*) or cosmological principles (earth, air, fire, and water; the hot, the cold, the dry, and the wet). Of the four doctors who are said to have focused on "elements," Petron, Philistion, and Polybus are all said to have identified cosmological principles as the basic constituents of human beings, while Menecrates, their near contemporary, focused on bodily compounds.[20]

For our purposes, we can focus on the entries for Petron and Philistion in the *Anonymus Londiniensis*. In these reports, we are told that the elements are just one of several factors that can bring about disease. Petron is said to have attributed diseases to *either* residues or elements, while Philistion supposedly identified three causes of disease: (1) the elements, (2) the physical condition of the body, and (3) external causes (XX.1–50, trans. Jones, modified):

> Petron of Aegina says that our bodies are composed of a pair of elements, the cold and the hot, and to each of these he assigns a partner, to the hot the dry and to the cold the wet, and out of these are our bodies composed. He says that diseases may arise through the residues of nutriment: whenever the belly, not [taking in?] what is commensurate but [too much?], cannot digest it,[21] the result is that diseases occur. He also derives diseases from the aforesaid elements,

---

digestion is commonplace in the Hippocratic Corpus (see pp. 105–106). At Arist. *HA* 511b9–10, the "residues" are defined as feces, phlegm, yellow bile, and black bile.

[20] Polybus is almost certainly to be identified as the author of *On the Nature of the Human Being* (on which see pp. 68–69). In this text, he claims that our bodies contain blood, phlegm, yellow bile, and black bile, which are themselves composed of the hot, the cold, the dry, and the wet. Menecrates, meanwhile, is said to have claimed that humans are composed of four elements, two hot (blood and bile) and two cold (*pneuma* and phlegm) (*Anon. Lond.* XIX.19–XX.1). For more on Menecrates, see Squillace (2012, 2015).

[21] There is a textual problem with lines 10–12, which Manetti (2011) prints as ὅταν ἀσύμμετρα ἡ κοιλία μὴ λ[| … απληρω δὲ μὴ κατεργάσηται | αὐτά. In her critical apparatus, Manetti notes that the string απληρωδε could also be read as απληιωδε. Diels (1893a) suggests the following reading: ὅταν, ἃ σύμμετρα, ἡ κοιλία μὴ λ[α-][[βοῦσ]α, πλείω δέ, μὴ κατεργάσηται | αὐτά ("whenever the belly, not taking in what is commensurate, but too much, cannot digest it"), which at least accords with what we find elsewhere in both the Hippocratic Corpus and the *Anonymus Londiniensis* (see pp. 105–106). Even without Diels's supplements, it seems safe to conclude that lines 10–12 refer to a situation in which nutriment enters the belly but cannot be digested because of some sort of incompatibility. This incompatibility could be *quantitative* (e.g., a flooding of the belly with more nutriment than it can handle) or *qualitative* (e.g., the consumption of foods and drinks that are raw, compacted, cold, strong, at odds with one another, or otherwise difficult for the belly to overpower). Both of these notions can be encompassed by the term *summetria* ("proportionality"), since even qualitative differences can impart a "power" to foods that is greater than the "power" of the belly to digest them. Compare *Aff.* 47, 6.254–258 L.

when they are irregular [ἀνώμαλα].²² But about the differentiation of diseases he says nothing with precision. As to bile, he expresses a rather peculiar view, saying that it is produced as the result of diseases. For whereas the others say that diseases come from bile, he says that bile is furnished by diseases. This thinker is in virtual agreement with Philolaus,²³ in that he thinks that the presence of bile is not natural. In this respect he agreed with Philolaus, in all other respects he †has views of his own†.²⁴

Philistion thinks that we are composed of four "forms" [ἰδέαι],²⁵ that is, of four elements – fire, air, water, earth. Each of these too has its own power [δύναμις]; of fire the power is the hot, of air it is the cold, of water the wet, and of earth the dry. According to him diseases occur in many ways, but speaking quite generally and in outline we may call them three: (1) because of the elements; (2) because of the condition of our bodies; (3) because of external causes. The elements cause disease when the hot and the wet are in excess, or when the hot becomes less and weak. External causes are of three kinds: (1) injuries and wounds; (2) excess of heat, cold, and so on; (3) change of heat to cold, or of cold to heat, or of nutriment to what is unsuitable and corrupt.²⁶ The condition of the body is a cause of disease in the following way. When, he says, the whole body breathes well and the breath passes through unhindered, health is the result. For breathing takes place not only by way of mouth and nostrils, but also over all the body. When the body does not breathe well, diseases occur, and in different ways [διαφόρως]. For when breathing is checked over all the body a disease ... [*text breaks off*]

As with any doxographical report, it is important to begin by considering the methodology that guided the composition of these entries. As Manetti (1990: 223) observes, these reports in the *Anonymus Londiniensis* about writers who focused on "elements" (στοιχεῖα) tend to be divided into three parts: (1) the elements of the body, (2) the "starting points"

---

²² On the potential meaning of this adjective, see note 45 of this chapter.

²³ On the medical interests of Philolaus, see Lloyd (1963), Huffman (1993: 289–306), and Manetti (1990, 1999b).

²⁴ The final word in this passage is corrupt, but it may be something like αὐτονοεῖ or αὐτολογεῖ.

²⁵ For this use of the term "form" (ἰδέα), compare *VM* 15.1, 1.604 L., 19.6, 1.618 L., *Genit.-Nat. Puer.* 3.1, 7.474 L., 11.1, 7.484 L., *Morb. IV* 32.1, 7.542 L., and *Carn.* 13.3, 8.600 L. The underlying idea is one of classification: fire, air, water, and earth are the four "types" or "classes" of matter. Compare Gillespie (1912: esp. 201) *contra* Taylor (1911: 250).

²⁶ For the attribution of diseases to food that is "unsuitable and corrupt," see pp. 54–55. For the claim that sudden changes give rise to disease (another common belief in the Hippocratic Corpus), see *VM* 10–11, 1.590–594 L., *Aër.* 11, 2.50–52 L., *Aph.* 2.51, 2.484 L., 3.1, 4.486 L., *Acut.* 26–37, 2.278–302 L., 45–49, 2.318–332 L., *Hum.* 15, 5.496 L., *Nat. Hom.* 9.5, 6.56 L., 11.6, 6.60 L., 16.2, 6.72 L., *Morb. Sacr.* 10.3–5, 6.378–380 L., *Aff.* 44, 6.254 L., *Vict.* 38.5, 6.534 L., 68, 6.594–604 L., *Oct.* 12.1–3, 7.456 L., *Th.* 7.87.1, and Arist. [*Pr.*] 1.3–4, 859a9–27, 1.15, 861a1–9, 1.27, 862b11–15.

(ἀρχαί) of disease, and (3) the "differentiations" (διαφοραί) of disease, which Manetti defines as "why the different kinds of disease can be explained in accordance with point (2)." This formulaic structure explains why the doxographer observes that Petron "says nothing with precision" about the "differentiation" of diseases (περὶ δὲ τῆς διαφορᾶς τῆς κατὰ τὰς νόσους οὐδὲν διακριβοῖ, *Anon. Lond.* XX.14–16). This comment does not mean that Petron did not go into detail about different diseases. Instead, the doxographer is simply noting that Petron did not formulate a clear statement about how the differences between individual diseases can be attributed to the differences in the application of his common "starting points." In the testimony for Hippocrates, for example (quoted on pp. 92–93), the doxographer notes that Hippocrates attributed all diseases to "breaths" (φῦσαι), but he then adds that differences in the quantity and temperature of breaths are what makes the resulting diseases differ from one another (VI.31–42). In the entry for Philolaus, the doxographer similarly notes that Philolaus attributed all diseases to blood, bile, and phlegm, but in addition to these "starting points of diseases" (ἀρχὰς τῶν νόσων), he also cited "co-operating factors" (συνεργά) such as "excesses of heat, of nutriment, of chill, and also defects of these or of things like these" (XVIII.47–XIX.1, trans. Jones).[27] Petron may well have described many different diseases, explaining the specific physiological processes that give rise to each. However, the doxographer was unable to extract from Petron's writings a clear generalization about secondary factors that work in tandem with his common "starting points," and which would thereby account for the variations that exist between different classes of disease.

The final portion of Petron's testimony illustrates another important point about the methodology of this doxographer. As we see in his remark about bile, the doxographer is not just compiling a passive summary of earlier views but is actively comparing these opinions with one another, placing different thinkers side by side in order to emphasize their points of

---

[27] For another example of what it means to account for the "differentiation" of diseases, see *Flat.* 2, 6.92 L.: "Of all diseases, the type is the same while the location differs [ὁ μὲν τρόπος ωὑτός, ὁ δὲ τόπος διαφέρει]. It is because of the diversity of their locations that diseases seem to bear no resemblance to each other, but of all diseases there is one and the same class and cause." Here, the author identifies *pneuma* as the "one cause" (i.e., the "starting point") of all diseases, while the differences that exist between individual diseases are attributed to the location of that *pneuma* within the body. In chapter 15, the author further observes that all factors other than *pneuma* are "accessory and contributing causes" (συναίτια καὶ μεταίτια), mirroring the reference to "co-operating factors" (συνεργά) that we find in the testimony for Philolaus. I will discuss both of these passages more fully in Chapter 3.

agreement and clash. As I noted earlier, Aristotle viewed doxography as an important first step for the development of original theories. At the beginning of *On the Soul*, he writes,

> For our study of soul it is necessary, while formulating the problems of which in our further advance we are to find the solutions, to call into council the views [δόξαι] of those of our predecessors who have declared any opinion on this subject, in order that we may profit by whatever is sound in their suggestions and avoid their errors. (403b20–24, trans. Smith *apud* Barnes)

To the frustration of modern historians, ancient doxographers seldom treat earlier thinkers on their own terms. The doxographer has little concern for anachronism, whether that applies to their use of terminology or even the specific questions that they ask. Even if a particular line of inquiry would never have occurred to an earlier thinker, the doxographer will nevertheless still read older texts for "answers" to these questions, since doxography is not just about cataloging what has come before but also, and more importantly, about considering what remains to be done.[28]

Because doxographers were reading their sources with specific questions already in mind, we need to exercise extreme caution when making use of their texts. These reports from the *Anonymus Londiniensis* are in no way complete records of what Petron and Philistion actually wrote. Much has surely been omitted, and we cannot even assume that all the details in these reports go all the way back to the authors themselves. These testimonies have passed through at least two filters – the author of the *Anonymus Londiniensis* and his Peripatetic source – and given what we know about the rest of this doxography, there is a good chance that these reports contain at least a moderate amount of distortion. One way to test this doxographer's reliability is to consider his statements about Plato, whose entry in the *Anonymus Londiniensis* can be checked against the surviving text of the *Timaeus*.[29] In the *Timaeus*, Plato divides diseases into three classes, of which the third is further subdivided into diseases due to *pneuma*, phlegm, or bile (τὸ μὲν ὑπὸ πνεύματος, τὸ δὲ φλέγματος, τὸ δὲ χολῆς, 84c–d). In reporting this phrase, the doxographer says that Plato attributed disease to "the breaths that arise from residues, or bile, or phlegm" (ἢ π[α]ρ[ὰ τὰς] φύσας [τὰς ἐκ τῶν πε]|ριττωμ[άτων ἢ παρ]ὰ

---

[28] On the character and purpose of ancient doxography, see the essays collected in Mansfeld and Runia (2010).

[29] For a full consideration of how the *Anonymus Londiniensis* makes use of the *Timaeus*, see Manetti (1999a: 119–125, 1999c).

χολὴν ἢ φλέγμα, XVII.46–XVIII.1), significantly altering the reference to *pneuma* in order to emphasize his own interest in the "residues" of food. Just after this passage, Plato describes how *pneuma* enters the body by way of the lungs and then says that it creates disturbances in the vessels when its normal channels are blocked. At no point in this section does Plato actually talk about digestion. In another section, the doxographer invokes an analogy between the intestines and winding rivers, even though no such analogy appears in the *Timaeus* (XVI.21–31). We also find a Stoic reference to "the ruling faculty" (τὸ ἡγεμονικόν) at XVI.38, another Stoic reference to three types of "blendings" (σύμφθαρσις, μῖξις, κρᾶσις) at XIV.12–32, and a change in the meaning of the noun *neura* from "tendons" to "nerves" at XVI.7–9, even though the true function of the nerves was not discovered until the Hellenistic period.[30] These distortions are a sobering reminder of the limitations that must attend our use of this doxography. Although there are some passages where the doxographer faithfully reports what Plato has to say, there are other points within the same text where Plato's thinking has been manipulated to align with later beliefs.

This observation is of critical importance for our reading of the *Anonymus Londiniensis*. We might ask, for example, whether Petron really did place the hot and the cold above their "partners," the dry and the wet, or whether this detail is merely a reflection of the doxographer's own preference to view the hot and the cold as more important than the dry and the wet.[31] Another point that warrants caution is Philistion's alleged construction of human beings out of fire, air, water, and earth. This detail has tended to be accepted without question, inspiring discussions of a "Sicilian" school of medicine with Empedocles at its head. We must bear in mind, however, that the *Anonymus Londiniensis* is Peripatetic in origin, and that Aristotle himself believed that everything is composed of fire, air, water, and earth. Since we have no other reports to corroborate this testimony, we must leave open the possibility that we are dealing with yet another distortion on the part of the doxographer. If Philistion did make extensive use of fire, air, water, and earth, it is curious that no other author from antiquity mentions this fact.[32] Galen frequently cites Philistion when listing ancient doctors who share his own beliefs, but he never invokes

---

[30] On the discovery of the nerves in the Hellenistic period, see Herophil. fr. 80–85 von Staden. For Stoic influence in the *Anonymus Londiniensis*, see Jones (1947: 2–3), Edelstein (1953: 1323), Mansfeld (1980a: 344), and Manetti (1990: 220, 232).

[31] For Aristotle's privileging of the hot and the cold over the dry and the wet, see Althoff (1992).

[32] The geographical grouping of Philistion with other "Italian" doctors at Gal. *MM* 10.5–6 K. hardly qualifies as a report about Philistion's doctrines.

Philistion's name in reference to this group of elements. Galen *does* include Philistion in his list of predecessors who all emphasized the hot, the cold, the dry, and the wet (*Nat. Fac.* 2.110–111 K.) and he also includes Philistion in a list of predecessors who believed that fire prevails in cases of fever (*Nom. Med.* 18.29–19.5 Meyerhof–Schacht). However, Galen never associates Philistion with the combination of fire, air, water, and earth, even though he cites other thinkers who utilized these elements (e.g., Empedocles, Plato, Aristotle, Theophrastus, Eudemus, Zeno, Cleanthes, Chrysippus) as "witnesses" for this doctrine on multiple occasions.[33] When Galen considers potential authors of the treatise *On Regimen*, he unproblematically cites Philistion on four separate occasions (see note 4 of this chapter), even though the central doctrine of *On Regimen* is that everything is composed of *two* elements (fire and water) rather than the four-element theory of fire, air, water, and earth. If these four elements were indeed central to Philistion's system, it seems difficult to claim that such a doctrine would simply have been overlooked, especially since at least some of Philistion's writings appear to have survived, in one form or another, until the Roman period.[34] Even in the testimony from the *Anonymus Londiniensis*, it is not fire, air, water, and earth but rather the hot, the cold, the dry, and the wet that play a determining role in pathogenesis. Perhaps Philistion briefly mentioned fire, air, water, and earth to illustrate the inherent properties of these substances but he then made the hot, the cold, the dry, and the wet the de facto first principles of his system.[35] Or maybe this is an instance where the doxographer let his own beliefs about the cosmos influence his reading of the text.[36] Philistion may have

---

[33] Compare especially Gal. *SMT* 11.460 K. and *Adv. Jul.* 18a.269 K. On this point, we might concede that Galen would have preferred to list philosophers rather than medical writers, although one imagines he would have found additional support for his system by citing more than just Hippocrates as a medical writer who also utilized these elements.

[34] Not only does Galen frequently invoke Philistion as a supporting "witness" (μάρτυς) for his own doctrines but specific citations of Philistion's views on both anatomy and dietetics can also be found in Pliny the Elder, Rufus of Ephesus, and Athenaeus, all of whom seem to have been directly consulting his work. Pliny includes Philistion in his list of sources for books 20–21 and 23–27 of the *Natural History*, while Rufus of Ephesus specifically comments on Philistion's use of the Doric dialect when discussing his anatomical vocabulary. Athenaeus, for his part, provides a long paraphrase from Philistion's writings on dietetics (quoted on pp. 57–58).

[35] Compare the brief mention of the Empedoclean elements at *Nat. Hom.* 1.1, 6.32 L., Meliss. DK 30 B8.2, and Diog. Apoll. DK 64 B2, none of whom ultimately adopt these four elements as the basis of their systems.

[36] Galen infamously tried to extract a belief in the four Empedoclean elements from *On the Nature of the Human Being*. Aristotle similarly tried to extract an implicit four-element theory from Parmenides (*GC* 330b13–15). For a modern example of misattributing a four-element theory to a cosmological doctor, see my discussion of *On Flesh* (pp. 178–180). Note also the emphasis on the

mentioned only a limited number of principles like fire and water, which the doxographer then expanded to conform to his own views. Alternatively, Philistion may have resembled Anaxagoras and the author of *On Flesh* in associating the hot with fire and the cold with earth, without actually claiming that fire and earth are the material elements from which other things are composed (see pp. 178–180). Another possibility is that Philistion took a stance similar to what we see in *On the Nature of the Human Being*, noting that *other* thinkers might talk about invisible substances such as fire, air, water, and earth but he would rather speak in terms of *perceptible* principles such as the hot, the cold, the dry, and the wet.[37] Or maybe he really did make use of the elements in his system but was simply eclipsed by Plato and Aristotle and therefore deemed unworthy of mention by later authors. There is only so much that we can do with this limited testimony, but it seems advisable to at least temper our expectation that fire, air, water, and earth would have played an important role in Philistion's system.

There are other passages where the doxographer is so vague as to make it extremely difficult to determine what his sources actually wrote. One such passage is the claim that Petron expressed a "rather peculiar" view about bile (περὶ δὲ τῆς χολῆς ἰδιώτερον παθολογεῖ, XX.16–17). In this passage, Petron is alleged to have said that bile "is furnished by the diseases themselves" (ὑπὸ τῶν νόσων αὐτῶν κατασκευάζεσθαι), whereas most other medical writers affirm that diseases arise from bile (XX.17–21). In the Hippocratic Corpus, it is often assumed that diseases are manifested by the *apokrisis* ("separating out") of harmful fluids like bile and phlegm.[38] For these authors, the question about whether "bile comes from diseases" or

---

[37] four elements at Heraclit. DK 22 B76 and Anaxag. DK 59 A1 (= D. L. 2.8), both of which might attract suspicion. A reference to four elements also appears at Xenoph. DK 21 A1 (= D. L. 9.19).

[37] *Nat. Hom.* 1.1, 6.32 L. (discussed on pp. 73–74). A similar view is attributed to the first-century physician Athenaeus of Attalia (Gal. *Elem.* 1.457–458 K.).

[38] The idea that part of a fluid will "separate out" (ἀποκρίνεσθαι) when the fluid is "set in motion" (κινεῖσθαι) or otherwise disturbed is attested as early as Anaximander (DK 12 A9–11). By the fifth century BCE, this concept was so well established that, as Lonie (1981: 99) observes, it seems to have simply been taken for granted by the writers who employ it. In the Hippocratic Corpus, the mechanism of *apokrisis* is deployed in a wide range of contexts. It persists even when medical writers disagree about the number and nature of the humors themselves. Lonie (1981: 100) suggests that "the ultimate basis of the principle was no doubt in everyday observation." In *Diseases IV*, the *apokrisis* that arises from overheating is compared to the churning of butter (51.1–3, 7.584–586 L.), while the *apokrisis* that arises from overcooling is compared to the curdling of milk (52.1–2, 7.590 L.). Lonie also compares "scum or foam forming on top of disturbed liquids," which is used to explain how semen "separates out" at *Genit.-Nat. Puer.* 1.2, 7.470 L. On the relationship between "separating out" and the definition of health as a form of "mixture" or "blending" (κρᾶσις), see Vlastos (1947: 156–157) and Schiefsky (2005: 248–250). I will address that connection later on in this chapter.

"diseases come from bile" would have boiled down to the question of what leads to a concentration of bile within the body.[39] What else Petron may have said about this topic is difficult to discern from such a limited report. Only slight help comes from the following sentence, in which the doxographer observes that Petron agreed with Philolaus in assuming that the presence of bile is not "natural" (οἰκείαν, XX.23). This adjective is poorly preserved in the papyrus, and Diels actually read it as ἀ[χρ]είαν ("useless"), apparently thinking of Aristotle's famous assertion that bile is a residue of unclean blood, serves no purpose, and is inherently harmful (*PA* 676b16–677b10). Assuming that Manetti's reading is correct, there are two ways in which we can interpret this reference. On the one hand, we might suppose that Petron thought that bile was "unnatural" in the sense that it was παρὰ φύσιν; that is, not a permanent, inborn component of human beings. In this way, Petron would have disagreed with the authors of *Diseases I*, *Diseases IV*, and *On the Nature of the Human Being*, all of whom claimed that bile, like the other humors, is always present in the body from the time of our birth.[40] If Petron did not think that bile was innate, he could have proposed that bile only arises from the food and drink that we consume,[41] or he might have thought that bile is only produced when some *other* humor (e.g., blood) undergoes transformation.[42] Another possible interpretation of this report is that Petron was discussing whether bile is permanently stored in some concentrated reservoir, just as phlegm is often said to have a permanent reservoir in the head. Some authors claimed that bile is stored within the liver or gallbladder,[43] but that view is far from universal. According to Aristotle, there was disagreement about whether

[39] For the ontological question of what actually constitutes a "disease" in the Hippocratic Corpus, see Pigeaud (1990).

[40] Compare *Morb. I* 2, 6.142 L. ("Bile and phlegm come into being together with [people] coming into being, and are always present in the body in greater or lesser amounts," trans. Potter, modified). A similar belief is expressed at *Morb. IV* 32.1, 7.542 L. and *Nat. Hom.* 5.3–4, 6.42–44 L. Compare also the reported view of Phasilas of Tenedos, who is said to have claimed that certain fluids in our bodies are "natural" (κατὰ φύσιν, *Anon. Lond.* XII.36–XIII.11).

[41] For the derivation of bile from food and drink, compare *Morb. IV* 33.2, 7.544 L., 36, 7.550–552 L., 40.1, 7.560 L., Erasistr. fr. 145 Garofalo, and Gal. *Nat. Fac.* 2.107–125 K.

[42] For the idea that bile arises from the transformation of another humor, compare *Anon. Lond.* XI.43–XII.8 (Thrasymachus of Sardis), *Nat. Hom.* 2, 6.34–36 L., and *Hebd.* 18.

[43] For example, Archil. fr. 234 West, Anaxag. DK 59 A105, *Morb. IV* 33.2, 7.544 L., 36, 7.550–552 L., 40.1, 7.560 L.; compare Lonie (1981: 285–286). In a divination scene at E. *El.* 827–828, Aegisthus inspects three parts of the liver: the λοβός ("lobe"), the πύλαι ("gates," traditionally identified as the portal vein), and the δοχαὶ χολῆς ("receptacles of bile," traditionally identified as the gallbladder). The same three terms also appear at Pl. *Ti.* 71a–d, where the liver is said to contain "bitterness" (i.e., bile). At *HA* 496b15–34, Aristotle similarly refers to the ἧπαρ ("liver"), the μεγάλη φλέψ ("large vessel"), and the χολή ("bile," another term traditionally identified as the gallbladder).

the gallbladder even exists in human beings (*PA* 676b30–36). Philolaus, with whom Petron is explicitly compared, is reported to have denied that bile is stored in either the liver or the gallbladder, and to have instead referred to this humor as a "serum of the flesh" (ἰχῶρα ... τῆς σαρκός, *Anon. Lond.* XVIII.37–38). Petron may have agreed with the common opinion that phlegm is concentrated in the head but thought that bile lacks a parallel reservoir within the body – an interpretation that might explain why only bile is mentioned in this passage.[44] In this instance, bile could still be a permanent, innate component of the body, but it would not be *concentrated* in the body, lurking instead in certain mixtures. It is even possible that Petron sought to redefine the very notion of disease, defining a "disease" as the condition that gives rise to a concentrated humor rather than the humor itself. Any of these interpretations (and perhaps others I have not even mentioned) are perfectly valid readings of this report. Which of these readings we ought to adopt, however, is impossible to determine from the vague language of this doxography.

Although the *Anonymus Londiniensis* is an imperfect source for reconstructing the beliefs of Petron and Philistion, we can nevertheless still use these testimonies to draw some conclusions about their systems. It is worth noting, for example, that Petron and Philistion are both said to have held that diseases arise in many ways, and that only one of these methods relates to an imbalance of elemental principles. Petron is said to have claimed that humans are composed of two elements, the hot and the cold, and that diseases can arise when these two elements are "irregular" (ἀνώμαλα).[45] Philistion, meanwhile, is said to have claimed that humans are composed

---

[44] As I will argue in Chapter 5, a similar view seems to have been held by the author of *On Flesh*, who claims that the brain is the "mother-city" of the "cold and glutinous" humor (= phlegm), while the "mother-city" of the "fatty" humor (= bile) is "the hot" (see pp. 193–197). By using the language of "mother-cities," the author implies that phlegm "separates out" from a preexisting reservoir (i.e., the brain), while bile does not have a single reservoir but rather "separates out" from the application of heat.

[45] For the doxographical use of this term, compare Diocl. fr. 51 van der Eijk: "Diocles says that most diseases arise through an irregularity (ἀνωμαλία) of the elements in the body and of the constitution (sc. of the air/climate)." Jones (1947) translates the adjective as "disproportionate," which would imply that diseases arise from a *quantitative* excess/deficiency in either the hot or the cold. However, the adjective ἀνώμαλος usually carries a wider sense of "uneven," "irregular," or even "abnormal." In the *Problemata*, a melancholic temperament is said to be ἀνώμαλος insofar as it is sometimes cold and sometimes hot (30.1, 954b8–10). Similarly, *On Humors* attributes some diseases to the "irregular" (ἀνώμαλος) alternation of heat and cold, comparing such alternations to what one experiences during the season of autumn (12, 5.492 L.). Thus, Petron may have supposed that diseases arise not from a purely *quantitative* excess/deficiency in the hot and the cold but from their *fluctuations* (like the sudden changes mentioned in the testimony for Philistion; cf. note 26 in this chapter). The adjective ἀνώμαλος might also point to *qualitative* changes in the nature of these substances (e.g., their concentration, fluidity, or density) or to the *displacement* of these substances from their usual

of fire, air, water, and earth. Each of these elements has a "power" – fire the hot, air the cold, water the wet, and earth the dry – and diseases can arise when some (but not all?) of these powers fall above or below some standard line: "when the hot and the wet are in excess, or when the hot becomes less and weak." The restriction of this imbalance to the hot and the wet is especially interesting. If these are in fact the only "powers" that Philistion cited as causes of disease, then he might have prioritized the same two elements (fire and water) as the author of *On Regimen*. As for Petron's assignments of "partners" to the hot and the cold (pairing the dry with the hot and the wet with the cold), these pairings are commonplace in early Greek medicine. *On the Nature of the Human Being* claims that bile is hot and dry while phlegm is cold and wet. Similarly, *On Regimen* attributes the hot and the dry to fire and the cold and the wet to water. Other common associations for these pairings include the oppositions of summer versus winter, youth versus old age, and the male versus the female.[46] If we can trust this testimony, then Petron might have invoked a similar range of associations.

In addition to pointing to imbalances in the hot, the cold, the dry, and the wet, Petron and Philistion are said to have attributed diseases to other causes. Interestingly, one of these causes is "the residues of nutriment" (τὰς περιττώσεις τῆς τροφῆς), suggesting that the division between "residues" and "elements" was not, in fact, as rigid as the doxographer's initial division might imply.[47] Petron is also said to have discussed the process by which bile is produced, while Philistion described the flow of *pneuma* through the body.[48] These references to humors and *pneuma* recall other testimonies on

locations (e.g., a downward flux of cold fluids from the head, or the intrusion of hot fluids into parts ill-equipped to receive them). It is important to remember that Greek thinkers tended to treat the hot and the cold as material substances rather than relative points on a temperature scale (note 22 on p. 13), so it is possible for "irregularities" in these substances to entail more than just a state of being "too hot" or "too cold."

[46] For these and other schematizations of the hot, the cold, the dry, and the wet, see Lloyd (1964).

[47] Of course, if the testimony on Plato is any lesson, we should not read too much into this statement.

[48] On Philistion's reported belief that "breathing takes place not only by way of mouth and nostrils, but also over all the body" (i.e., through the skin), compare *Aph.* 5.63, 4.556 L., *Epid.* VI 6.1, 5.322 L., *Morb.* I 25, 6.190 L., *Vict.* 9.1, 6.482 L., 64.3, 6.580 L., *Alim.* 28, 9.108 L., *Hebd.* 52, Emp. DK 31 B100, Pl. *Ti.* 79c–e, Thphr. *Sud.* 2, *Anon. Lond.* VI.20–21, Gal. *HVA* 17b.420 K., and *Anon. Bruxell.* 17. Scholars used to believe that skin-breathing was a hallmark of "Sicilian" medicine, passed down from Empedocles to Plato via Philistion (cf. Wellmann 1901: 71; Jaeger 1938: 214; Harris 1973: 17–18; note also Lloyd 1968: 88). Furley and Wilkie (1984: 3–9) have stressed, however, that this belief in skin-breathing was not restricted to southern Italy, while van der Eijk (2001: xxxv–xxxvi) suggests that the entire notion of a "Sicilian school" of medicine may simply be a modern construct, similar to the now debunked division of the Hippocratic Corpus into "Coan" and "Cnidian" texts. Compare Vlastos (1947: 158n26) and Thivel (1981: 56–57).

Petron and Philistion, in which they are said to have discussed the powers of certain foods to promote humors and *pneuma*, and to have given treatments that transform, purge, or otherwise target bodily fluids.

In the report on Philistion, there is an especially important point about multiple levels of causation. On the one hand, the elements create diseases "when the hot and the wet are in excess, or when the hot becomes less and weak." But what leads to such conditions? To account for these imbalances, Philistion is said to have identified three classes of "external things" (τὰ ἐκτός): (1) wounds and injuries, (2) excess of heat, cold, and so on, and (3) changes from one quality to another, including not only changes between heat and cold but also changes in nutriment to what is "unsuitable and corrupt." This distinction between "external" and "internal" causes recalls a passage from *Diseases I*, in which the author asserts that "all diseases arise in us either from things inside the body [τῶν μὲν ἐν τῷ σώματι ἐνεόντων], viz. bile and phlegm, or from things outside [τῶν δὲ ἔξωθεν], viz. exertions, wounds, the hot overheating, and the cold overcooling" (2, 6.142 L.). Strikingly, the first two "external things" from Philistion's account are the same "outside things" that are listed in *Diseases I*. The "exertions" and "wounds" in *Diseases I* recall Philistion's "wounds and injuries," while "the hot overheating" and "the cold overcooling" recall Philistion's "excess of heat, cold, and so on." Elsewhere in *Diseases I*, the author also mentions the effects of food and drink. However, whereas Philistion is said to have included nutriment that is "unsuitable and corrupt" among his "external things," the author of *Diseases I* claims that food and drink influence the humors "from inside" (ἔσωθεν, 23, 6.188 L., trans. Potter):[49]

> Fever arises from the following: when bile or phlegm becomes heated, from this all the rest of the body, too, is heated, and this is called fever. Both bile and phlegm are heated from inside [ἔσωθεν] by the foods and drinks out of which they are nourished and grow, from outside [ἔξωθεν] by exertions and wounds, and by heat that makes them too hot, and cold that makes them too cold; they are also heated by seeing and hearing, but least of all by these.

Another parallel for Philistion's testimony can be found in *On Affections*. In this text, the author resembles both Philistion and the author of *Diseases*

---

[49] On the distinction between "external" and "internal" causes, compare Thphr. *CP* 5.8.2, who classifies the deficiency and excess of food as an "internal" cause of disease but notes that, "as some assert" (ὥς τινές φασιν), the deficiency and excess of food arises "from the external things" (ἀπὸ τῶν ἔξωθεν). In the end, Theophrastus concludes that it makes no difference whether we label the deficiency and excess of food an "internal" or "external" cause of disease. If Philistion did use a term like "external things" (τὰ ἐκτός), he may have been one of the thinkers to whom Theophrastus refers in this passage.

I insofar as he includes wounds, excesses in heat and cold, and improper food and drink in his list of external factors that can initiate disease. He also resembles both of these authors insofar as he states that these factors engender disease through excesses in the hot, the cold, the dry, and the wet (1, 6.208 L., trans. Potter, modified):

> All diseases arise in human beings from bile and phlegm; the bile and phlegm provide diseases when, inside the body, one of them becomes too wet, too dry, too hot, or too cold; the bile and phlegm suffer these things from foods and drinks, from exertions and wounds, from smell, sound, sight, and sexual intercourse, and from the hot and the cold; this happens when any of the things mentioned are applied to the body at the wrong time, against custom, in too great amount and too strong, or in insufficient amount and too weak.

It is interesting that all of these passages include the hot and the cold at two different levels of pathogenesis. For all of these thinkers, the hot and the cold are *themselves* said to create excesses in the hot, the cold, the dry, and the wet. Presumably, the reason for this repetition is that diseases will arise from excessive heat, cold, dryness, and moisture *within* the body, but one way in which such internal changes can arise is from the *external* application of heat and cold. If the weather becomes too hot or too cold, for example, the external temperature will make the internal parts of the body hotter, cooler, drier, or moister. When these parts become too hot, too cold, too dry, or too wet, they will then initiate a series of physiological changes (e.g., the "separating out" of one humor from the rest) that eventually gives rise to disease.[50]

In the above-quoted passages from *Diseases I* and *On Affections*, diseases are also attributed to seeing and hearing (and sometimes also smell and sexual intercourse). These factors are not mentioned in the testimony for Philistion. Instead, Philistion is said to have cited an additional "internal" factor – the flow of *pneuma* through the body. It should be pointed out, however, that *pneuma* was often considered an agent of sensation. Alcmaeon, for example, is said to have described both hearing and smell in terms of *pneuma* entering the body and traveling through "channels" (DK 24 A5), comparing the entire process to "respiration" in a manner quite similar to the reference to "breathing" in the testimony for Philistion. A similar description of sensation can be found in *On Regimen*. In this text,

---

[50] For the idea that external imbalance can engender internal imbalance, compare Arist. [*Pr.*] 1.1, 859a2–3: "Why is it that great excesses cause diseases? Is it because they *engender* excess or defect, and it is in these after all that disease consists?" (trans. Forster *apud* Barnes, my emphasis).

the author claims that both sight and hearing occur when sensory material enters the body's vessels and strikes against the soul, defining the entire process as a form of "natural exercise" that encourages the movement of the soul through its circuits (61, 6.574–576 L.). When he first introduces the topic of disease agents in his discussion of pains in the chest (11, 6.158 L.), the author of *Diseases I* cites "air being mixed with the innate heat" (ἠέρος ἐπιμιγνυμένου τῷ συμφύτῳ θερμῷ) in the same place where he later refers to sight and hearing, perhaps suggesting that he, too, associates sight and hearing with the movement of *pneuma* through the body.[51] The testimony on Philistion breaks off before we learn the various ways in which he claimed that *pneuma* could give rise to disease. However, the parallels with *Diseases I* and *On Affections* suggest that sensory activities such as sight, smell, and hearing could have been one of the disease agents that he included in his narratives of pathogenesis.[52]

Another factor to account for are the humors. What role did they play in Philistion's system? Other testimonies report that Philistion mentioned good and bad humors in his writings on dietetics. We may also recall his giving of the name "eagles" to the temporal vessels, which suggests an interest in vascular anatomy,[53] as well as Galen's inclusion of Philistion in a list of medical writers who applied the hot, the cold, the wet, and the dry to the formation of the humors (*Nat. Fac.* 2.110–111 K.). It therefore seems likely that bodily fluids would have played *some* role in Philistion's explanations of disease. To judge from the parallels with *Diseases I* and *On Affections*, both of whose authors claim that diseases arise when bile and phlegm become too hot, too cold, too wet, or too dry, Philistion could have

---

[51] At *Morb. I* 25, 6.190 L., the author recalls Philistion's notion of "skin-breathing" when he writes that sweating occurs when moisture mixes with *pneuma* and thereby passes out of the body. At *Morb. I* 4, 6.146 L., the author further notes that "If the brain is shaken and suffers damage as the result of a blow, the patient immediately loses his speech, sight, and hearing" (trans. Potter), which could possibly be attributed to the blockage of *pneuma* if the author adopts a view similar to what we see at either *Morb. Sacr.* 6–7, 6.370–374 L., 16, 6.390–392 L., or *Morb. II* 4a.2, 7.10–12 L.

[52] For additional ways in which *pneuma* can give rise to disease, see my discussion of *On Breaths* in Chapter 3.

[53] In *On Head Wounds*, the author notes that each temple contains a "hollow and powerful vessel" (2.4, 3.190 L.) and that one may safely incise any vessel in the head *except* the temporal vessels, for their incision will produce spasms on the opposite side of the body (13.5, 3.234 L.). This observation is repeated at *Art.* 30, 4.142 L., *Coac.* 184, 5.624 L., 488, 5.696 L., and *Prorrh. I* 121, 5.550–552 L., and it is supported by the vascular anatomy of *Nat. Hom.* 11.3, 6.58–60 L., where each temporal vessel is said to pass to the opposite side of the body. As we have already noted, Philistion is said to have discussed the movement of *pneuma* through the vessels, which may have been connected to his discussion of the "eagles." For the attribution of throbbing temples to the presence of *pneuma* within the vessels, see *Flat.* 8.7, 6.102–104 L. Contrast this with *Loc. Hom.* 3.2, 6.280 L., where the constant throbbing of the temples is attributed to two streams of blood that flow in opposite directions and collide with one another.

likewise included the humors in his claim that diseases arise "when the hot and the wet are in excess, or when the hot becomes less and weak." In the Hippocratic Corpus, humors are often said to cause problems when they become too hot or too cold.[54] Hippon of Croton is even said to have put this interaction in general terms, observing that the moisture in our bodies "changes through excess of heat and excess of cold, and so brings on diseases" (*Anon. Lond.* XI.35–38, trans. Jones). As for Philistion's reference to an excess of the "wet," this can be associated with any number of conditions, all of which are frequently mentioned in the Hippocratic Corpus: (1) the "saturating" and/or "melting" of phlegm, flesh, or other bodily components, which can in turn flow to other parts of the body, (2) the flooding of the belly with excess nutriment, or (3) the "separating off" (ἀπόκρισις) of one humor from the rest, which then becomes concentrated, draws more fluids to itself, and finally enters a state of "dominance" (ἐπικράτεια). All of these are conditions that commonly appear in medical systems of this era, and they are all conditions in which the "wet" may be said to have entered a state of excess.[55] To connect the humors with his elemental theory, Philistion could have made a move similar to what we see in *On the Nature of the Human Being*. In this text, the author presumes that the humors respond to external factors like heat and cold because separate substances labeled the "hot," the "cold," the "dry," and the "wet" are immanent in the humors themselves (7, 6.46–50 L.).

To conclude this discussion of Petron and Philistion, I would like to compare one final passage that invokes a multitiered approach to pathogenesis. This passage purports to summarize the beliefs of Alcmaeon of Croton, an early Greek thinker whose status as a doctor has been the source of some debate.[56] Like Petron and Philistion, Alcmaeon is said to have

---

[54] On Greek doctors' tendency to speak in general terms about the effects of heat and cold on bodily fluids, see pp. 184–189.

[55] The author of *On Breaths* finds it important to account for all of these conditions when he tries to prove that *pneuma* is the common cause of all diseases, discussing the melting of flesh at 12, 6.108–110 L., the flooding of the belly at 7, 6.98–100 L., and the separating off of one humor from the rest at 10, 6.104–108 L. Like the author of *On Breaths*, Philistion may have wanted to group these conditions under a single, overarching principle. Hence, he would have identified "excessive wetness" as a common feature of these ailments, and then used this common feature to place all of these conditions within one and the same class. For the attribution of diseases to a *combined* excess of heat and moisture, see Arist. [*Pr.*] 1.23, 862a17–26.

[56] Compare Mansfeld (1975) with Perilli (2001). Diogenes Laertius observes that Alcmaeon wrote primarily on medical topics (DK 24 A1), while Galen never refers to Alcmaeon as a doctor, instead grouping him with Melissus, Parmenides, Empedocles, and other thinkers who wrote "on nature" (DK 24 A2). Of course, as we will see over the course of this study, the two categories of "doctor" and "cosmologist" need not be mutually exclusive. For the problematic question of when Alcmaeon was writing, see Huffman (2021).

combined an interest in cosmology with investigations into anatomy, physiology, and the nature of health and disease. He also recalls these figures insofar as he is said to have defined the maintenance of health as the balance of opposing "powers" (δυνάμεις) like the hot, the cold, the dry, and the wet, and to have invoked these factors within a complex narrative of pathogenesis that considers both "external" and "internal" causes of disease (DK 24 B4, trans. Laks and Most, modified):

> Alcmaeon says that the containing cause of health is equality among the powers [τὴν ἰσονομίαν τῶν δυνάμεων] – wet, dry, cold, hot, bitter, sweet, and the rest – while the single rule among these [τὴν ἐν αὐτοῖς μοναρχίαν] is productive of disease, for the single rule of each member of a pair is destructive. And sickness occurs, with regard to the agent, from excess of heat or cold; with regard to the origin, from abundance or lack of nourishment; and with regard to place, blood, marrow, or the brain; it is also sometimes produced by external causes [τῶν ἔξωθεν], certain kinds of water, the country, blows, dearth, and other causes similar to these, while health is the proportionate mixture [σύμμετρον κρᾶσιν] of the qualities.

It is noteworthy that Philistion's three "external" factors – injuries, the hot and the cold, and food and drink – can all be found in this passage. It is also interesting that Alcmaeon is said to have talked not only about the hot, the cold, the dry, and the wet but also about other opposites like the bitter and the sweet. I will come back to this second observation at a later point in this chapter. I will also come back to the notion of a "proportionate mixture" (σύμμετρος κρᾶσις), wherein health is defined as a form of "equality" (ἰσονομία) while diseases arise from the "single rule" (μοναρχία) of one substance over the rest.[57] For the time being, suffice it to say that Alcmaeon provides yet another parallel for the complex systems of pathogenesis that we find attested for both Petron and Philistion. These are all systems in which pairs of opposites (e.g., the hot, the cold, the dry, and the wet) play an important role in the production of disease. However, they do not play the only role, and they do not prevent the consideration of physiological processes involving the humors, *pneuma*, or the "powers" of food and drink. As we move ahead in our investigation, it will be useful to keep these observations in mind. Petron and Philistion both developed their own theories about the elements, placing special emphasis on the hot, the cold,

---

[57] For the purpose of this study, we do not need to wade into the contested question of whether the terms "equality" and "single rule" originated with Alcmaeon himself. While most scholars believe that Alcmaeon employed some kind of political metaphor, Mansfeld (2018: 262–285) has argued that the specific terms *isonomia* and *monarchia* are a doxographical intrusion. For a good overview of the question, with bibliography, see Huffman (2021).

the dry, and the wet. At the same time, they also studied topics that are more conventionally identified as "medical," apparently believing that a knowledge of first principles is important, but not necessarily the only thing that a doctor should bear in mind.

1.2 Plato's *Symposium*

Let us now turn to the second indirect source for the cosmological doctors: the speech of Eryximachus in Plato's *Symposium*. Composed in the early fourth century BCE (most scholars suggest ca. 385–380 BCE), the *Symposium* has a dramatic date of 416 BCE.[58] In the setup to the dialogue, we are told that Agathon, a tragic poet, has just won first place at a local festival. To celebrate his victory, Agathon has invited a veritable who's who of Athenians to his home: Phaedrus, a young aristocrat and an avid student of the sophists; Pausanias, Agathon's lover and an apparent expert in laws and customs; Aristophanes, a comic poet; Eryximachus, a doctor; and Socrates, a philosopher. The dialogue centers around six speeches (a seventh by Alcibiades is appended at the end), each of which is delivered by a different participant in the symposium. All six speeches are in praise of *eros*, the divine embodiment of "love" or "desire," and in a manner befitting the topic and setting, all but the speech of Socrates is delivered in a playful, semi-serious manner. The speech of Eryximachus is the third in the sequence. It follows the speeches of Phaedrus and Pausanias, both of whom define *eros* as the attraction between two human beings. Phaedrus praises *eros* because it spurs us to act nobly when under the scrutiny of our lovers. Pausanias, meanwhile, claims that there are in fact two forms of *eros*, one "heavenly" and one "vulgar," of which the heavenly *eros* involves the noble attraction one feels toward intelligent young men, while the vulgar *eros* lacks any claim to nobility, as it focuses on the body in preference to the mind. At the conclusion of Pausanias's speech, Aristophanes is slated to speak next. He comes down with a case of the hiccups, however, and must cede his turn to Eryximachus.[59]

---

[58] On the evidence for the *Symposium*'s date of composition, see Bury (1932: lxvi–lxviii) and Dover (1980: 10). The reference to Agathon's victory at the Lenaia confirms a dramatic date of 416 BCE.

[59] Many scholars have commented on this unusual detail, which suggests a pun on Eryximachus's name ("Belch-Fighter"). Some think the scene is meant to ridicule Eryximachus's speech, either because Aristophanes will supposedly be hiccupping, sneezing, and holding his breath while Eryximachus is talking (although no such interruptions are actually mentioned in the text), or because the swapping of turns between Aristophanes and Eryximachus emphasizes an unflattering juxtaposition between the speech of Eryximachus and that of Aristophanes, who does in fact appear to lampoon the specifically Empedoclean aspects of the doctor's account. If Eryximachus is supposed to remind us of Empedocles, however, we should just as much emphasize the

From what we can tell, Eryximachus was an actual person who flourished toward the end of the fifth century BCE. He was a doctor, the son of a doctor, and perhaps the grandson of one as well,[60] and he has the distinction of being the only physician to be dramatically portrayed in Plato's dialogues. Both he and his father Acumenus seem to have traveled in elite circles. In the *Protagoras*, whose dramatic date is usually set between 430 and 420 BCE,[61] Eryximachus is present in the house of Callias, a wealthy aristocrat and admirer of the sophists. In this dialogue, Eryximachus briefly appears alongside Phaedrus, Andron, and a number of non-Athenians, all of whom are asking Hippias, a famous sophist, questions about "astronomical matters concerning nature and the things on high" (περὶ φύσεώς τε καὶ τῶν μετεώρων ἀστρονομικὰ ἄττα, 315c). In the *Phaedrus*, we learn that Eryximachus and Phaedrus are good friends (268a) and that Phaedrus also knows Eryximachus's father (227a). In the *Symposium*, Eryximachus is again identified as Phaedrus's friend (176d–177d), and he is greeted by a drunken Alcibiades as "the noblest son of the noblest and soberest father" (214b). Such familiarity with members of the Athenian elite suggests a high status for both Eryximachus and his father. It may have also led to their downfall, however, as we learn in Andocides's *On the Mysteries*. In this speech, we are told that a certain Eryximachus (almost certainly our doctor) was among those accused in 415 BCE of mutilating the herms (1.35), while an Acumenus (again, almost certainly his father) joined Phaedrus and Alcibiades among those accused of profaning the Eleusinian mysteries (1.17–18).

For our purposes, we cannot take anything that Eryximachus says in the *Symposium* as a reliable record of what the real-life doctor actually believed. Not only is his speech a literary creation but it is also presented, within the framework of the dialogue, as a response to what initially takes the form of a rhetorical game.[62] It is unknown whether the real-life Eryximachus ever wrote anything of his own, or even whether he

---

juxtaposition between the speech of Pausanias and that of Eryximachus. In Eryximachus's speech, Pausanias plays the role of a wayward thinker who must be shown the true nature of things. In precisely the same way, Empedocles had earlier addressed another thinker, also named Pausanias, who likewise needed to extend his thinking to the "whole" as distinct from the "parts." Thus, the repositioning of the speech of Eryximachus just after that of Pausanias would draw our attention to this similarity between Eryximachus and Empedocles, making Eryximachus not simply the butt of a joke but a stand-in for one of Plato's most important intellectual predecessors.

[60] On his father, see Nails (2002: 1–2, s.v. Acumenus). The name Acumenus literally means "Healer" (< ἀκέομαι) and may suggest that medicine was already the family profession at the time of his birth.

[61] On the dramatic date of the *Protagoras*, see Denyer (2008: 66).

[62] On the rhetorical exercise whereby a speaker composes a eulogy on some mundane, undeserving, or otherwise paradoxical subject, see Burgess (1902: 157–166), Pease (1926), and Nightingale (1995: 100–102). The seriousness of Eryximachus's speech is not a topic that needs to be addressed here. Some have read the speech as tongue-in-cheek, but Levin (2014) cautions against such a view.

propounded original theories. The doxographical tradition has nothing to say about him, save the claim, elsewhere attributed to Hippocrates and Democritus, that "sexual intercourse is a minor epilepsy" (τὴν συνουσίαν μικρὰν ἐπιληψίαν, Stob. 3.6.44).[63] Although the speech of Eryximachus cannot provide direct evidence for the personal views of the real-life physician, it is nevertheless invaluable insofar as it purports to mimic the arguments of a cosmological doctor. The choice of *eros* as the first principle of all things is not otherwise paralleled in the Hippocratic Corpus, but the specific attributes that Eryximachus assigns to this principle, as well as the methods he uses to argue his points, would have reminded Plato's audience of actual doctors, doctors who must have been fairly well known for the parody to have any effect.

Eryximachus begins his speech by accepting Pausanias's division of *eros* into two types. The good, "heavenly" *eros* is healthy (186b, 188a), well ordered (187d, 188a, 188c), temperate (188a, 188d), just (188a, 188d), and pious (188d), while the bad, "vulgar" *eros* is diseased (186b, 187e, 188b), disorderly (188b), undisciplined (186c, 187e), insolent (188a), unjust (188a), and impious (188c). Eryximachus differs from Pausanias in terms of the scope of his encomium, claiming that *eros* "exists not only in the souls of human beings toward beautiful people, but also toward many other things and in other things, in the bodies of all animals, in what grows in the earth, and in practically all that is" (186a). He also differs in his emphasis on the *technai*, the "arts" or "crafts" in which expert knowledge is applied to some practical end.[64] Eryximachus begins with medicine "so that we

---

[63] Hippocrates: Macr. 2.8.15. Democritus: DK 68 B32. The doxographers who attribute this fragment to Democritus sometimes use the term "apoplexy" instead of "epilepsy" and include the explanation that "a human being rushes out of a human being and is wrenched away, being divided off by a sort of blow." In the Hippocratic Corpus, "apoplexy" is usually characterized by paralysis, while "epilepsy" is characterized by a violent shaking of the body. Although opinions differ on the etiology of these conditions, one commonly attested explanation is that both epilepsy and apoplexy arise from some kind of blockage of *pneuma* in the vessels (*Acut. App.* 7, 2.404–406 L., *Flat.* 13–14, 6.110–114 L., *Morb. Sacr.* 7, 6.372–374 L.). By writing that "sexual intercourse is a minor epilepsy," the original author of this statement may have speculated that sexual intercourse also involves a "stoppage" within the vessels (cf. LSJ s.v. ἐπιληψία I, ἐπιλαμβάνω II.3), which allows the seed to gradually build up until the *pneuma* finally ejects it all at once. At *GA* 737b27–738a6, Aristotle directly rebuts thinkers who claim that the generative seed is discharged with the help of *pneuma*, and who cite as their evidence the observation that, during sexual intercourse, this discharge is accompanied by a holding of the breath. Another close parallel can be found at [*Pr.*] 2.1, 866b9–14, where a similar case of "stoppage" (ἐπιληψία) is said to create a situation in which perspiration gradually builds up beneath the skin before the *pneuma* emits it in a mass. For Aristotle's comparison of sleep to epilepsy, see *Somn.* 457a8–14.

[64] Many scholars have claimed that Eryximachus's emphasis on the *technai* suggests that the primary model for his speech is *On Regimen*, a text that similarly describes a series of crafts

may venerate the art" (186b), and he then describes the role of *eros* in music, astronomy, and divination. For each of these crafts, he claims that it is the duty of the craftsman to know the difference between good and bad *eros* and to be able to "diagnose" them correctly (διαγιγνώσκειν, 186c, 187c). Where possible, the craftsman must also gratify (χαρίζεσθαι) the good *eros* while rebuffing (ἀχαριστεῖν) the bad (186c–d, 187d, 188c), in the same way that a beloved might either "gratify" or "rebuff" a lover.

In his section on medicine, Eryximachus discusses the extent to which *eros* guides his professional thinking. Beginning with the *phusis* ("constitution, nature") of human beings, he notes that the double *eros* is to be found in the bodies of all people. "It is generally agreed," he says, "that what is healthy in the body is different and dissimilar from what is sick, and what is dissimilar longs for and desires dissimilar things" (186b). To put it another way, he claims that, in any given patient, there are some substances that are healthy and others that are diseased, and that these substances are encouraged by different things. This discussion of healthy substances that "desire" good things and unhealthy substances that "desire" bad things has never been definitively explained.[65] In all likelihood, it relates to a pair of beliefs that are frequently invoked in early Greek medicine. The first is the belief that nutritive juices are distributed through the body by a principle of "like to like." Nutrition occurs when each part of the body, through some inherent power, literally *attracts* its appropriate humor to itself. The author of *On Regimen* describes this process in general terms: "When the body has been dried out and foods of all sorts fall upon it, it draws to itself [ἕλκει ... αὐτὸ ἑωυτῷ] what is fitting for each part from each of the several foods" (66.8, 6.588 L.). A similar description of "like-to-like" attraction can be found in *On Flesh*, where the "thinnest and wettest"

---

while making arguments about the cosmos. Given the prevalence of craft analogies in early Greek thought, however, this seems to be a hasty conclusion. The author of *Diseases I* broadly states that anyone who wants to engage in debates about medicine must know "to which of the other arts medicine has similarities, and to which it has none" (1, 6.142 L., trans. Potter). Moreover, it must be emphasized that *On Regimen* uses these craft analogies to argue that the *technai* are themselves reflections of human nature, while Eryximachus uses them to argue a very different thesis, viz. that *eros* governs all things. As we will see in Chapter 3, Eryximachus's speech has more in common with *On Breaths* than it does with *On Regimen*, especially in its claim that a single principle wields more "power" (δύναμις) than anything else.

[65] For some previous attempts, see Konstan and Young-Bruehl (1982), Rowe (1999), and Hunter (2004: 57).

humors are said to be drawn into the vessels and then distributed to each part of the body (13.2–3, 8.600 L.):

> The vessels from the intestines' belly [τῆς νηδύος τῶν ἐντέρων, a pre-Herophilean term for the duodenum?],[66] into which the food and drink are collected and then heated, draw [ἕλκουσι] the thinnest and the wettest part. … When the nutriment arrives at each part, it renders the particular form of that part. For it is through being irrigated by the nutriment that everything increases.[67]

The second belief that Eryximachus seems to be referencing in this passage is the notion that diseases are normally manifested in the form of concentrated humors, and that these humors can spontaneously grow hot and thereby attract further moisture to themselves. The end result of this attraction is to "feed" the fires of disease, just as nutritive juices are said to "feed" a healthy body. In *Diseases I*, we are told about an ailment in which the concentrated humor "produces severe pains, becomes heated, and, because of its heat, attracts to itself [ἄγει ἐφ' ἑωυτό] phlegm and bile from the nearby vessels and flesh" (26, 6.192 L., trans. Potter, modified). A similar case appears in *Diseases II*, where the blood in the head is said to be heated by bile and phlegm, after which "the head, in consequence of its being overheated, attracts to itself [ἕλκει ἐφ' ἑωυτήν] bile that has been set in motion in the body, and the thickest part is vomited up, while the thinnest part is drawn to itself" (3.2, 7.10 L., trans. Potter, modified). In both passages, a specific substance within the body possesses an inherent, attractive force that literally *draws* nutritive fluids to itself.

On their own, these parallels provide a good explanation for Eryximachus's invocation of two forms of *eros*, one "healthy" and one "diseased," that exist within the body and are encouraged by different

---

[66] On Herophilus's renaming of the duodenum, see von Staden (1989: 165). For the phrase "intestines' belly," a significant repetition can be found at *Cord.* 11.1, 9.90 L. ("feeding, as it were, from the intestines' belly"). Although editors tend to emend both passages (cf. Duminil 1998: 256n53), it is unlikely that the same error would have occurred in both texts. The duodenum does in fact look like a smaller stomach, and the Greeks at this time were well aware of the fact that the first section of the small intestine tends to contain food while the second, the jejunum, is found empty. The Greek term for the jejunum is νῆστις, literally "fasting." At *Carn.* 13.2, 8.600 L., the author refers to vessels that draw food from "the intestines above the jejunum" (τῶν ἐντέρων τῶν ἄνωθεν τῆς νήστιος), while Galen also writes about vessels that extend to the duodenum in *On Anatomical Procedures* (13.1). Compare also the common designation of the calf as the "leg's stomach" (γαστροκνημία) in the Hippocratic Corpus.

[67] For other references to this principle of nutrition by "like to like," see *Morb. I* 12, 6.160 L., *Vict.* 7.1–2, 6.480 L., *Morb. IV* 33–34, 7.544–548 L., Emp. DK 31 B90, Pl. *Ti.* 81a, and the comprehensive study of Müller (1965a).

things. The healthy parts use an inherent, attractive force to acquire the necessary fluids for nutrition and growth, while a concentrated humor uses a similar force to feed a disease.[68] The parallel is strengthened even more, however, when we observe that the "nourishment" of the body and the "nourishment" of morbid humors were frequently considered *side by side* in the therapeutic process. This is because practicing doctors often thought about disease in terms of a battle between the body and a concentrated humor.[69] In this conceptual framework, both the body and the concentrated humor were thought to have a certain "strength" (ἰσχύς). The patient's outcome, meanwhile, depends on whether the healthy parts or the humor ultimately "gains the upper hand" (κρατεῖν, ἐπικρατεῖν). In the Hippocratic Corpus, it is often said that doctors must strengthen the "healthy parts" (τὰ ὑγιεινά) in order to give the body the nourishment it needs to win the battle against concentrated humors. If a patient's body is strong (ἰσχυρός), it is more likely that the patient will recover. If a patient's body is weak (ἀσθενής), it is more likely that the patient will succumb. In addition to strengthening the body, Greek doctors also instructed their colleagues to avoid any treatments that might strengthen the disease. This is especially clear in the many passages where doctors are told to prescribe foods of certain qualities while carefully avoiding others. "Have the patient eat all the acidic and salty foods and drink harsh Coan wine, as dark as possible," writes the author of *Internal Affections*, "but have him abstain from the foods that are sweet" (25, 7.232 L.). In another text (*Acut. App.* 1.1–3, 2.394–396 L.), a patient suffering from "pungent and bilious serums" (δριμέας καὶ χολώδεας ἰχῶρας) is specifically told to avoid food that is "pungent" (δριμύ), presumably because the pungent food will exacerbate the equally pungent humor. Timing was also an important factor, as doctors were advised against giving food when a disease was at its

---

[68] For other references to the attractive force of concentrated humors, see *Flat.* 10.3, 6.106 L., *Morb. I* 13, 6.160 L., 15, 6.166 L., 20, 6.176–178 L., 27, 6.194–196 L., 29, 6.198–200 L., *Haem.* 1.1, 6.436 L., *Morb. II* 10.1, 7.18 L., and *Int.* 47, 7.282 L., and compare *Morb. II* 8.2, 7.16 L., 11.1, 7.18 L. For the attractive power of heat, see Gundert (1992: 461). On the parallelism between the "nourishment" of the body and the "nourishment" of disease, see *VM* 6.1, 1.582 L., 14.6, 1.604 L., *Aph.* 7.66, 4.598 L., *Flat.* 7.1, 6.98 L., *Morb. I* 6, 6.150 L., 23, 6.188 L., *Aff.* 50, 6.260 L., *Loc. Hom.* 38.2, 6.328 L., 43.1–2, 6.336 L., *Morb. Sacr.* 18.2, 6.394 L., *Morb. IV* 35–38, 7.548–556 L., 46.3, 7.572 L., 46.5, 7.574 L., 49.3–4, 7.580 L., 51.4–9, 7.586–588 L., *Carn.* 16.3, 8.604 L., and *Hebd.* 19, 24.

[69] For some explicit references to this struggle, see *VM* 3.4–5, 1.576–578 L., 14.3–6, 1.602–604 L., *Acut. App.* 5.1, 2.402 L., 33.2, 2.464 L., *Aff.* 16, 6.224 L., 22, 6.232–234 L., *Morb. II* 8.2, 7.16 L., and *Morb. IV* 46.3, 7.572 L., 46.5, 7.574 L. For a more general discussion of military metaphors in the Hippocratic Corpus, see von Staden (1990: 97–102). At *Vict.* 2.4, 6.472 L., the two combatants are specifically identified as the "healthy" and the "diseased," closely matching Eryximachus's language.

height,[70] and some even debated whether patients should be starved from the onset or else given some initial food, the idea being that, as long as the disease is still relatively weak, their bodies would benefit from an influx of additional strength.[71] In *On Ancient Medicine*, the author stresses that one must distinguish foods that nourish the body from foods that nourish the disease, writing that "those of the sick to whom gruels are not suited, but rather opposed, see their fever and pains become more acute if they take them, and it is clear that what they have taken provides nourishment and growth for the disease, but wasting and weakness for the body" (6.1, 1.582 L., trans. Schiefsky, modified). The so-called appendix to *On Regimen in Acute Diseases* also contains a passage that refers to this struggle between what is "healthy" and what is "diseased" (5, 2.402 L., trans. Potter, modified):

> Those who undertake to resolve swellings at the beginning of diseases, by using purgative medications, draw off nothing of what is stretched and swollen – for the affection does not go away as long as it is raw – but consume the healthy elements that are resisting the disease [τὰ δ' ἀντέχοντα τῷ νοσήματι καὶ ὑγιεινά]. The body weakens and the disease gains the upper hand [ἀσθενέος δὲ τοῦ σώματος γινομένου τὸ νόσημα ἐπικρατεῖ], and when the disease wins out over the body, such a thing is incurable.

In this passage, the author explicitly refers to a conflict between the disease (τὸ νόσημα) and the healthy parts (τὰ ὑγιεινά), in which the weakening of the healthy parts will cause the disease to "gain the upper hand" (ἐπικρατεῖ). The disease can only be defeated when its concentrated humor is no longer "raw," a process that occurs when the healthy parts acquire enough strength to initiate "coction" (πέψις) and literally "cook" the humor's power away.[72] On the basis of these parallels, we can provide a reasonable explanation for Eryximachus's claim that there are two forms of *eros*, one healthy and one diseased, that exist within the body and are encouraged by different things. If his contemporaries were to hear this statement, they would have assumed that Eryximachus is thinking about doctors who "gratify" (i.e., nourish) the healthy parts of the body at the same time that they "rebuff" (i.e., starve) a disease. Since the nourishment

---

[70] On this point, see especially *Acut. App.* 54, 2.502–504 L., *Aph.* 1.10, 4.464 L., and *Hum.* 6, 5.484–486 L.

[71] The question is put in precisely these terms at Arist. [*Pr.*] 1.50, 865a35–37. See also *Acut.* 7, 2.238–240 L., 26, 2.278–280 L. As Lonie (1977: 248) observes, "the general practice of the Hippocratic writers was to give no solid food until after the crisis," although gruels could be administered in cases where such nourishment was deemed helpful and safe.

[72] On the concept of "coction," see p. 52.

of both healthy and morbid parts involves the spontaneous attraction of humors through a principle of "like to like," the parts themselves may be viewed as possessing either a healthy or a diseased form of *eros*.

It is the job of the doctor, Eryximachus continues, to increase what is healthy and to diminish what is diseased, gratifying the former while rebuffing the latter. Whoever can differentiate good and bad *eros* is a "master of the healer's art" (ἰατρικώτατος), while whoever knows how to implant *eros* when it is absent and take it away when it is present is a "good workman" (ἀγαθὸς δημιουργός, 186c–d). Eryximachus then appears to switch gears, mentioning another instance in which medicine depends on *eros*. It is necessary, he says, for the practicing physician to establish "love" (ἔρως) and "unanimity" (ὁμόνοια) between natural opposites: "cold and hot, bitter and sweet, dry and wet, and all things of such a sort" (186d). In this case, Eryximachus no longer distinguishes between a good and bad *eros* but associates the absence of *eros* with the production of disease. In this way, he resembles Petron and Philistion insofar as he associates health with the right balance between pairs of opposing powers, while diseases arise when one of these powers falls above or below some standard line. The testimonies on Petron and Philistion limit these powers to the hot, the cold, the dry, and the wet, while Eryximachus recalls Alcmaeon in his addition of the bitter, the sweet, and "all things of such a sort." It was by knowing how to balance such opposites, he claims, that Asclepius first composed the art of medicine. Eryximachus then draws an analogy with two other crafts, noting that "all of medicine is governed by this god [sc. *eros*], as too is gymnastics and agriculture" (186e–187a).

This sudden shift in Eryximachus's definition of *eros* from "desire" to a sort of "friendship" has long puzzled modern scholars. In the first instance, *eros* is divided into the healthy and the sick, while in the second, *eros* is always healthy, representing the wholesome equilibrium between two opposing powers.[73] In their discussion of this passage, Konstan and Young-Bruehl (1982: 42) suggest that these two definitions of *eros* might be combined along the following lines: "Healthy bodies have desires for things which tend to preserve the proper concord of their elements, while sick bodies will find pleasure in the consumption of foods or other substances that are harmful to their disposition." It should

---

[73] I borrow the terms "desire" and "friendship" from Konstan and Young-Bruehl (1982), who employ the Greek terms *epithumia* and *philia*. Dover (1980: 105) views the shift as typical of Eryximachus's incoherence, while Rowe (1999: 55–60) tries to show that no actual shift occurs.

be noted, however, that Konstan and Young-Bruehl do not cite any parallels from the Hippocratic Corpus to support this interpretation. Their explanation also conflicts with the everyday observation that healthy people are fully capable of desiring unhealthy foods, while sickness tends to lead to an aversion to *any* food, not an increased appetite for rich, unhealthy foods.[74]

If we want to give some sense to this passage, I suggest that we read the shifting definition of *eros* as an attempt to incorporate two distinct aspects of treatment:[75] it is the disharmony between the opposites that creates the diseased *eros*, while treatment should involve (1) the purging of this diseased *eros* and (2) the restoration of the opposites to their initial state of harmony. To translate this abstract language into physiological terms, consider the following case. A patient falls ill after excessive drying creates an *apokrisis* ("separating out") of bile within the body. This concentration of bile then stagnates, grows hot, and attracts further humors to itself. To cure the patient, the doctor must purge the concentrated bile, since this is the primary cause of the patient's discomfort. At the same time, the doctor must also prescribe a moistening regimen, as the illness was initially set in motion by a case of over-drying. In this example, note how the two-pronged treatment maps onto Eryximachus's description of *eros*. The bile contains the bad, diseased *eros* that can draw even more humors to itself. The over-drying, meanwhile, is the disharmony between the opposites. Both senses of *eros* are essential to the healing process, with one embodying the illness itself and the other the initiating cause.

Another, almost certainly simultaneous explanation for this shifting definition of *eros* is that Eryximachus divides the humors into opposing pairs, much like the common polarity between bile and phlegm.[76] As we will see in our discussion of *On Ancient Medicine*, medical writers often assert that the body enjoys health when the humors maintain an even "blending" (κρᾶσις), while diseases arise from the "separating off" (ἀπόκρισις) of one humor from the rest. Thus, the

---

[74] In the Hippocratic Corpus, "loss of appetite" (ἀποσιτία, ἀσιτία) is frequently cited as a symptom of disease. A variation on Konstan and Young-Bruehl's interpretation can be found in Hunter (2004: 57), who writes that "a body which is too cold (i.e., in which 'cold' has encroached on the space of 'warm' and thus caused unhealthy imbalance) will want more cold and reject the warmth which it needs for health. A good doctor can reconcile the two opposed qualities (186d1–5), can make them 'love each other.'" Like Konstan and Young-Bruehl, Hunter does not cite any parallels from the Hippocratic Corpus to support this interpretation. He also relies on an oversimplified model of pathology that is not attested for any Greek doctor of the Classical period.

[75] Note that Eryximachus is specifically talking about treatment in this passage.

[76] For the polarity between bile and phlegm, see p. 72.

very act of "separating off" could be envisioned as a sort of disharmony between opposites, while an even blending would be defined as a harmonious mixture between substances that, when taken separately, appear to be fundamentally at odds.[77] A theory of opposing humors would in fact explain why both Eryximachus and Alcmaeon invoke the sweet and the bitter alongside the hot, the cold, the dry, and the wet, as the Greeks typically viewed flavors such as the sweet and the bitter as biological juices, locating them in animals as well as plants.[78] That is not to say, of course, that the sweet and the bitter could not also have acted as triggering causes, implanting diseased *eros* in the same way that the hot, the cold, the dry, and the wet can give rise to an *apokrisis*. Eryximachus might have thought, for example, that whenever we consume food and drink that contains an excessive concentration of either the sweet or the bitter, these humors will create a disturbance in the body that will eventually cause one of the humors to separate out.

In the rest of his speech, Eryximachus discusses the role of *eros* in music, astronomy, and divination. In each section, he comes back to medicine as the standard for viewing these other crafts. In the same way that medicine is governed by *eros*, he says, so too is music (ὥσπερ ἐκεῖ ἡ ἰατρική, 187c; πάλιν γὰρ ἥκει ὁ αὐτὸς λόγος, 187d; ὥσπερ ἐν τῇ ἡμετέρᾳ τέχνῃ, 187e). He again invokes medicine in his transition to celestial matters, noting that "in music, in medicine, and in all other things, both human and divine, we must, insofar as it is permitted, be on the watch for either sort of *eros*" (187e). His interest in "astronomy" extends only to the question of what seasons produce health and what engender disease (188a–b), and even religion comes to resemble medicine, as Eryximachus observes that the interactions between humans and gods "concern nothing other than the preservation and healing of *eros*" (188c).[79] In the section on astronomy,

---

[77] Compare Empedocles's theory that the elements separate off and mix together under the influence of "love" and "strife." In the verbatim fragments, Empedocles uses the same terms for "separating off" (ἀποκρίνεσθαι, B9.4) and "mixing together" (κρῆσις, B21.14) that Greek doctors applied to the humors.

[78] Compare *Nat. Hom.* 6.3, 6.44–46 L., *Morb. IV* 30.5, 7.534 L., 34.4–5, 7.546–548 L., and the humoral system of *On Ancient Medicine*. Note also *Nat. Hom.* 2.2, 6.34 L., where the humors are said to have the properties of being "sweet, bitter, white, black, and so on," and *Vict.* 56.2, 6.566 L., where bitter foods are said to lose their "power" (δύναμις) and "strength" (ἰσχύς) when mixed with foods that are sweet.

[79] Note also Eryximachus's assertion that the task of the seer is to keep watch over *eros* and to "doctor" it when necessary (ἰατρεύειν, 188c).

Eryximachus makes some interesting remarks about the pathogenic qualities of the hot, the cold, the dry, and the wet (188a–b):

> When the things I have just mentioned – the hot and the cold, both dry and wet – hit upon the orderly *eros* and acquire harmony and a temperate mixture, they come bearing prosperity and health to human beings, to the other animals, and to plants, and they commit no injustice. But when the insolent *eros* gains the upper hand regarding the seasons of the year, they inflict much destruction and injustice. For pestilences tend to arise from such things, as do many other diseases, not like one another, both for animals and for plants.

This passage contains the same double definition of *eros* that we have already seen in Eryximachus's discussion of the body, combining a notion of *eros* as form of "desire," which can be either good or bad, healthy or diseased, with a notion of *eros* as a form of "friendship," which is *always* healthy, since diseases are produced by its absence. In his discussion of medicine, Eryximachus had already implied that the body acquires a diseased form of *eros* from the loss of "love" and "unanimity" between natural opposites. This loss of "love" and "unanimity" is presumably to be understood as both the *apokrisis* ("separating off") of one humor from the rest and an imbalance in external factors like the hot, the cold, the dry, and the wet, which can in turn give rise to an *apokrisis*. In his discussion of the seasons, the unhealthy *eros* "gains the upper hand" (ἐγκρατέστερος ... γένηται) when the harmonious mixture (κρᾶσις) of the hot, the cold, the dry, and the wet is disrupted. As a result, there is a concentration in the hot, the cold, the dry, or the wet that can in turn give rise to a disease. The major difference between this passage and Eryximachus's earlier comments on human nature is that whereas the unhealthy *eros* is said to be contained within the *body* in the section on medicine, it is now said to be found within the *seasons*. Presumably, Eryximachus views the "blending" of the seasons as analogous to humoral *krasis*. The hot, the cold, the dry, and the wet can become concentrated and "gain the upper hand" in the same way that diseases arise when one of the body's humors becomes more concentrated and thereby "gains the upper hand" over the rest.[80]

In his discussion of health and disease, Eryximachus assumes that his audience is familiar with such concepts as like-to-like attraction, the "blending" (κρᾶσις) and "separating out" (ἀπόκρισις) of humors within

---

[80] For a similar analogy between the seasons and the humors, see *Hum.* 13, 5.492–494 L., where the author notes that the seasons, like the humors, can experience both crises and relapses. Plato himself will return to this comparison between bodies and seasons at *Lg.* 10.906c.

the body, and the need for doctors to nourish the healthy parts while simultaneously starving peccant humors. These notions were shared by many doctors in the Classical period, and they suggest that what makes Eryximachus stand out from his contemporaries is not his understanding of human physiology but rather his interest in interpreting this framework through a principle that applies to the universe as a whole. Indeed, it cannot be stressed enough that Eryximachus's entire speech is driven by a single goal: to prove that *eros* is a universal principle. As he notes in his opening remarks (185e–186b):

> Well, since Pausanias made a fine beginning to his speech but did not satisfactorily finish it off, I think it is necessary that I should try to append a conclusion to his account. For I think he did well to divide *eros* in two, but that *eros* exists not only in the souls of human beings toward beautiful people, but also toward many other things and in other things, in the bodies of all animals, in what grows in the earth, and in practically all that is [ὡς ἔπος εἰπεῖν ἐν πᾶσι τοῖς οὖσι], I think I have seen from medicine, our art, how great and wonderful is the god, and how he extends over everything both human and divine.

Eryximachus repeatedly emphasizes the universality of *eros* (the adjective πᾶς appears thirteen times over the course of his speech). He reprises this thesis in his concluding remarks, noting that "the undivided *eros*, taken as a whole, has a wide, a strong, nay an absolute power" (188d). It is this emphasis on the universal power of *eros* that defines Eryximachus as a cosmologist. Interestingly, he claims to have acquired this insight "from medicine, our art" (ἐκ τῆς ἰατρικῆς, τῆς ἡμετέρας τέχνης, 186a), suggesting that he views the search for first principles as a natural pursuit for the practicing doctor.

To "prove" that *eros* is a universal principle, Eryximachus constructs a simple argument from induction. He compiles a list of (seemingly disparate) cases in which *eros* can be found, and he then argues that the apparent differences between medicine, gymnastics, agriculture, music, astronomy, and divination, coupled with the parallelism in how *eros* is manifested in each, qualify as sufficient proof that *eros* "extends over everything both human and divine" and is present "in animals, in plants, and in practically all that is." As we will see, this mode of argument from induction, whereby universal principles are "proven" by drawing analogies across a wide range of cases, was very popular among the cosmological doctors. It can be found in *On Breaths*, *On Flesh*, and *On Regimen*, and it suggests that even though the speech of Eryximachus advances a thesis that is not otherwise attested, his style of argumentation would have nevertheless been recognizable to Greek readers of the fourth century BCE.

At this point, I would like to draw one final comparison between the speech of Eryximachus and the testimonies on Petron and Philistion. As we have already noted, all three doctors show an interest in pairs of opposites (the hot and the cold, the dry and the wet, the sweet and the bitter, etc.), and they all hold that diseases can arise when one of these opposites is incommensurate with the other. At the same time, none of these physicians seems to have reduced the art of medicine to a simple opposition between elemental forces. Petron and Philistion are said to have devoted a good deal of attention to anatomy and physiology, discussing the production and transformation of both humors and *pneuma* within the body. In his treatment of fever patients, Petron does not treat "opposites with opposites," but he actually begins by *warming* the patient up. Afterwards, he purges the peccant humors and then restores the patient's strength, removing what is harmful and increasing what is beneficial. Similarly, Eryximachus claims that doctors must increase what is healthy and diminish what is diseased (186c–d). In this passage, he specifically says that doctors should "take away" (ἐξελεῖν) bad *eros* and "implant" (ἐμποιῆσαι) good *eros*, using language that could easily be applied to the traditional method of purging diseased humors and then restoring the patient's strength. As we noted earlier, this method of removing bad *eros* and implanting good *eros* is qualitatively different from Eryximachus's subsequent discussion of how doctors must establish "love" (ἔρως) and "unanimity" (ὁμόνοια) between natural opposites. For Eryximachus, the balance between opposites is essential to maintaining health, but it is not the only factor that doctors should bear in mind. When dealing with the "separating out" of one humor from the rest, the most common treatment is not to combine it with its opposite but rather to remove the diseased matter in its entirety.

1.3 *On Ancient Medicine*

As we will see in later chapters, Petron, Philistion, and Eryximachus were not the only Greek doctors from the Classical period to combine cosmological principles with a more traditional model of pathogenesis. *On the Nature of the Human Being, On Breaths, On Flesh,* and *On Regimen* all combine their speculations about the cosmos with widely attested beliefs about humors and *pneuma*. Before we turn to these texts, however, I would like to discuss one more secondhand report: the treatise *On*

Ancient Medicine.[81] Preserved in the Hippocratic Corpus, *On Ancient Medicine* has usually been dated to around 420–400 BCE. Maucolin (2009: 8–12) has rightly observed, however, that it could have conceivably been written as much as fifty years after this point. Even more so than the texts of the cosmological doctors themselves, *On Ancient Medicine* has long guided our assumptions about what cosmological medicine is all about. As we will soon see, however, this text provides at best an incomplete picture of what the cosmological doctors were doing, and an overreliance on its testimony will ultimately hinder our understanding of how these doctors came to be.

Our first hint that *On Ancient Medicine* may be less than reliable is the fact that the author is openly hostile to the cosmological doctors. In particular, he claims that their theories about human *phusis* – theories that resemble the work of "Empedocles or others who have written, concerning nature, what a human being is from the beginning, how it originally came to be, and from what it was compounded" (20.1, 1.620 L.) – "tend toward philosophy" (τείνει ἐς φιλοσοφίην, 20.1, 1.620 L.), and that their emphasis on *hupotheseis* (ὑποθέσεις) like the hot, the cold, the dry, and the wet is unnecessary for a genuine "craft" (τέχνη) like medicine, although such principles may be required for discussing obscure and irresolvable matters such as "the things on high or under the earth" (1.3, 1.572 L.). According to the author of *On Ancient Medicine*, it is important to separate the practical, falsifiable knowledge of the "crafts" from the impractical, unfalsifiable speculations of "philosophy." Making the former depend on the latter, the author argues, not only combines two fundamentally incompatible modes of thought but also runs the risk of destroying any progress that doctors have already made.

A great deal of attention has been paid to what this author means by *hupotheseis*. The etymological sense of the word is "basis" or "foundation," in the sense of something that is "established at the beginning of a process ... and which underlies and guides all subsequent activity" (Schiefsky 2005: 112). In *On Ancient Medicine*, the term seems to carry two basic meanings: (1) a "foundational principle" and (2) an unproven "assumption." *Hupotheseis* are "foundational principles" insofar as they underlie all aspects of a medical system. According to the author of *On Ancient Medicine*, some medical theorists reduce the entire art to a small number of principles like

---

[81] In this section, all translations from *On Ancient Medicine* will be adapted from Schiefsky (2005).

the hot, the cold, the dry, and the wet. These theorists claim that all diseases arise from these principles, and they treat them by opposing the hot with the cold, the cold with the hot, the dry with the wet, and the wet with the dry. In addition to functioning as "foundational principles," *hupotheseis* are also unproven "assumptions." They are merely postulated for the sake of constructing explanations, and they cannot be subjected to any test to either confirm or reject their validity.[82]

Whereas Petron, Philistion, and Eryximachus all combine their first principles with a more traditional model of pathogenesis, the author of *On Ancient Medicine* directly contrasts the use of *hupotheseis* with a humoral model of disease. He points out that there is no such thing as the hot, the cold, the dry, and the wet that exists purely in itself (αὐτό τι ἐφ' ἑωυτοῦ, 15.1, 1.604 L.). What the human body actually contains are "humors" (χυμοί) such as the sweet, the acid, the salty, the bitter, and "myriad other things having powers of all kinds" (14.4, 1.602 L.). When one of these humors is "separated out" (ἀποκρίνεσθαι), the patient becomes diseased. Health is restored when the concentrated humor is either purged from the body or is blended with other humors.[83]

For the author of *On Ancient Medicine*, it is not the hot, the cold, the dry, or the wet that harms human beings. Instead, it is "the strength of each thing and that which is more powerful than the human constitution . . . the strongest of the sweet being the sweetest, of the bitter the bitterest, of the acid the most acidic, and of each one of all the things present, the extreme degree" (14.3, 1.602 L.). The body has its own "power" (δύναμις) that normally keeps these humors mixed together. When one of these humors becomes too concentrated, however, its own strength overcomes that of the body.[84] What happens when one of these humors "separates out" depends on the nature of the humor and its location in the body, as well as the constitution of the individual patient. In many cases, the concentrated humor produces pain, heat, and inflammation, and it can also eat away the flesh and give rise to ulceration.[85]

---

[82] *VM* 1.3, 1.572 L. On the arbitrariness of *hupotheseis*, note also 1.1, 1.570 L.: "having laid down as a foundational principle hot, cold, wet, dry, *or anything else they want* [ἢ ἄλλο τι ὃ ἂν θέλωσιν]."

[83] For the definition of health as an even blending (κρᾶσις) of the humors, see *VM* 14.3–6, 1.600–604 L., 16.1, 1.606–608 L., 18–19, 1.614–620 L. For the view that flavors such as the sweet, the acid, the salty, and the bitter are biological juices, see p. 46.

[84] On this struggle between opposing powers, in which either the body or the concentrated humor "gains the upper hand," see *VM* 3.5, 1.578 L., 4.2, 1.580 L., 5.4, 1.582 L., 7.2, 1.584 L., 11.1, 1.594 L. This is the same theory we find reflected in the speech of Eryximachus.

[85] *VM* 18–19, 1.612–620 L.

Sometimes, the humors do not stay in one place but rather flow to other parts of the body. This movement of humors is called a "flux" (ῥεῦμα), and it produces different complaints depending on the place to which it flows. The author of *On Ancient Medicine* holds that diseases can be cured only when the concentrated humor is either purged from the body or is blended with other humors. Both remedies are assisted by a process known as "coction" (πέψις), a form of "cooking" or "ripening" whereby the peccant humor grows thicker (παχύτερον) and better mixed (μεμιγμένον μᾶλλον), and which parallels the "cooking" and "ripening" of meat, fruits, and other foods.[86] In chapter 19, the author also refers to the notion of a "crisis" (κρίσις); that is, the decisive "turning point" in a disease, which was often presumed to occur at regular intervals called "critical days," and which, if favorable, was considered the time when a concentrated humor has ripened to the point that it can be removed all at once.[87] The author holds that just as cooking involves more than a simple replacement of the cold with the hot, the dry with the wet, so too is the process of coction irreducible to these four *hupotheseis*. "All these [sc. humors] at first send forth salty and moist and acrid discharges (and in such things diseases have their strength), but when they become thicker and more ripe and free of all acridness, then and only then do the fevers cease as well as the other things that harm the human being" (19.2, 1.616 L.).

For the author of *On Ancient Medicine*, there are many different types of humors, and so there must also be many different types of treatment. When it comes to *hupotheseis*, however, the author assumes that the doctors who make use of these principles can only think in terms of the hot, the cold, the dry, and the wet. With each food, they identify one as "hot," another "cold," another "dry," and another "wet."

> But if one hot thing happens to be astringent, another insipid, and yet another causes disturbance – for there are also many other hot things, which have many other powers opposed to one another – surely it will make a difference which of them is administered: the hot and astringent, or the hot and insipid, or that which is at once cold and astringent (for there is also such a thing), or cold and insipid. (15.3, 1.606 L.)

---

[86] *VM* 18.2, 1.614 L.; compare 19.1–2, 1.616 L., 19.6, 1.618 L.

[87] *VM* 19.6, 1.618 L. On the concepts of "coction," "crisis," and "critical days," which are closely related to one another and explicitly utilized in over twenty different works in the Hippocratic Corpus, see Jones (1923a: li–lv), Bourgey (1953: 236–251), Langholf (1990a: 79–135), and Schiefsky (2005: 279–283).

In each of these cases, the hot and the cold are merely "present as an auxiliary [συμπάρεστι], having strength in accordance with the strength of the leading factor [ῥώμης μετέχον, ὡς ἂν τὸ ἡγεύμενον]" (17.3, 1.612 L.). When treating patients who suffer from a fever, it will do no good to simply oppose the fever with cooling agents. Instead, the doctor must purge, concoct, or otherwise transform the humor that is at the root of these symptoms, since it is only by removing the concentration of what is "both bitter and hot, acid and hot, salty and hot, and myriad other combinations" (17.2, 1.612 L.) that the patient will return to a state of health.[88]

To judge from the testimony of *On Ancient Medicine*, the proponents of *hupotheseis* do nothing but treat the hot with the cold, the cold with the hot, the dry with the wet, and the wet with the dry. As Schiefsky (2005: 112–113) observes,

> At the beginning of chapter 13 the author remarks that the opponents, who "pursue the τέχνη from a ὑπόθεσις" are committed to the assumptions that the cause of any disease is one of the ὑποθέσεις (hot, cold, wet, or dry) and that the proper therapy is to treat the cause with its opposite. … Hence any disease may be treated *simply* by determining which of the ὑποθέσεις is its cause and attempting to counteract it by its opposite [my emphasis].

In chapter 17, the author argues that fevers are not due *simply* to the hot (οὐ διὰ τὸ θερμὸν ἁπλῶς) and that the hot is not the *only* cause of this condition (οὐδὲ τοῦτ' εἴη τὸ αἴτιον … μοῦνον; cf. ὑπὸ ψύχεος … μόνου, 18.3, 1.614 L.), again implying that his opponents discard any consideration of the humors in favor of a radically simplified method of arriving at diagnoses and treatments. As we have already noted, however, such radical reductionism is not attested for either Petron or Philistion, and it is also incompatible with the speech of Eryximachus in Plato's *Symposium*. In fact, as we will see in later chapters, the cosmological doctors actually *agreed* with this author, claiming that diseases are primarily manifested in the form of concentrated humors, and that the doctor must purge, concoct, or otherwise transform such humors in order to restore a patient's health.

Because the author of *On Ancient Medicine* presumes that his opponents simply treat the hot with the cold, the cold with the hot, the dry with the wet, and the wet with the dry, he presents several objections to the use of *hupotheseis* that his opponents would not have found particularly difficult to rebut. Consider, for example, the following passage, in which the author

---

[88] On this section, compare the similar remarks about cooling agents at *Morb. III* 17, 7.156 L.

constructs a scenario that he thinks his opponents will be unable to explain (13, 1.598–600 L.):

> But I wish to return to the account of those who pursue their researches in the art according to the new method, from a foundational principle [ἐξ ὑποθέσιος]. For if it is something hot or cold or dry or wet that harms the human being, and if the one who treats correctly must render aid with the hot against the cold, the cold against the hot, the dry against the wet, and the wet against the dry, give me a person whose constitution is not strong, but rather weak. Let this person eat wheat he picks up from the threshing floor, raw and unprepared, and raw meats, and let him drink water. If he follows this regimen I know very well that he will suffer many terrible things: for he will experience pains, his body will be weak, his cavity will be ruined, and he will not be able to live for long. Now what assistance should be prepared for a person in such a state? Hot or cold or dry or wet? One of these, clearly: for if what causes the harm is one or another of these, it must be removed by its opposite, as their account has it. In fact the surest and most obvious remedy is to do away with the regimen he was following and to give wine to drink. These changes must restore him to health, at least if his condition has not been completely ruined by following the bad regimen for a long time. What then are we to say? That his suffering was due to the cold and they helped him by administering these hot things, or the reverse? I think I have created a fine dilemma for the one who is asked this question.

Before we consider the potential rebuttals to this argument, I would like to point out that the cosmological doctors were fully capable of attributing certain ailments to indigestion. We have already seen the testimonies in which Petron is said to have held that diseases arise "whenever the belly, not [taking in?] what is commensurate but [too much?], cannot digest it" (*Anon. Lond.* XX.10–12), while Philistion is said to have attributed some diseases to nutriment that is "unsuitable and corrupt" (*Anon. Lond.* XX.42) and to have classified different varieties of bread on the basis of whether they are easier or more difficult to digest. In *On Regimen*, digestibility is a central concern in the author's food catalogue.[89] At one point, he even writes specifically about foods that are "raw" (ἔνωμα), noting that "raw things cause colic and belching, because what ought to be digested by the fire is dealt with by the belly, which is too weak for the substances that enter it" (56.8, 6.570 L., trans. Jones). There is also a passage from *On the Nature of the*

---

[89] For example, *Vict.* 40.2, 6.536 L. (barley bread passes easily because it is quickly digested), 46.1, 6.544 L. (beef is difficult to digest because it has thick and abundant blood), 54.2, 6.558 L. (radishes stagnate in the belly and are hard to digest), 55.2, 6.562 L. (sweet apples are difficult to digest; acidic and ripe apples less so). Compare also the cases of indigestion at 74.1, 6.614–616 L., 75.1, 6.616 L., and 79.1, 6.624 L.

Human Being that not only deals with indigestion but actually prescribes the same remedies that we find in *On Ancient Medicine*. After noting that patients whose stools contain undigested matter are not adequately "cooking" the food in their bellies, the author writes that "the food of such should be well-baked bread crumbled into wine, and their drink should be as undiluted and as little as possible" (22.2, 6.82 L., trans. Jones) – the same prescriptions of wine and well-baked bread that we see in *On Ancient Medicine*.[90]

The main problem with the above-quoted passage is that it discounts any overlap between *hupotheseis* and humoral theory. The author assumes that causal reductionism is the same as therapeutic reductionism, and that anyone who prioritizes the hot, the cold, the dry, and the wet must simultaneously be rejecting such notions as *apokrisis*, flux, coction, and crisis. It is important to note, however, that *hupotheseis* and humoral theory do not have to be mutually exclusive. A doctor could claim that the hot, the cold, the dry, and the wet engender diseases by *initiating* the separating out of one humor from the rest. If a Greek doctor adopts such a theory, there is nothing to prevent him from assuming that a patient can get sick from eating something that already contains a concentrated humor, as would be the case in the above-quoted passage. Even if an ancient doctor were to make the stronger claim that *all* diseases, without exception, are caused by the hot, the cold, the dry, or the wet, he could still find a way to apply this theory to the scenario described above. One might claim, for instance, that raw food requires a longer period of digestion, since "what ought to be digested by the fire is dealt with by the belly." As the raw food takes more time to digest, the contents of the belly grow hotter than normal, and this heat then initiates the separating out of one humor from the rest.[91]

The author of *On Ancient Medicine* would have made a stronger case if he had used the above-quoted argument to oppose the claim that the hot, the cold, the dry, and the wet are the material elements from which all things are composed. Even on this point, however, his opponents would not have lacked

---

[90] A similar remedy can be found at *Vict.* 79.2, 6.624 L., where the author is also discussing indigestion.
[91] On the heating that arises from stagnant moisture in the belly, see *Hum.* 11, 5.490 L., *Vict.* 46.3, 6.546 L., and compare the reference to "those things that produce heat when they are digested" at *Genit.-Nat. Puer.* 26.2, 7.526 L. On the power of heat to initiate an *apokrisis*, see *Aër.* 9.4, 2.38 L., *Epid. VI* 6.1, 5.322 L., *Nat. Hom.* 12.6, 6.62 L., *Morb. I* 25, 6.190–192 L., *Vict.* 62.2, 6.576 L., 70.2, 6.608 L., *Int.* 30, 7.244 L., *Nat. Mul.* 15, 7.332 L., *Genit.-Nat. Puer.* 1.2, 7.470 L., 30.12, 7.538 L., *Morb. IV* 51, 7.584–590 L., and *Mul. II* 119, 8.258 L. In *On Affections* the consumption of food and drink "in too great an amount and too *strong* [ἰσχυρότερα]" appears in a list of factors that are explicitly said to create diseases by heating, cooling, drying, or moistening bile and phlegm (1, 6.208 L.). This same author also claims that bile and phlegm create problems when they "separate out" and become concentrated (e.g., 16, 6.224 L.), clearly showing that an emphasis on the hot, the cold, the dry, and the wet does not have to be at odds with more traditional theories about the humors.

a response. Consider, for example, the following two passages, in which the author stresses the inability of *hupotheseis* to account for two forms of "cooking":

> Has the person who prepares bread [i.e., the person who transforms raw, unprocessed wheat into edible bread] removed from wheat the hot, the cold, the dry, or the wet? For that which has been given over to fire, moistened with water, and treated in many other ways, each of which has its own power and nature, has lost some of its properties but gained others through blending and mixing. (13.3, 1.600 L.)

> But undergoing coction, changing, thinning, or thickening into a kind of humor through kinds many and varied – for which reason both crises and the reckoning of time are of great importance in such diseases – such modifications hot and cold are the least likely of all these things to undergo: for in this case there could be neither putrefaction nor thickening. How then can we say that there are blends of them that are different, the one from the other, each with its own power, since the hot will not lose its heat except when mixed with the cold, nor indeed will the cold lose its coldness except when mixed with the hot? (19.6, 1.618 L.)

In these passages, the author assumes that his opponents can only *replace* one *hupothesis* with its opposite (i.e., they can only exchange the hot for the cold, the cold for the hot, the dry for the wet, or the wet for the dry). In the first passage, they can only explain the baking of bread as the *removal* of the hot, the cold, the dry, or the wet, while in the second, they can only explain coction and putrefaction by replacing the hot with the cold or the cold with the hot. Such simple exchanges are easy to refute, but they do not exhaust the options that would have been available to the author's opponents. The proponents of *hupotheseis* could have claimed, for example, that coction occurs when a "passive" substance (e.g., moisture) is altered by an "active" substance (e.g., heat). Aristotle in fact defines coction as what happens to everything when its constituent moisture is mastered by the hot (*Mete.* 379b32–33), while *On the Nature of the Human Being* reports that some doctors postulated a unitary substance that "changes its form [ἰδέη] and power [δύναμις] under the compulsion of the hot and the cold, becoming sweet, bitter, white, black, and so on" (2.2, 6.34 L.). The author of *On Flesh* gives a similar explanation for putrefaction, claiming that the "fatty" and the "glutinous" arose when the hot "putrefied" the cold that is contained within the earth (3, 8.584–586 L.).[92] Such passages clearly show

---

[92] On the ability of heat to initiate putrefaction, see also *Aër.* 15.1, 2.60 L., *Acut.* 66.2, 2.368 L., *Aph.* 5.22, 4.538 L., *Liqu.* 6.5, 6.134 L., *Int.* 10, 7.190 L., *Genit.-Nat. Puer.* 24.2, 7.520 L., and *Morb. IV* 51.7,

that coction and putrefaction could be incorporated into a system that postulates nothing more than the hot, the cold, the dry, and the wet. The author of *On Ancient Medicine* deserves credit for seeing the weakness in these theories, but his opponents would not have found his objections particularly compelling, primarily because he discounts the range of interactions that one might attribute to "active" and "passive" substances.

The author of *On Ancient Medicine* oversimplifies the theories of his opponents, assuming that they do nothing but replace the hot with the cold, the cold with the hot, the dry with the wet, and the wet with the dry. The net effect of this oversimplification is that this text is an unreliable witness to what the cosmological doctors were doing. If we follow its testimony too closely, we will get a distorted picture of what this phenomenon is all about. For a good example of this author's unreliability, consider the following passage, in which the author implies that the proponents of *hupotheseis* ignore the fine distinctions that exist between different varieties of bread (14.1–2, 1.600 L.):

> Now I know this too, of course, that it makes a difference to the human body whether bread is made from pure or unsifted flour, from unwinnowed or winnowed wheat, whether it is kneaded with much water or with little, thoroughly kneaded or not kneaded at all, well-baked or undercooked, and myriad other differences in addition to these. The same holds for barley cake as well; the powers [δυνάμιες] of each kind are great and no power is at all like any other. But how could the person who has not examined these matters, or who despite his examination is ignorant of them, have any knowledge of the affections that come upon the human being? For by each one of these things the human being is affected and altered in one way or another, and a person's whole life depends on them, whether he is healthy, recovering from illness, or sick.

This passage is especially ironic if we compare it with the above-mentioned testimonies on Philistion. Philistion was widely recognized as an authority on dietetics, and Athenaeus even provides a detailed summary of the fine distinctions that he drew between different varieties of bread (3.83, trans. Olson, modified):

> Philistion of Locri says that bread made with top-quality flour promotes physical strength more than bread made of coarse-ground flour does; he ranks bread made with coarse-ground flour second, and bread made with ordinary flour after that. Bread made with very fine meal produces worse *chulos* ["juice, humor"] and is less nourishing. Warm bread of all sorts is

---

7.586–588 L. Similar explanations of qualitative change appear in the *Anonymus Londiniensis*; see especially XI.43–XII.8 (Thrasymachus of Sardis) and XI.23–43 (Hippon of Croton).

more easily digested and more nourishing than bread that has cooled, and produces better *chulos*; it also promotes the production of *pneuma* and is easily distributed through the body. Bread that is quite old and very cold is less nourishing, arrests the movement of the bowels, and produces bad *chulos*. Bread baked within the coals is heavy and difficult to digest because it is baked unevenly. Oven bread and kiln bread are difficult to break down and digest. Brazier bread and bread made in a frying-pan are easier to excrete, because oil has been mixed into them, but are harder on the stomach because of their greasiness. Baking-shell bread is rich in good characteristics of all sorts, for it produces good *chulos*, is easy on the stomach, and is easily digested, broken down, and distributed through the body, because it neither arrests the movement of the bowels nor distends them.

In this passage, Philistion does not simply assert that one variety of bread is "hot," another "cold," another "dry," and another "wet." Instead, he observes that certain types of bread are easier or more difficult to digest, more or less nourishing, and either relax or constrict the bowels. He also refers to breads that produce good or bad humors and breads that promote and repress *pneuma*, clearly showing that a theory of first principles can coexist with a more traditional model of pathogenesis. Similar observations can be made about two other texts, *On Regimen* and *On Affections*, both of whose authors give a central role to the hot, the cold, the dry, and the wet. These authors also write about different varieties of bread (*Vict.* 40–44, 6.536–542 L., *Aff.* 52, 6.260–262 L.), and, like Philistion, they describe the "powers" of food and drink in such a way that they clearly have more complex understandings of health and disease than *On Ancient Medicine* would lead us to believe.

So why does the author of *On Ancient Medicine* misrepresent the systems of his opponents? Why does he write as if they rejected more traditional approaches to pathogenesis and thought exclusively in terms of the hot, the cold, the dry, and the wet? Part of the explanation comes from the author's tendency to favor a highly restricted definition of what it means to be a "cause." In chapter 19, the author contrasts the use of *hupotheseis* with his own general theory of human *phusis*. While describing how humors create problems when they "separate out" and then move throughout the body, the author notes, "One must of course consider these fluxes to be the cause [αἴτιον] of each condition, since their presence is necessarily accompanied by that condition in a certain form, while when they change into another blend it ceases" (19.3, 1.616–618 L.). In this passage, the author describes two criteria that allow him to say that humoral fluxes are the "cause" of a disease. First, these fluxes *necessarily* produce a disease whenever they are present. Second, their removal *always* leads to the removal of the disease. When the author writes about the use of *hupotheseis*, he presumes that his opponents adopt this same definition of a cause. They assume that diseases *necessarily* arise when the hot, the cold, the wet, and the dry are in excess, and that the removal of these excesses will *always* lead to the removal of the disease. The author ignores the possibility that his opponents could have viewed their *hupotheseis* as procatarctic causes; that is, as remote causes that initiate a process but whose effects are not always stopped by their removal. He also ignores the possibility that they may have invoked accessory causes in conjunction with their *hupotheseis*, causes that ensure a disease will be produced only when the hot, the cold, the dry, and the wet interact with the body under a specific set of circumstances.[93]

On Ancient Medicine's treatment of causation is reminiscent of a position later endorsed by Erasistratus, who preferred to describe the "cause" of a fever as whatever necessarily produces a fever whenever it occurs (fr. 211 Garofalo, trans. Allen):

> Most people both now and earlier have sought the causes of fevers by wishing to hear and learn from the ill whether their illness had its origin in being chilled or exhausted or in repletion or some other cause of this kind, in this way neither truly [*vere*] nor profitably [*conferenter*] investigating the causes of disease. For if cold were a cause of fever, then those who have been chilled the more would suffer the greater fever. But this is not what happens: rather there are some who have faced extreme danger from freezing, and when rescued have remained unaffected by fever. The same thing happens in regard to exhaustion and repletion: many people who experience far worse exhaustion and repletion than when some people have come down with a fever none the less escape the illness.

Galen wrote an entire treatise, *On Procatarctic Causes*, to challenge this position, although he is probably mistaken in his belief that Erasistratus rejects *all* procatarctic causes, as Allen (2000: 86) observes in his analysis of this fragment:

> Erasistratus is complaining about physicians who, on his view, put forward an item – one of the so called procatarctic causes – as if it furnished

---

[93] For "accessory and contributing causes," see pp. 116–119. On the various levels of causation in Greek medicine, see Vegetti (1999), Pelling (2000: 84–85), and Hankinson (2001, 2018). At 1.1, 1.570 L., the author seems to acknowledge multiple levels of causation when he claims that his opponents narrow down "the starting point of the cause" (τὴν ἀρχὴν τῆς αἰτίης) of diseases and death for human beings. However, the rest of his arguments presuppose that his opponents think *exclusively* in terms of the hot, the cold, the dry, and the wet.

a complete explanation when it manifestly fails to do so. Erasistratus could also believe that there is an especially important factor in the explanation of fevers which deserves to be privileged as the cause because it explains, or plays the principal part in explaining, why fevers arise when and as they do, something that his opponents' causes signally fail to do. ... Erasistratus may also have been moved by the not unreasonable thought that without a deeper understanding of the aetiology of fevers we shall not be in a position to evaluate claims made on behalf of heating, chilling, repletion and the like.

Although the author of *On Ancient Medicine* does not address the issue as directly as Erasistratus, he may have been motivated by a similar set of concerns, believing that doctors should prioritize internal processes over external triggers. Not only are the internal processes *directly* relevant to treatment but an excessive emphasis on external triggers can also lead the doctor astray. In chapter 21, the author complains about the *post hoc, propter hoc* reasoning of doctors who think that whatever their patients did before falling ill must be the "cause" of their affection:

I know that the majority of doctors, like lay people, if patients happen to have done anything unusual on a particular day, either by bathing or walking or eating something different – whether all these things are better done or not – none the less assign the responsibility to one of them, not knowing the cause [τὸ αἴτιον] and perhaps depriving the patient of what is most beneficial. One must not do this, but rather know what will be the effect of an additional bath taken at the wrong time or of fatigue. For the same suffering never arises from either of these, nor indeed from repletion nor from food of one kind or another. Whoever does not know how each of these things stands in relation to the human being will be able neither to recognize their effects nor to make correct use of them.

Just after this passage, the author claims that what doctors should really consider is

which affections come upon the human being from powers [δυναμίων] and which from structures [σχημάτων]. What do I mean by this? By "power" I mean the acuity and strength of the humors; by "structures" I mean all the parts inside the human being, some hollow and tapering from wide to narrow, others also extended, others solid and round, others broad and suspended, others stretched, others long, others dense, others loose in texture and swollen, others spongy and porous. (22.1, 1.626 L.)

In other words, the doctor should pay more attention to what is happening *inside* the body than to what affects it from the outside, since it is only by thinking about internal physiology that the doctor will know what must be done. The same external trigger will not always have the same effect, but the same internal state will always demand the same action. By rebutting the proponents of *hupotheseis* as if their principles performed the same functions as the humors, the author demonstrates that any discussion of disease must consider what is happening within the body.

On the one hand, then, the author of *On Ancient Medicine* misrepresents his opponents because he assumes that their discussions of the hot, the cold, the dry, and the wet must follow the same strong definition of what it means to be a "cause" that he attributes to the humors. At the same time, the author also mischaracterizes his opponents because he is committed to another hard and fast distinction that is not, in fact, as inviolable as he thinks. This distinction concerns two strategies for advancing the medical art: (1) by making it more complex and (2) by making it simpler. In his opening remarks, the author complains that the proponents of *hupotheseis* oversimplify the medical art, narrowing down the causes of disease to "one or two" principles like the hot, the cold, the dry, or the wet (1.1, 1.570 L.). In response, the author claims that *hupotheseis* are unnecessary because medicine has long had its own "starting point and method" (ἀρχὴ καὶ ὁδός, 2.1, 1.572 L.). This method can be traced back to the earliest period of human civilization, and it is responsible for all discoveries that doctors have ever made. "The art of medicine would never have been discovered," the author writes, "nor would anyone have sought for it – for there would have been no need for it – if it were beneficial for the sick to follow the same regimen and diet as the healthy, taking the same foods and drinks and following the same regimen in other respects, and if there were not other things better than these" (3.1, 1.574 L.). Just as Eryximachus observes that "what is dissimilar longs for and desires dissimilar things" (186b), so the author of *On Ancient Medicine* stresses that different types of patients require different modes of treatment. Medicine has advanced, the author asserts, as doctors have made finer and finer distinctions between different classes of patients, recognizing that a doctor's success rests primarily on his ability to distinguish one type of patient from another.

The author of *On Ancient Medicine* presents *hupotheseis* as an attempt to replace this method of advancing the medical art by dividing and subdividing patients into different groups. For as long as can be remembered, doctors have always made discoveries by drawing more precise distinctions between different classes of individuals: humans differ from animals, the sick from the healthy, and specific categories of the sick from those with different "constitutions" (φύσεις) and "physical states" (διαθέσεις).[94] Each of these groups requires a different mode of treatment, and medicine has grown more effective as doctors have determined what is "fitting" (ἁρμόζων) for each class.[95] With the introduction of "foundational principles," by contrast, the author implies that some doctors are now trying to move medicine in the opposite direction. Instead of increasing the complexity of the art, they are "narrowing down the starting point of the cause of diseases and death for human beings, laying down the same one or two things as the cause in all cases" (1.1, 1.570 L.). Such reductionism, the author holds, runs counter to the interest of doctors in identifying the *differences* between individual patients. Medicine has always improved by growing more complex, and there is no reason to reject this time-tested method in favor of "foundational principles" that are the same in every case.

This emphasis on dividing patients into groups, and then adapting treatments to the particular needs of each group, carries over into the author's second polemic, in which he takes issue with accounts of human *phusis* that focus on the genesis and elemental constitution of human beings. In chapter 20, the author writes that there are some doctors and "sophists" who claim that anyone who intends to practice medicine correctly must first have a knowledge of what a human being is. In particular, they claim that doctors should know "what a human being is from the beginning, how it originally came to be, and from what it was compounded" (20.1, 1.620 L.), even though such accounts have no practical purpose but rather "tend toward philosophy" (τείνει ἐς φιλοσοφίην). Here, the term "philosophy" is used in its etymological sense of "wisdom-loving," the idea being that such knowledge has no practical use but is merely pursued for its own sake.[96] Doctors should know about human *phusis*, the author writes,

---

[94] On the distinctions between patients with different "constitutions" (φύσεις) and "physical states" (διαθέσεις), see *VM* 3.4–5, 1.576–578 L., 5.4, 1.580–582 L., 6.2, 1.582–584 L., 7.2, 1.584 L., 8.2, 1.586 L., 12.1, 1.596 L., 13.1, 1.598 L. Generally speaking, the author uses the term *phusis* to refer to a physical condition that is always present, while *diathesis* denotes a condition that is only temporary (e.g., an illness). Hence, we would say that humans differ from other animals in terms of their *phuseis*, while the healthy differ from the sick in terms of their *diatheseis*.

[95] *VM* 3.4, 1.576 L., 5.1, 1.580 L.

[96] On the history of the term "philosophy," see Schiefsky (2005: 300–302) and Laks (2006: 55–81). The sense of "wisdom-loving" also appears in the earliest attestations of the verb φιλοσοφεῖν at Hdt. 1.30.2 and Th. 2.40.1. For similar distinctions between practical knowledge and the impractical chattering of purveyors of "wisdom," see *Fract.* 1–2, 3.412–422 L., *Art.* 14, 4.120 L., 44, 4.188 L., and Isoc. 13.7–8; compare also Arist. *Metaph.* 982b11–21 with Nightingale (2004: 187–252). Especially close to the sense of "philosophy" in *On Ancient Medicine* is what Callicles says to Socrates at Pl. *Grg.*

but only in terms of how the same things, administered in the same way, will have different effects on different constitutions. To illustrate this point, the author observes that a single foodstuff could simultaneously be harmful to some patients and beneficial to others, as we see in the case of cheese (20.5–6, 1.624 L.):

> Cheese . . . does not harm all human beings in the same way: there are some who can eat their fill of it without being harmed at all, and it even provides a wondrous strength to those whom it benefits; but there are others who have difficulty coping with it. Hence the natures of these people differ, and the difference concerns the very thing in the body that is hostile to cheese and is stirred up and set in motion by it. Those in whom such a humor happens to be present in greater quantity and to exert more power in the body will naturally suffer more. But if cheese were bad for human nature in general, it would harm all people.

The author's hostility toward cosmological accounts of human *phusis* is similar to his hostility toward *hupotheseis*. Broadly understood, this author's approach to medicine consists of dividing and subdividing patients into groups, and then considering how treatments should be adapted to each. When his opponents introduce a small set of principles that apply to all patients, to all diseases, and to all things in general, the author suggests that they are simultaneously rejecting the fine distinctions that exist between individual cases.

A good parallel for this author's complaint about *hupotheseis* can be found in *On Fractures*. In this text, the author warns against "wisdom-mongering doctors" (οἱ ἰητροὶ σοφιζόμενοι; cf. *On Ancient Medicine*'s ἰητροὶ καὶ σοφισταί, 20.1, 1.620 L.) who indiscriminately apply the same treatment in every case (1–2, 3.412–422 L., trans. Withington, modified):

> Indeed, those who have no preconceived idea [οἳ μὲν οὖν μηδὲν προβουλεύονται] make no mistake as a rule, for the patient himself holds out the arm for bandaging in the position impressed on it by conformity with nature [φύσις]. The wisdom-mongering doctors are just the ones who go wrong. In fact the treatment of a fractured arm is not difficult, and is almost any practitioner's job, but I have to write a good deal about it because I know practitioners who have got credit for wisdom by putting up arms in positions which ought rather to have given them a name for ignorance. And many other parts of this art are

484c–486d. Gorgias's characterization of "philosophical speeches" at *Hel.* 13 also stresses the impracticality and unreliability of such exchanges.

judged thus: for they praise what seems outlandish [ξενοπρεπές] before they know whether it is good, rather than the customary [σύνηθες] which they already know to be good; the bizarre [ἀλλόκοτον] rather than the obvious [εὔδηλον]. ... [One such doctor made his patient hold a broken arm] as the archers do when they bring forward the shoulder, and he put it up in this posture, persuading himself that this was its natural position [τὸ κατὰ φύσιν]. He adduced as evidence the forearm bones, and the surface also, how it has its outer and inner parts in a direct line, declaring this to be the natural disposition of the flesh and tendons [οὕτω δὲ ἔφη καὶ τὰς σάρκας καὶ τὰ νεῦρα πεφυκέναι], and he brought in the art of the archer as evidence. This gave an appearance of wisdom to his discourse and practice, but he had forgotten the other arts and all those things which are executed by strength or artifice, not knowing that the natural position varies in one and another [ἄλλο ἐν ἄλλῳ τὸ κατὰ φύσιν σχῆμά ἐστιν], and that in doing the same work it may be that the right arm has one natural position and the left another. For there is one natural position in throwing the javelin, another in using the sling, another in casting a stone, another in boxing, another in repose. How many arts might one find in which the natural position of the arms is not the same, but they assume postures in accordance with the apparatus each man uses and the work he wants to accomplish! As to the practiser of archery, he naturally finds the above posture strongest for one arm. ... But there is nothing in common between putting up fractures and archery. For, first, if the operator, after putting up an arm, kept it in this position, he would inflict much additional pain, greater than that of the injury, and again, if he bade him bend the elbow, neither bones, tendons, nor flesh would keep in the same position, but would rearrange themselves in spite of the dressings. Where, then, is the advantage of the archer position? And perhaps our wisdom-mongerer [σοφιζόμενος] would not have committed this error had he let the patient himself present the arm.

Like the author of *On Ancient Medicine*, the author of *On Fractures* advocates treatments that are "in accordance with the nature" (κατὰ φύσιν) of the patient. This procedure will change from one case to the next, but the patient will hold his arm in such a way as to show what is needed in each case. The "wisdom-mongering" doctors, on the other hand, make use of preconceived notions (προβουλεύονται; cf. *On Ancient Medicine*'s *hupotheseis*). They simply formulate some universal principle about the "nature" (φύσις) of human beings (cf. οὕτω δὲ ἔφη καὶ τὰς σάρκας καὶ τὰ νεῦρα πεφυκέναι) and then appeal to this principle when applying the same treatment in every case. Like the author of *On Ancient Medicine*, the author of *On Fractures* complains that his opponents are dispensing with a methodology that has been proven over time (σύνηθες) and whose principles are open to the senses (εὔδηλον), replacing this with treatments that are outlandish and bizarre (ξενοπρεπές, ἀλλόκοτον). Adding insult to injury, these "wisdom-mongering" doctors draw on fields of learning that have nothing to do with medicine. The author of *On Fractures* criticizes a doctor who invokes the art of archery when setting broken bones. In response, he observes that "there is nothing in common between putting up fractures and archery," a phrase that recalls *On Ancient Medicine*'s assertion that "whatever has been said or written about 'nature' by a sophist or doctor pertains less to the *techne* of the doctor than to that of the painter" (ἧσσον νομίζω τῇ ἰητρικῇ τέχνῃ προσήκειν ἢ τῇ γραφικῇ, 20.2, 1.620 L.).[97]

Of course, if there really *were* doctors who insisted on setting every broken arm in the position of an archer, then the author of *On Fractures* would be justified in criticizing such doctors for not adapting their treatments to fit the needs of individual patients. Similarly, if there really *were* doctors who did nothing but treat the hot with the cold, the cold with the hot, the dry with the wet, and the wet with the dry, then the author of *On Ancient Medicine* would be right to criticize these doctors for oversimplifying the medical art. It should be noted, however, that beyond the polemic in *On Ancient Medicine*, we have no evidence that any Greek doctor from the Classical period actually simplified medicine to this extent. Such radical reductionism cannot be found in the testimonies on Petron and Philistion, in the speech of Eryximachus, or, as we will see, in the surviving works of the cosmological doctors.[98] In fact, as I will argue in Chapter 2, the

---

[97] The idea seems to be that just as it would be ridiculous for the *techne* of the painter to rely on cosmological theories, so too is it unnecessary for medicine, another *techne*, to be rooted in "philosophy." For a different interpretation, see Schiefsky (2005: 306–310), who follows Müller (1965b) in reading ἡ γραφικὴ τέχνη as "the art of writing treatises." It seems impossible, however, for ἡ γραφικὴ τέχνη to be translated in this way, as (1) the *technai* are traditionally named for their practitioners (cf. ἰατρική < ἰατρός, μαντική < μάντις, ῥητορική < ῥήτωρ) and (2) a "writer of treatises" is not a γραφεύς but a συγγραφεύς. For the common pairing of medicine and painting as quintessential *technai*, see Pl. *Prt.* 311c–312d, *Grg.* 448b–c, 450a–d, and Arist. *EN* 1180b35, 1181a21–b3. Note also the inclusion of these activities alongside other *technai* at *De arte* 11.7, 6.22 L., Pl. *Plt.* 299b–e, *Grg.* 503e–504a, *Ion* 531e–533a, and *Lg.* 10.889d.

[98] Lloyd (1963: 121) similarly observes that "the author of *VM* refers to pathologists who apparently reduced the causes of diseases to such opposites alone, and this extreme form of the doctrine is found neither in the Hippocratic Corpus nor in the account of medical theories in *Anon. Lond.*" Lloyd goes on to assume, however, that there may have been other theorists who constructed such systems but are simply unattested. While we of course cannot fully discount such a possibility, I will argue over the next few chapters that such a combination of both causal and therapeutic reductionism runs

cosmological doctors actually *agreed* with this author when it came to dividing patients into groups, considering the "nature" of each group, and adapting their treatments to fit the needs of individual situations. Far from replacing one system with another, the cosmological doctors were building on the very approach to clinical decision-making that *On Ancient Medicine* claims they were rejecting.

counter to the very pressures that gave rise to cosmological medicine in the first place. A far more likely conclusion is that the author of *On Ancient Medicine* is simply exaggerating the position of his opponents, a tactic that is certainly not unprecedented in intellectual debates.

CHAPTER 2

On the Nature of the Human Being

2.1 The Hot, the Cold, the Wet, and the Dry

In Chapter 1, we examined three indirect sources for the cosmological doctors: (1) the *Anonymus Londiniensis*, (2) the speech of Eryximachus in Plato's *Symposium*, and (3) *On Ancient Medicine*. We observed that Petron and Philistion speculated about the elemental constitution of human beings, that they attributed some diseases to an imbalance in the hot, the cold, the dry, and the wet, and that they also cultivated more traditional theories regarding the humors, *pneuma*, and the "powers" of food and drink. We also saw that Eryximachus uses an argument from induction to demonstrate that *eros* is a universal principle, and, like Petron and Philistion, he seems to combine a theory of opposites with a more traditional model of pathogenesis. Finally, we noted that *On Ancient Medicine* is an unreliable witness to what the cosmological doctors were doing. The author writes as if these doctors were exclusively treating the hot with the cold, the cold with the hot, the dry with the wet, and the wet with the dry, when in fact they seem to have *agreed* with this author, at least insofar as they recognized the importance of identifying and then purging harmful humors from the body.

At this point, it is difficult to say much more about the cosmological doctors. None of these sources give us detailed information concerning the structure of their systems, let alone any indication as to why these doctors would have created such systems in the first place. We would like to know, for example, why the cosmological doctors thought they *needed* to combine the first principles of the universe with a humoral model of disease. What limitations did they think they were addressing by constructing such systems, and what might their systems tell us about the priorities of Greek doctors in the fifth and fourth centuries BCE? Fortunately, the Hippocratic Corpus contains four texts that can help us answer these questions. These are *On the Nature of the Human Being, On Breaths, On Flesh*, and *On Regimen*. Over the rest of this study, I will examine each of these texts, providing a general outline of their systems. I will also consider what these texts can tell us about the cosmological doctors as a group. I will begin with *On the Nature of the Human Being*, a text whose system is presently the best understood of those expounded by a cosmological doctor. I will start by summarizing this author's beliefs about the elements, the humors, and the role of the doctor in both treating and preventing disease. I will then show that this text is incompatible with the two central complaints in *On Ancient Medicine*: (1) that the cosmological doctors dispensed with humoral theory in favor of exclusively treating the hot with the cold, the cold with the hot, the dry with the wet, and the wet with the dry, and (2) that these same doctors rejected the division and subdivision of patients into groups in favor of a handful of *hupotheseis* that are the same in every case.

There is a strong case to be made that *On the Nature of the Human Being* was written by Polybus of Cos, a famous doctor who flourished around 400 BCE. Polybus was the son of a certain Apollonius, but he was better known in antiquity as the student and successor of Hippocrates. According to Galen, Polybus stayed on Cos for his entire life, eventually taking over leadership of Hippocrates's school.[1] Other sources claim, with varying degrees of believability, that he married Hippocrates's daughter,[2] that he provided his mentor with seven books on medicine from the Egyptian city of Memphis,[3] that Hippocrates sent him to provide treatment to Greek cities during the plague,[4] and that he was the author of not only *On the Nature of the Human Being* but also the treatise *On the Eight Months' Child.*[5] We do not know the criteria that ancient editors used when attributing *On the Nature of the Human Being* to Polybus. Galen, for his

---

[1] Gal. *Opt. Med.* 1.58 K., *HNH* 15.11–12 K., *Sept. Part.* 2, p. 344.59–64 Walzer.
[2] *Thess. orat.* 9.420 L., Gal. *Diff. Resp.* 7.960 K.   [3] *Vita Hippocratis Bruxellensis* 39–40.
[4] *Thess. orat.* 9.420 L. Contrast Gal. *Opt. Med.* 1.58 K.
[5] *On the Nature of the Human Being*: Gal. *HNH* 15.11 K., 15.171–172 K. *On the Eight Months' Child*: Gal. *Sept. Part.* 2, p. 344.49–59 Walzer, *Hipp. Epid. II* p. 300 Wenkebach and Pfaff, Clem. Alex. *Strom.* 6.16.139, Plu. [*Placit.*] 908a–b, Gal. [*Hist. Phil.*] 19.331 K. Galen mentions two further treatises, *On Affections* and *On the Nature of the Child*, as the work of "either Hippocrates or Polybus" (*Hipp. Aph.* 18a.8 K., *Foet. Form.* 4.653 K.). This may, however, simply reflect his interest in claiming that these texts are "at least Hippocratic, if not by Hippocrates himself." See *Diff. Resp.* 7.959–960 K. and *HNH* 15.11–12 K. for Galen's belief that Polybus did not deviate from the teachings of Hippocrates, and *Hipp. Off. Med.* 18b.666 K. for a similar reference to "either Hippocrates or Thessalus" as the author of *In the Workshop*. On the attribution of *On the Eight Months' Child* to Polybus, see Grensemann (1968), who argues for its acceptance. For rebuttals, see Jouanna (1969) and Joly (1970: 158–162) with the response of Grensemann (1974: 431–433). For more on Polybus's life, see Nutton (2007b) and Manetti (2008d).

part, argues that chapters 1–8 are by Hippocrates, 9–15 by an anonymous interpolator, and only 16–22 by Polybus. It is important to remember, however, that Galen had a professional interest in attributing chapters 1–8 to Hippocrates, while his arguments for identifying chapters 9–15 as an interpolation no longer stand up to critical scrutiny.[6] The modern case for identifying Polybus as the author of this text depends on two pieces of evidence. First, Aristotle quotes chapter 11 of *On the Nature of the Human Being* in his *History of Animals*, attributing it to Polybus (512b12–513a7). Second, the *Anonymus Londiniensis*, which draws on a Peripatetic source, summarizes chapters 1–4 in its entry on Polybus (XIX.1–18). Since only a few decades separate Aristotle from Polybus, it is reasonable to assume that the physician from Cos was indeed the author of this text. Few authorities, in fact, would have been better positioned to identify this author, as Aristotle was himself the son of a doctor and deeply interested in medical science. In light of these testimonies, I will refer to the author of *On the Nature of the Human Being* as "Polybus" from this point forward. Although my arguments will not rely on this identification, the name "Polybus" will provide a useful shorthand for denoting the author of this text.

Like the other cosmological doctors we have encountered so far, Polybus places the hot, the cold, the dry, and the wet at the center of his medical system. In chapter 3, he claims that all things are composed of these four substances, referring to their interactions as "the nature of humans/animals and of all other things" (τῆς φύσιος ... καὶ τῶν ἄλλων πάντων καὶ τοῦ ἀνθρώπου, 3.2, 6.38 L.; τῶν ζῴων ... ἡ φύσις καὶ τῶν ἄλλων πάντων, 3.4, 6.38 L.). Because these four substances are neither created nor destroyed, Polybus does not believe in generation or destruction in the usual sense of these terms. Instead, he describes "generation" as a form of mixture (κρῆσις, 3.1, 6.38 L.; cf. μίσγηται, 3.1, 6.38 L.), while "destruction" is merely dissolution. In chapter 3, Polybus writes that "each must return to its own nature when a human body dies, wet to wet, dry to dry, hot to hot, and cold to cold" (3.3, 6.38 L.). He also observes that "to the same thing from which each was composed, that is where it departs" (3.4, 6.38 L.), implying that the hot, the cold, the dry, and the wet are constantly combined, separated, and recombined to create everything in the universe. This belief that all things are composed of four substances, which are both mixed and separated without ever being destroyed, has reminded many scholars of

---

[6] On the unity of *On the Nature of the Human Being*, see note 15 of this chapter. This unity persists even if we assume, with Langholf (2004), that some parts of this text were adapted from other sources.

Empedocles. Like Polybus, Empedocles postulated that all things are composed of four elements (fire, air, water, and earth), and he likewise attributed "creation" and "destruction" to the mixing and dissolution of these fundamental principles. Polybus takes an unusual turn, however, when he sets the following requirement for generation (3.1, 6.38 L., trans. Jones, modified):

> If the combination of hot with cold and of dry with wet be not proportioned and equal to one another [μετρίως πρὸς ἄλληλα . . . καὶ ἴσως], but the one constituent is much in excess of the other [τὸ ἕτερον τοῦ ἑτέρου πολλὸν προέξει], and the stronger is much stronger than the weaker [τὸ ἰσχυρότερον τοῦ ἀσθενεστέρου], generation will not take place.

With this statement, Polybus seems to assert that, for generation to occur (i.e., for the hot, the cold, the wet, and the dry to come together and form a stable compound), all four substances must be present *simultaneously*, and that these four substances must also be present in roughly equal proportions. Such a stipulation is difficult to reconcile with the system of Empedocles, who is happy to claim that stable compounds can be created from imbalanced mixtures. At DK 31 B96, Empedocles claims that bones are composed of two parts earth, two parts water, and four parts fire. Not only does this mixture include one element (fire) that is "much in excess" when compared with the other two, but a fourth element (air) is completely absent from this mixture.

Polybus's stipulation that generation requires components that are "proportioned and equal to one other" is certainly unusual. However, it becomes easier to understand when we compare this view with his statements about health and disease. In chapter 4, Polybus identifies the specific "nature" of human beings as the combination of four humors: blood, phlegm, yellow bile, and black bile. Like the universe, animals, and human beings in general, each of these humors is composed of four substances – the hot, the cold, the dry, and the wet – and they each acquire a particular "aspect" (ἰδέα) and "power" (δύναμις) from minor imbalances in their elemental mixture (5.2, 6.40–42 L.). Polybus believes that diseases arise when there is a "separating out" of one humor from the rest. As he writes in the opening of chapter 4 (trans. Jones, modified):

> The body of the human being has in itself blood, phlegm, yellow bile, and black bile; these are the nature of his body, and it is on account of these that he feels pain or enjoys health. Now he enjoys the most perfect health when these are duly proportioned to one another in respect of power and quantity [μετρίως ἔχῃ ταῦτα τῆς πρὸς ἄλληλα δυνάμιος καὶ τοῦ πλήθεος], and when

they are most perfectly mixed together. Pain is felt when one of these, in a smaller or greater quantity, is isolated in the body without being blended with all the others.

This passage closely recalls the definition of disease that we find in *On Ancient Medicine*. In both texts, diseases are attributed to a "separating out" of certain humors whereby the "power" or "strength" of one humor overpowers that of the rest.[7] *On Ancient Medicine* counts these humors as "myriad" (14.4, 1.602 L.) and defines them primarily by their taste. Polybus, meanwhile, reduces the humors to four, defining them as blood, phlegm, yellow bile, and black bile.[8] Interestingly, Polybus repeats the same phrase, "proportioned to one another" (μετρίως πρὸς ἄλληλα), that appears in his discussion of the elements, again defining such a balance in terms of both power (δύναμις; cf. τὸ ἰσχυρότερον τοῦ ἀσθενεστέρου) and quantity (πλῆθος; cf. τὸ ἕτερον τοῦ ἑτέρου πολλὸν προέξει). Just as the isolation of one humor is detrimental to human health, so too is the concentration of an element detrimental to coming to be. If this mechanism of humoral *apokrisis* does in fact lie behind Polybus's theory of generation, then our author has taken an intriguing stance regarding the relationship between medicine and cosmology. By asserting that both the elements and the humors must exist in a proportionate "blending" for the continued wellbeing of whatever they inhabit, Polybus takes a requirement for *health* and makes it a requirement for *being*.[9]

In chapter 7, Polybus describes the tendency of each humor to increase and diminish during the year. Phlegm is cold and wet, and it increases during the winter. Blood is hot and wet, and it increases during the spring. Yellow bile is hot and dry, and it increases during the summer. Black bile is cold and dry, and it increases during the fall. Polybus claims to have come to this conclusion after observing the cyclical nature of disease: "It is in winter that the sputum and nasal discharge of human beings is fullest of

---

[7] On the "power" (δύναμις) and "strength" (ἰσχύς) of concentrated humors, see also *Nat. Hom.* 8.1, 6.52 L.

[8] There are some passages, however, in which Polybus seems to associate the humors with tastes. In chapter 2, he describes different humors as being "sweet or bitter, white or black," while in chapter 6, he compares the purging of humors to the process by which plants draw from the earth "the acid, the bitter, the sweet, the salt, and so on." The author of *On Ancient Medicine* likewise refers to "bile" at 19.5, 1.618 L., suggesting a similar flexibility in terminology.

[9] Compare *Nat. Hom.* 2.3, 6.34 L. (discussed on p. 74), where Polybus uses the inability to account for pain as his first argument against material monists who claim that humans are composed of a single humor. This suggests that Polybus was indeed thinking about the creation of pain when he contemplated the nature of the elements.

phlegm; at this season mostly swellings become white, and diseases generally phlegmatic" (7.3, 6.46 L.). "It is chiefly in spring and summer," meanwhile, "that humans are attacked by bloody stools and by hemorrhage from the nose, and they are then hottest and red" (7.4, 6.48 L.). Finally, it is in the summer and autumn that "humans vomit bile without an emetic, and when they take purges the discharges are most bilious" (7.5, 6.48 L., trans. Jones, modified; cf. 15.5, 6.68 L.). Connections between winter and phlegm, summer and bile are very common in the Hippocratic Corpus.[10] The association of blood with spring and black bile with autumn is less common, though not unparalleled.[11] Most scholars now agree that Polybus built his four-humor system on top of a familiar polarity between bile and phlegm. Within this polarity, bile could be associated with the hot, the dry, summer, fire, youth, and the male, while phlegm could be associated with the cold, the wet, winter, water, old age, and the female.[12] In *On the Nature of the Human Being*, Polybus explicitly refers to oppositions between fire and water (5.2, 6.42 L.), summer and winter (5.4, 6.42 L., 7.5, 6.48 L., 8.1, 6.50 L., 16–18, 6.72–76 L., 20, 6.78–80 L., 22.1, 6.82 L.), youth and old age (9.3, 6.52–54 L., 17.3–4, 6.74–76 L.), and the male and the female (9.3, 6.54 L., 21.2, 6.82 L.). In all but the reference to fire and water (where such qualities are presumably self-evident), he explicitly associates the first member of each pair with the hot and the dry, the second with the cold and the wet.

Polybus frequently relies on analogies to draw connections between disparate phenomena. The number four is especially important in his system, as it connects the four elements, the four humors, and the four seasons of the year. Toward the end of chapter 7, he asserts that just as all objects must contain a simultaneous blending of the hot, the cold, the dry, and the wet, so too must the body contain a simultaneous blending of blood, phlegm, yellow bile, and black bile. Even though the four humors ebb and flow, all four must be present at all times. Polybus justifies this principle by claiming that the hot, the cold, the dry, and the wet are

---

[10] For example, *Aër.* 7.2, 2.26 L., *Acut. App.* 1.1, 2.394 L., *Aph.* 3.21, 4.494–496 L., 3.23, 4.496 L., *Epid. V* 71–72, 5.246 L., *Epid. VII* 82, 5.438 L., *Hum.* 14, 5.496 L., *Aff.* 14, 6.220–222 L., and *Int.* 28, 7.240 L., 30, 7.244 L., 35, 7.252 L., 38–39, 7.260–262 L.

[11] Blood in spring: *Epid. I* 14–17, 2.640–650 L., *Aph.* 3.20, 4.494 L., *Hum.* 14, 5.496 L.; compare *Epid. III* 4.6, 3.76 L., *Int.* 32, 7.248 L. Black bile in autumn: *Aph.* 3.22, 4.496 L., *Epid. IV* 16, 5.154 L., *Epid. VI* 1.11, 5.272 L., *Int.* 27, 7.236 L., 34, 7.252 L.

[12] For the identification of bile as hot and phlegm as cold, compare Arist. [*Pr.*] 1.29, 862b28. A scheme of blood, phlegm, bile, and black bile is also suggested by *Epid. III* 14, 3.96–98 L., *Epid. VI* 5.8, 5.318 L., and *Int.* 30–34, 7.244–252 L.; compare also Arist. *HA* 511b1–10 with van der Eijk (1990: 52–53). In all, bile and phlegm are cited side by side in over twenty different Hippocratic works.

mutually dependent: "none in fact of these would last for a moment without all the things that are present in this cosmos, but if one were to fail all would disappear, for by the same necessity all things are constructed and nourished by one another" (7.8, 6.48–50 L.). Polybus does not elaborate on this point, but he seems to believe that opposite principles depend on one another. The hot, for example, would depend on the cold, the dry on the wet, and so on. As we will see, this principle of opposite-interdependence can also be found in *On Regimen*. It explains the cyclical dominance of each element (for it would be impossible for any one element to sustain perpetual dominance without running out of fuel), and it also implicitly demands that a single element not exist on its own.

Polybus's insistence that all four humors must be present at all times, and that these four humors mirror the four roots of all things, ultimately leads him to oppose all thinkers who claim that the body is constructed of a single element. He begins his treatise with a two-part polemic, in which he first dismisses those who assert that humans are composed entirely of "air, fire, water, earth, or anything else not obviously present in human beings" (1, 6.32–34 L., trans. Jones, modified). As we have already noted, Polybus will later assert that all things are composed of the hot, the cold, the dry, and the wet. He therefore seems to draw an empirical distinction between (1) air, fire, water, and earth and (2) the hot, the cold, the dry, and the wet, dismissing unprovable theories about air, fire, water, or earth while simultaneously believing that substances labeled the "hot," the "cold," the "dry," and the "wet" are open to perception and accordingly fall within the limits of what a doctor is permitted to discuss. Some scholars have overlooked this empirical distinction and have thus downplayed the role of cosmological thinking in Polybus's system. Jouanna even claims that Polybus wishes to affirm "the autonomy of medicine in relation to cosmology."[13] In reality, Polybus is not arguing against the formulation of cosmological principles. Instead, he is only arguing against rooting such principles in substances whose presence cannot be confirmed through the senses. For a similar sentiment, we may compare Herodotus's dismissal of those who claim that the Nile flows from Oceanus, a mythical river that was once believed to encircle the earth. Herodotus asserts that "the person who spoke of Oceanus, transporting his tale into the realm of the obscure, cannot be submitted to scrutiny. For I, at least, do not know that any river called Oceanus exists" (2.23). In this passage, Herodotus is not rejecting all forms of speculation about the Nile. Instead, he only rejects those theories

---

[13] Jouanna (1965: 207), repeated at Jouanna (2002: 224).

that he considers irredeemably obscure, preferring to focus on explanations that appeal to verifiable phenomena. In *On the Nature of the Human Being*, Polybus similarly treats verifiability as a demarcating line between his own discussion of human beings and other speculations about the body. Other people may wish to talk about things that are not obviously present in human beings, but such discussions of human *phusis* extend beyond the limits of medicine (προσωτέρω ἢ ὅσον αὐτῆς ἐς ἰητρικὴν ἀφήκει, 1.1, 6.32 L.). Implicit in this statement is the same contrast between impractical "wisdom loving" (φιλοσοφία) and practical "craft knowledge" (τέχνη) that we see in *On Ancient Medicine*. Polybus and the author of *On Ancient Medicine* come to different conclusions about the hot, the cold, the dry, and the wet, but they both believe in a dividing line between medicine and other fields.

After dismissing those who assert that humans are composed entirely of air, fire, water, or earth, Polybus turns to a second group: those who claim that humans are composed of a single humor. In response to these theorists, whom Polybus identifies as "doctors" (ἰητροί), he offers two rebuttals. First, he claims that a one-humor theory cannot be reconciled with the existence of pain, which, as we have already seen, Polybus attributes to the "separating out" of one humor from the rest.[14] Even if a one-humor theory could account for pain, he adds, there would be no variation in either diseases or their treatments. Instead, all cures would be one and the same, whereas experience shows us that "there are many forms of diseases and also many modes of treatment" (πολλαὶ μὲν ἰδέαι τῶν νοσημάτων, πολλὴ δὲ ἡ ἴησις, 2.3, 6.34–36 L., trans. Jones). Polybus's second rebuttal of one-humor theories draws on his observation that the humors ebb and flow in unison with the seasons. If humans were composed of a single humor, he contends, then there should be a single season in which the body is entirely blood, bile, or phlegm (2.4, 6.36 L.). No such season exists, however, so the humors cannot be one.

2.2   Remote and Proximate Causes

Polybus's general discussion of human *phusis* extends through the end of chapter 7. In the second part of this text, chapters 8–15, he offers a series of precepts on pathology and treatment.[15] One key concept that arises from

---

[14] For a similar argument that a unity cannot feel pain, see Meliss. DK 30 B7.4–6. An opposing view was expressed by Diogenes of Apollonia (DK 64 B2), who alleged that nothing can suffer harm *unless* all things are one substance. For Polybus's possible engagement with Melissus, see Jouanna (1965).

[15] Jouanna (2002: 22–38) has persuasively demonstrated the continuity of this section with the rest of *On the Nature of the Human Being*. In coming to this conclusion, he was preceded by Schöne (1900)

this section is the notion of humoral flux. Polybus defines the origin of disease as the "separating out" of one humor from the rest. Once a humor separates out, however, it does not necessarily stay in one place. Instead, the humor can move throughout the body, eventually becoming stuck in one part or another. In chapter 10, Polybus observes that a disease that originates and then flows from a stronger part of the body is more difficult to treat than one that originates and then flows from a weaker part. In chapter 11, he describes four pairs of vessels that descend from the head, noting how they extend to the eyes, the ears, the spine, the hips, the lungs, the spleen, and other parts – all places to which humors were commonly thought to flow and get stuck.[16] In chapter 12, he describes three fluxes that originate in the flesh and produce different ailments depending on the place to which they flow, while in chapter 13, he observes that "diseases which originate from a scanty flux and whose causes are easily diagnosed offer the surest prognoses." Finally, in chapter 14, Polybus offers advice on how to determine the starting point of a flux that terminates in the bladder. The presence of blood in the urine, for example, will mark an affection that originates in the vessels, while small pieces of flesh will indicate that the affection has started in the kidneys.

and Deichgräber (1971: 105–112). Of particular note are the many verbal parallels listed at Jouanna (2002: 30–37). In both sections, the humors are designated with the periphrasis "the things inside the body" (τῶν ἐν τῷ σώματι ἐνεόντων, 7.1, 6.46 L. ~ τῶν ἐν τῷ σώματι ἐνεόντων, 15.5, 6.68 L.). In both sections, black bile is called the "stickiest" of the humors (γλισχρότατον, 7.2, 6.46 L. ~ γλισχρότατον, 15.5, 6.68 L.), objects are said to become hot when they are moved "with force" (βίη, 7.2, 6.46 L. ~ πρὸς βίην, 12.6, 6.64 L.), and analogous formulas are used to describe the tendencies of certain humors to attack at specific times of year or stages of life (οἱ ἄνθρωποι τοῦ ἦρος καὶ τοῦ θέρεος μάλιστα ὑπό τε τῶν δυσεντεριῶν ἁλίσκονται, 7.4, 6.48 L. ~ φθινοπώρου μάλιστα οἱ ἄνθρωποι ἁλίσκονται ὑπό τῶν τεταρταίων, 15.5, 6.68 L.; ἡ δὲ χολὴ τοῦ θέρεος κατέχει τὸ σῶμα καὶ τοῦ φθινοπώρου, 7.5, 6.48 L. ~ ἡ δὲ ἡλικίη αὕτη ὑπὸ μελαίνης χολῆς κατέχεται, 15.5, 6.68 L.). The importance of the number four continues in this section, with references to four pairs of vessels that descend from the head (11.1, 6.58 L.) and four types of fevers that arise from bile (15.1, 6.66 L.). Both sections also illustrate an interest in establishing principles that remain the same regardless of other variables (καὶ νέου ἐόντος καὶ γέροντος, καὶ τῆς ὥρης ψυχρῆς ἐούσης καὶ θερμῆς, 2.5, 6.36 L. ~ καὶ τῶν νεωτέρων καὶ τῶν πρεσβυτέρων, καὶ γυναικῶν καὶ ἀνδρῶν, 9.3, 6.52–54 L.), and both are structured around Polybus's theory of four humors, with chapter 11 referencing both the painful accumulation of blood in the body (11.6, 6.60 L.) and the four pairs of vessels that convey phlegm from the head (11.1–4, 6.58–60 L.), while chapter 15 attributes three types of fevers to bile (15.2–4, 6.66–68 L.) and one to black bile (15.5, 6.68 L.). This is on top of the already noted references to Polybus as the author of both chapters 1–4 (*Anon. Lond.* XIX.1–18) and chapter 11 (Arist. *HA* 512b12–513a7). All these details, and others cited by Jouanna, are sufficient to trust the continuity of this section with what has come before. As for the *internal* coherence of chapters 8–15, a list of further parallels can be found at Jouanna (2002: 30).

[16] On the typical destinations of humoral fluxes, see *Loc. Hom.* 10, 6.294–296 L. and *Gland.* 11–14, 8.564–570 L.

Polybus repeatedly stresses the importance of tracing diseases to their source. In chapter 13, he observes that patients should be treated "by opposing the cause [πρόφασις] of the disease, for in this way you will remove that which is providing the disease to the body." A similar emphasis on tracing diseases to their source can be found in *On Places in the Human Being* (31, 6.324 L., trans. Craik, modified):

> One should treat ailments from their source [ἀπ᾿ ἀρχῆς]. In all cases which arise from flux, first arrest the flux. In all cases from another cause, arrest the source of the illness, and treat it. Then draw off the matter which has flowed together, if it is copious; if it is slight, restore the patient by regimen.[17]

For Polybus, the "cause" (πρόφασις) of a disease denotes any factor that can initiate the "separating out" (ἀπόκρισις) of one humor from the rest. Such causes include the changes in the seasons, the consumption of food and drinks, and either idleness or physical activity.[18] In chapter 8, Polybus observes that diseases that arise during one part of the year tend to depart in the season with opposite qualities. He then generalizes this principle in chapter 9, noting that all factors that can initiate an *apokrisis* are cured by applying their opposite (trans. Jones, modified):

> Furthermore, one must know the following: that diseases due to repletion are cured by evacuation, and those due to evacuation are cured by repletion; those due to exercise are cured by rest, and those due to idleness are cured by exercise. To know the whole matter, the physician must set himself against what is established – diseases, constitutions, seasons, and ages; he must relax what is tense and make tense what is relaxed. For in this way the diseased part would rest most, and this, in my opinion, constitutes treatment.

It is important to note that even though Polybus claims that the "cause" of a disease should be treated by applying its opposite, he never reduces all cures to a simple opposition between the hot, the cold, the dry, and the wet. Instead, Polybus actually agrees with the author of *On Ancient Medicine*, stressing the importance of identifying and then purging diseased humors from the body. In chapter 5, he refers to the use of drugs to

---

[17] For similar assertions that doctors should treat diseases at their "source," see *Acut.* 43–44, 2.314–318 L., *Epid. II* 4.5, 5.126 L., *Epid. VI* 3.20, 5.302 L., *Flat.* 1.4, 6.92 L., *Aff.* 25, 6.236 L., *Loc. Hom.* 1.3, 6.276–278 L., *Mul. I* 62, 8.126 L., Pl. *Ti.* 88a, and Diod. 1.82.1–2.

[18] On the history of the term *prophasis*, which sometimes (but not always) denotes not simply a "cause" in the general sense but more specifically an external, visible, or initiating cause, see Deichgräber (1933) and Rawlings (1975). In *On the Nature of the Human Being*, Polybus may well be drawing on this more specialized sense of *prophasis* as an "initiating" or "triggering" cause. Note his definition of a disease's *prophasis* as "that which is providing the disease to the body" (τὸ τὴν νοῦσον παρέχον τῷ σώματι) at 13.1, 6.64 L.

purge phlegm, yellow bile, and black bile. In chapter 11, he gives instructions on the practice of venesection. In chapter 15, he refers to the need to wait for a "crisis" (κρίσις); that is, the period at which a concentrated humor has ripened to the point that it can be removed all at once. Some diseases reach their crises more quickly than others. They do this, he says, because their fevers are continuous and thus "cook" the humors more rapidly (15.2, 6.66 L.), while other diseases last longer because their fevers are interrupted by periods of intermission, and because the humor at the root of the affection is "very sticky" (γλισχρότατον, 15.5, 6.68 L.) and thus more difficult to remove. In the above-quoted passage, Polybus says that the doctor should oppose the cause of a disease "for in this way the diseased part would rest most" (οὕτω γὰρ ἂν μάλιστα τὸ κάμνον ἀναπαύοιτο, 9.2, 6.52 L.). In other words, the doctor should put a stop to whatever is causing the humors to "separate out." By taking away the source of the *apokrisis*, the doctor will create a situation in which the offending humor is no longer being nourished. This starving of the disease will in turn allow the strength of the body to surpass that of the humor, eventually reaching a state of "dominance" (ἐπικράτεια) that is a prerequisite for concocting peccant humors.[19]

When coction and crisis are the keys to restoring health, treatment cannot be reduced to a simple opposition between the hot, the cold, the dry, and the wet. In fact, if the doctor's primary goal is to concoct and then purge harmful humors from the body, it will sometimes make more sense to treat "fire with fire," just as Petron is said to have covered fever patients with blankets so as to encourage the production of heat. We should note, however, that these principles of coction and crisis only apply *after* a humor has separated out. Before a concentration arises, Polybus is more than happy to treat opposites with opposites, as we see in chapters 16–22. In this third and final section, Polybus provides general precepts on how to adapt a patient's regimen to ward off disease.[20] He begins by giving instructions on how to respond to changes in the seasons: in winter, patients should consume food and drinks that will make them both dry and hot, while in summer, they should make themselves as wet and cold as possible. Spring and autumn, meanwhile, are transitional periods. During these seasons,

---

[19] On the view that humors are overcome by means of coction, and that the body must have more "strength" than the humor before such coction can occur, see p. 43. "Rest" (ἀνάπαυσις) is also mentioned as a prerequisite for coction at *VM* 11.1, 1.594 L. and *Morb. III* 16, 7.152 L.

[20] Modern scholars have sometimes tried to separate chapters 16–22 as an independent treatise entitled *Regimen in Health*. Here, too, however, there are close verbal parallels between these chapters and what has come before, as has been powerfully demonstrated by Jouanna (2002: 35–38).

one should gradually replace the previous regimen with its opposite, slowly moving from hot to cold, from cold to hot, from dry to wet, or from wet to dry.[21] In addition to counteracting the effects of each season, Polybus also gives prescriptions for different ages and constitutional types. Those whose constitution is soft and fleshy should employ a drier regimen for most of the year, "for the nature of these constitutions is wet" (17.1, 6.74 L.), while those whose constitution is compact and thin should adopt a moister regimen, since their bodies are naturally dry. Polybus offers further prescriptions for the young and the old, women, and athletes. All of these groups have certain predispositions toward the hot, the cold, the dry, and the wet, and they should each counteract their individual imbalances by adopting a regimen with opposite qualities.

Toward the end of chapter 17, Polybus writes in general terms about this mode of disease prevention: "When prescribing regimens, one should do so with an eye to the age, the season, the year, the district, and the physical constitution, opposing whatever is being established [τοῖσι καθισταμένοισι], be it heat or cold." According to Polybus, all diseases arise from a separation of the humors, but the humors are themselves separated by heat, cold, dryness, or moisture, which can in turn come from a variety of sources, including the climate, physical activity, and the consumption of food and drinks. For similar multitiered models of pathogenesis, we may compare the various systems we encountered in Chapter 1. For all of these thinkers, diseases are manifested by the "separating off" of one humor from the rest. This separation, in turn, arises when the humors are disturbed in some manner. According to the speech of Eryximachus, an *apokrisis* can coincide with the changes in the seasons, as the shifts in both temperature and precipitation cause the humors to be heated, cooled, dried, or moistened to an excessive degree. Like the authors of *Diseases I* and *On Affections*, Philistion and Alcmaeon also held that heating, cooling, drying, and moistening can arise from various "external things," including wounds and injuries, an excess in the hot or the cold, or food and drink. Polybus seems to fall in line with these thinkers who refer to both "internal" and "external" causes of disease. He believes that the hot, the cold, the dry, and the wet are intermediate factors between an external, triggering cause and the internal "separating off" of one humor from the rest.[22]

---

[21] On the need to act gradually so as to avoid sudden changes, see note 26 on p. 23.

[22] For yet another instance of a multitiered model of pathogenesis, where heat and cold are intermediate factors between an external cause and humoral *apokrisis*, see *Morb. II* 11, 7.18 L.: "First, the head

Contrary to what we read in *On Ancient Medicine*, the choice between *hupotheseis* and humoral theory was never mutually exclusive. Instead of replacing one system with the other, the cosmological doctors actually combined these two systems into one, targeting both the humors themselves and the various factors that could set these humors in motion. What allowed them to do this was their distinguishing the proximate cause of a disease (i.e., an *apokrisis* of the humors) from its remote cause (i.e., the heating, cooling, drying, or moistening of the humors). The cosmological doctors only treated opposites with opposites when they targeted the remote cause. The proximate cause, meanwhile, was still treated by identifying and then purging diseased humors from the body. When a patient is already ill, it is necessary to treat both the remote and proximate causes. Not only does this remove the offending humor but it also removes the external trigger that might otherwise threaten a relapse. When a patient is still healthy, on the other hand, the job of a doctor is much simpler. He only needs to maintain a healthy state by opposing remote causes with their opposites.

2.3 Commonality and Difference

To conclude this discussion of *On the Nature of the Human Being*, I would like to address one final misconception about the cosmological doctors. As we noted in Chapter 1, the author of *On Ancient Medicine* opposes these doctors because he thinks they reject the time-tested method of dividing and subdividing patients into different groups. This method is necessary, he asserts, because the same treatments, administered in the same way, will have different effects on different patients – as we see in the case of cheese. There are some who have a *phusis* that is amenable to cheese, and others whose *phusis* is not. The proponents of *hupotheseis*, by contrast, are trying to do away with such distinctions. They merely speculate about the common *phusis* of all human beings, focusing on "foundational principles" that are the same in every case.

The author of *On Ancient Medicine* writes as if the cosmological doctors emphasize universal principles at the expense of particular details. Polybus, however, combines these two emphases in one and the same system. He not only describes the common nature of all human beings but also stresses the importance of considering the age and physical constitution of each

draws phlegm out of the body; it does this on becoming heated, and it becomes heated from foods, drinks, sun, cold, exertions, and fire" (trans. Potter).

patient, as well as the season of the year and the geographical location. In chapters 16–22, Polybus gives instructions on how to adjust a patient's regimen to ward off disease. In this section, he divides patients into different classes, and he then assigns to each class a "constitution" (εἶδος). This method of dividing patients into groups, and then assigning to each group a "constitution," is the same procedure that is endorsed in *On Ancient Medicine*. Polybus also writes in chapter 9 about the importance of adapting one's treatments to fit the needs of individual situations. In this chapter, he begins by describing diseases that are caused by the *pneuma* that we breathe. When a disease afflicts all patients indiscriminately, "both younger and older, men as much as women, those who drink wine as much as those who drink water, those who eat barley cake as much as those who live on bread, those who take much exercise as well as those who take little," then the cause must be the *pneuma* that we breathe, since this is "most common" (κοινότατον) to all groups (9.3, 6.52–54 L., trans. Jones). "But when diseases of all sorts occur at one and the same time," he continues (9.4, 6.54 L., trans. Jones, modified),

> it is clear that in each case the particular regimen is the cause, and that the treatment carried out should be that opposed to the cause of the disease, as has been set forth by me elsewhere, and should be by change of regimen. For it is clear that, of the regimen the patient is wont to use, either all, or the greater part, or some one part, is not suited to him. This one should learn and change, and carry out treatment only after examination of the patient's age, constitution, the season of the year, and the fashion of the disease, sometimes taking away and sometimes adding, as I have already said, and so making changes in drugging or in regimen to suit the several conditions of age, season, constitution, and disease.

In this passage, Polybus refers to regimens that are "suited" or "unsuited" to particular individuals. He claims that doctors should classify patients according to a wide range of variables, and that they should consider these variables when adapting their treatments to fit the needs of each particular case. The same idea is expressed at 9.1–2, 6.52 L., in which Polybus notes that the doctor must set himself against "what is established" (trans. Jones, modified):

> Furthermore, one must know the following: that diseases due to repletion are cured by evacuation, and those due to evacuation are cured by repletion; those due to exercise are cured by rest, and those due to idleness are cured by exercise. To know the whole matter, the physician must set himself against what is established [τοῖσι καθεστηκόσι] – diseases, constitutions, seasons, and ages; he must relax what is tense and make tense what is relaxed. For in

this way the diseased part would rest most, and this, in my opinion, constitutes treatment.

In these two passages, Polybus is specifically talking about what the doctor should bear in mind *after* a humor has separated out. With these two lists, we may compare the list that appears in chapter 17, in which Polybus describes the adaptations that must be made *before* a disease has occurred (17.5, 6.76 L.):

> When prescribing regimens, one should do so with an eye to the age, the season, the year, the district, and the physical constitution, opposing whatever is being established [τοῖσι καθισταμένοισι], be it heat or cold.

These lists contain overlapping elements, specifically the patient's age and constitution and the season of the year, with the only major difference being that when a doctor is treating a patient in whom one of the humors has separated out, he must also consider "the fashion of the disease" (τῆς νούσου τὸν τρόπον, 9.4, 6.54 L.; cf. νοσήμασι, 9.2, 6.52 L.), a factor that would presumably include the identity of the morbid humor, its quantity and quality, the specific part it has overpowered, and any secondary events such as fluxes and ulceration.

Contrary to what *On Ancient Medicine* implies about the cosmological doctors, Polybus puts significant emphasis on the differences between individual patients. This concern for individualization can even be found when he writes about the shared nature of all human beings (2.5, 6.36 L., trans. Jones, modified):

> I for my part will prove that what I declare to be the constituents of a human being are, according to both convention and nature, always alike the same, whether the patient be young or old, or whether the season be cold or hot.

In this passage, Polybus emphasizes that blood, phlegm, yellow bile, and black bile are "always alike the same" (αἰεὶ ταὐτὰ ἐόντα ὁμοίως). It makes no difference "whether the patient be young or old, or whether the season be cold or hot," a phrase that illustrates a simultaneous concern for both commonality and difference. Despite what *On Ancient Medicine* might lead us to believe, the investigation of high-level commonalities is not incompatible with a concern for individual differences. Rather, it is to say that there are some deep similarities across all human beings, similarities that persist even when all other variables change.

Polybus is not merely concerned with the differences between individual cases. He also tries to find *commonalities* that transcend these various differences. We have already seen this interest in commonality in his discussion of diseases that arise from the *pneuma* that we breathe. It does not matter whether a patient is young or old, male or female, a drinker of water or a drinker of wine, an eater of barley cake or an eater of bread, one who exercises much or one who only exercises a little. When *pneuma* is the cause of an epidemic, all patients will suffer the same disease because they all breathe the same body of air. A similar interest in commonality and difference can be seen in chapter 12. In this chapter, Polybus describes three affections that appear to be very different, but in fact have a common *arche*. When a male patient who used to be active stops exercising and puts on weight, his flesh will eventually melt, and this melting releases humors. These humors, in turn, will produce a different affection depending on the place to which they flow. If they flow into the intestines, the patient's stools will become bloody. If they flow into the chest, the patient will cough up pus. If they flow into the bladder, they will turn into a white sediment and be expelled with the urine. In all three cases, the symptoms are very different, but the "starting point" remains the same. The doctor is not actually dealing with three different diseases, but there is in fact one and the same source that can be targeted with medical treatment.

The greatest commonality of all, of course, is the shared nature of everything in the universe. Just a few steps below this, we find the shared nature of all human beings. As we will see in the following chapters, the authors of *On Breaths*, *On Flesh*, and *On Regimen* all show a similar interest in commonality and difference. They all emphasize the differences between individual cases, as well as the high-level commonalities that transcend these various differences.

CHAPTER 3

On Breaths

3.1 A Rhetorical Game?

The next text that I would like to consider is unusual among the works of the cosmological doctors. What makes this text unusual is not its author's views on human physiology, or even his theory about the cosmos. Instead, what sets *On Breaths* apart is the simple fact that many scholars have doubted both its seriousness and the possibility that it could have ever been written by a practicing doctor. *On Breaths* makes use of Gorgianic rhetoric, including end-rhyme, antithesis, and carefully balanced phrases, all of which would place it within the short period of time when such stylings had been devised but were not yet dismissed as excessive (by a generous estimation, between 430 and 370 BCE).[1] Many scholars familiar with the works of Gorgias, especially his *Encomium to Helen* and *On What Is Not*, have assumed that just as Gorgias concludes the *Helen* by calling it "an amusement for myself" (ἐμὸν δὲ παίγνιον), so the goal of *On Breaths* is not to make a genuine contribution to medical knowledge but to illustrate the author's ability to sustain an unusual and paradoxical thesis. Jones (1923b: 222) writes that the author of *On Breaths* "shows no genuine interest in medicine, nor do his contentions manifest any serious study of physiology or pathology." Nelson (1909: 100) concedes that the author's medical knowledge is "not to be underestimated," but he also thinks the author is more likely to have been a sophist than a practicing doctor. More recently, Thivel (1981: 146), Langholf (1986, 1990b), Jouanna (1988), Thomas (1993), and Cross (2018) have all pushed back against this tendency to view *On Breaths* as little more than a rhetorical *jeu d'esprit*. They

---

[1] So Jouanna (1988: 48–49); compare Nelson (1909: 98–99, 103). Cicero (*Orat.* 175–176) claims that these stylistic embellishments were first restrained by Isocrates, who opened his first school of rhetoric on Chios around 393 BCE.

maintain that the author could well have been a serious doctor, working in a period when doctors and laymen publicly debated both the nature of the cosmos and the foundations of the medical art. Other scholars have either contended or at least conceded that *On Breaths* may be the work of a practicing doctor, although many still find it hard to believe that this text could have ever been written by a physician, let alone that it belonged to the "mainstream" of Greek medicine.[2] For what it is worth, the author himself asserts that his proposal (i.e., that all diseases are caused by *pneuma*) will be directly relevant to treatment: "If someone knows the cause [αἰτίην] of the disease, he will be able to administer what is beneficial to the body, opposing the disease with the use of contraries" (1.4, 6.92 L.). The author also asserts that this targeting of a disease's cause is a form of "medicine" (ἰητρική) that is "most in accordance with nature" (μάλιστα κατὰ φύσιν, 1.4, 6.92 L.), and that "whoever does this best [i.e., whoever best identifies the cause of a disease and opposes it with contraries] is the best physician, while whoever most falls short of this most falls short of the art" (1.5, 6.92 L.). This final statement provides a close parallel with the speech of Eryximachus in Plato's *Symposium*, as the Athenian doctor similarly asserts that whoever can differentiate good and bad *eros* is a "master of the healer's art," while whoever knows how to implant *eros* when it is absent and take it away when it is present is a "good workman" (186c–d). Before I discuss this text in depth – after which I think it will become clear that *On Breaths* is not the intellectual outlier that many scholars have supposed – let me begin with a few general observations that will help us put this work in perspective.

First, it is fair to say that much of the hesitance to view *On Breaths* as the serious work of a practicing doctor has not been motivated by a careful study of this text, but is rather the product of a gut reaction, fueled in no small part by an implicit hostility toward the cosmological doctors and toward their perceived intellectual inferiority.[3] Modern scholars have long

---

[2] For the continued resistance to view *On Breaths* as the serious work of a practicing doctor, see Kühn (1956: 57–58), Lloyd (1968: 90n57, 1979: 88, 1987: 15–16, 1991a: 136), Kerferd (1981: 58), Smith (1983: 282), Lichtenthaeler (1991), Longrigg (1993: 93), López Férez (1997: 122–123), Cooper (2004: 21n24), and Walshe (2016: 24).

[3] Compare Jones (1923b: 222n1), who asserts that the intellect of the author of *On Breaths* "is distinctly of an inferior type." Similarly, Longrigg (1983: 255–256) writes that "Those [medical] treatises revealing philosophical influence tend, by and large, to be eclectic and of a somewhat low intellectual merit." Of course, the standards employed by these scholars have little to do with the methods and motivations of the authors they are describing. Such value judgments have long obfuscated the historical project of understanding the cosmological doctors, leading to a peculiar status quo in which these fully surviving texts, illustrating what seems to have been a significant development in Classical Greek medicine, are often marginalized in discussions of early Greek thought.

been embarrassed by these authors, labeling them as "confused" and even detrimental to the medical art. It cannot be denied, however, that many Greek doctors in the Classical period were genuinely interested in cosmology, and that they were serious in their attempts to isolate a small number of principles that might be considered the "cause" of all diseases. If other doctors from this period could trace all diseases back to fire and water, to the hot and the cold, or to a small number of humors like blood, bile, and phlegm, there is no reason for us to assume, a priori, that a practicing physician could not have identified *pneuma* as the root cause of all diseases. As we will see, the arguments of this text are strongly reminiscent of other works in the Hippocratic Corpus, especially those that combine an interest in "making the invisible visible" with a sophisticated approach to evidence and argument. *On Breaths* also has much in common with the speech of Eryximachus in Plato's *Symposium*, which employs arguments that must have been fairly representative of contemporary doctors for Plato to have included them in his dialogue.[4] Like Eryximachus, the author of *On Breaths* does not present his first principle as the material substance from which all things are composed, but rather frames it as a causal factor that has more "power" (δύναμις) than anything else.[5] The author's penchant for end-rhyme, antithesis, and carefully balanced phrases also finds parallels in Eryximachus's speech – as does his unabashed confidence in the validity of his argument – and, like Plato's doctor, the author supports his thesis with an argument from induction, illustrating the supremacy of *pneuma* in every class of disease. As we have already noted, arguments from induction were very popular among the cosmological doctors. In addition to the speech of Eryximachus, two passages from *On Flesh* and *On Regimen* are especially illuminating when compared with this text. In the final chapter of *On Flesh*, the author claims that all aspects of human life are governed by the number seven. In support of this thesis, he simply lists all the scenarios in which this number can be found: the embryo is fully articulated by the

---

[4] On the question of whether Plato was familiar with *On Breaths*, see Jouanna (1988: 38–39, 105n1). *On Regimen* is usually cited as the most likely model for Eryximachus's speech (e.g., Bury 1932: xxxii–xxxiii; Craik 2001b; Levin 2014: 80), but the structural parallels are even closer for *On Breaths*, whose overarching thesis about the universal "power" of *pneuma* is directly paralleled in Eryximachus's thesis about the universal "power" of *eros*.

[5] *Flat.* 3.2, 6.94 L., 4.1, 6.96 L., 15.1, 6.114 L.; compare Pl. *Smp.* 188d. Incidentally, *On Breaths*' silence regarding the elemental constitution of human beings speaks against the claim, very common in modern scholarship, that the author reworks the doctrines of either Anaximenes or Diogenes. For a rebuttal of the assumption that *On Breaths* was written by a follower of Diogenes, see Orelli (1998) and Laks (1998, 2008: 260–262). A similar observation vitiates the claim that the author of *On Breaths* would have fallen within the category of material monists whom Polybus attacks in *On the Nature of the Human Being*.

seventh day after conception (19.1, 8.608–610 L.), abstention from food and drink leads to death after seven days (19.2, 8.610–612 L.), the seven months' child tends to live while the eight months' child tends to die (19.3, 8.612 L.), diseases reach their crises on days that are multiples of seven, plus or minus half-seven (i.e., 4, 7, 11, 14, 18, 21, etc.) (19.4–5, 8.612–614 L.), and children acquire all their teeth by the time they have reached their seventh year (19.7, 8.614 L.). A similar argument from induction can be found in *On Regimen*. After describing the nature of fire and water and the process by which our bodies are formed, the author chides his fellow humans for failing to ascertain a divinely inspired analogy between the arts (τέχναι) and the body, according to which everything that we do in our daily occupations has some parallel in human physiology (11–24, 6.486–496 L.). To "prove" the existence of this universal principle,[6] the author simply catalogs the many ways in which the principle can be applied, all in the belief that the more parallels he cites, the more confidence we should place in the validity of his generalization. Throughout this section, the author writes in a riddling, Heraclitean style – a style far more peculiar than the rhetorical devices that appear in *On Breaths*. Nowadays, few scholars would assert that *On Regimen* could not have been the work of a practicing doctor, and so we have to ask why some readers have been so quick to deny this possibility to *On Breaths*.

One reason, of course, is the style of this text, which is designed to impress the ears with its sound effects and balanced phrases. On this point, however, it is helpful to remember the close relationship between form and content in early Greek prose, specifically how some Greek authors conveyed meaning not just through the logic of their arguments but also through their use of language. Cross (2018) has recently studied this matter as it pertains to the Hippocratic Corpus. Building off of Kahn's (1979) work on the language of Heraclitus, Cross has shown that the use of sound in medical texts is not simply an idle embellishment, but a key tool for establishing the author's authority, for exploring various notions of similarity and difference, and for reinforcing the logical arguments that the author is trying to make. Consider, for example, the opening of *On Breaths*, in which the author presents a series of oppositions between the doctor and the layman (1.1–3, 6.90 L.):

> Among the arts, there are some which are a cause of suffering [ἐπίπονοι] to those who possess them [τοῖσι μὲν κεκτημένοισιν], but very beneficial

---

[6] On the universality of this principle, note the author's concluding sentence: "In this way, *all* the arts [αἱ τέχναι πᾶσαι] have something in common with human nature" (24.3, 6.496 L.).

[ὀνήϊστοι] to those who consult them [τοῖσι δὲ χρεωμένοισιν], a common good for laymen, but painful for those who handle them. Among such arts there is, in particular, the one which the Greeks call medicine. For the doctor sees terrible things, touches unpleasant things, and in times of another's misfortune reaps pains for himself. Through the art, the sick are turned away from the greatest evils, diseases, pain, sufferings, death. For medicine stands opposed to all these. Of this art, it is difficult to discern what is bad, while it is easier to discern what is good. To know what is bad is possible for doctors only, and not for laymen. For they are not deeds of the body, but of the mind. For whatever one must do with the hands should be acquired through habit – for habit is a very fine school for the hands – while concerning the most obscure and difficult diseases, distinctions are based on opinion rather than craft, and in these cases experience differs very much from inexperience [διαφέρει δ' ἐν αὐτοῖσι πλεῖστον ἡ πεῖρα τῆς ἀπειρίης].

In this passage, the author reinforces his oppositional arguments with oppositional language, using symmetry and antithesis to distinguish the practitioner from the layman both logically and linguistically. A series of carefully constructed oppositions gradually build a case for viewing the doctor as a unique, even heroic, figure, who endures pain so another's pain may be removed, and who is superior to others on the topic of disease both in his experience and in the powers of his mind. This notion of superiority, of a gulf that exists between the doctor and the layman, is reinforced by the very placement of the words. In the first sentence, the rhyming symmetry between two four-syllable adjectives (ἐπίπονοι - ὀνήϊστοι) and two five-syllable participles that both start with a "k" sound (τοῖσι μὲν κεκτημένοισιν - τοῖσι δὲ χρεωμένοισιν) emphasizes from the start that we are dealing with a case of diametric opposition, where the similarity of sounds highlights a dissimilarity of meaning, and where the doctor and non-doctor are placed at either end of a pole with no middle ground in between. Here, we have no place for Aristotle's "educated person" (πεπαιδευμένος) who shares the ability of judgment (τὸ κρίνειν) with the expert in the art (*Pol.* 1282a3–7). Nor is there room for the intended reader of *On Affections*, who has studied enough medicine to know how to help himself "from his own mind" (ἀπὸ τῆς ἑωυτοῦ γνώμης) and who can "know and discern" (ἐπίστασθαι ... καὶ διαγινώσκειν) the things said and done by doctors (1, 6.208 L.). For the author of *On Breaths*, the "mind" (γνώμη) that can "discern" (γνῶναι) what is good and bad in medicine is the exclusive possession of the doctor. In the first sentence, the author carefully distinguishes those who "possess" the art (τοῖσι μὲν κεκτημένοισιν) from those who merely "consult" it (τοῖσι δὲ χρεωμένοισιν), while the echoing juxtaposition of "experience" and "inexperience" in the final clause (ἡ πεῖρα τῆς ἀπειρίης) reinforces the idea that the practicing doctor is the ultimate authority on disease, while all others should yield to his judgments. When it comes to "the most obscure and difficult diseases," the doctor is no mere handyman trained by habit. Instead, he is a thinking professional whose accumulated "experience" (πεῖρα) allows him to formulate an "opinion" (δόξα) that is superior to the opinions of non-doctors.

This opening is not simply some idle praise for the medical art, but a self-conscious attempt by the author to present himself as an authority on truth. With these accumulated oppositions, the author draws a clear distinction between himself and the layman, relying on his own experience as a practicing healer to give persuasive weight to the claims that are to follow. Such jockeying for authority is typical of medical writing in the late fifth century BCE. It was especially common in the *epideixis*, which was not simply, as Aristotle puts it, a speech of praise or blame, but a term that encompasses many forms of "display," including both public lectures and competitive debates.[7] In an *epideixis*, the speaker frequently begins by drawing a clear distinction between himself and rival claimants to authority. This practice informs the opening of *On Ancient Medicine*, in which the author distinguishes himself from his opponents in a manner reminiscent of *On Breaths*. Like the author *On Breaths*, the author of *On Ancient Medicine* presents himself as an expert on "the craft" (ἡ τέχνη). He clearly defines the parameters of medicine, carefully distinguishing it from investigations into "the things on high and under the earth" (1.3, 1.572 L.), and he also implicitly promotes his own authority by differentiating those practitioners who excel "in hand and in mind" (κατὰ χεῖρα καὶ κατὰ γνώμην) from those who are "lacking in both experience and knowledge" (ἄπειροί τε καὶ ἀνεπιστήμονες, 1.2, 1.570–572 L.). The bulk of the author's arguments are then rooted in further sets of mutually exclusive oppositions: *hupotheseis* versus humors, simplicity versus complexity, craft knowledge (τέχνη) versus wisdom-loving (φιλοσοφία), the old versus the new. This commitment to oppositional thinking is so strong that, as we have

---

[7] For Aristotle's limited definition of *epideixis*, see Cross (2018: 57–62). On medical *epideixeis* in the Classical period, see Lloyd (1979: 59–125), Jouanna (1984), Thomas (1993, 2000: 249–269, 2003), Demont (1993), and Schiefsky (2005: 36–46). As Cross (2018: 18) observes, the depiction of Eryximachus in Plato's *Symposium* is strongly indicative of "the engagement of doctors in public debates and displays of oratorical skill," an observation that seems to be corroborated by the texts of the Hippocratic Corpus. Diels (1911: 273–274) suggests that *On Breaths* could have formed part of the author's application to the post of public physician, a process for which doctors are known to have given public speeches: see Pl. *Grg.* 456b–c, X. *Mem.* 4.2.5, Cohn-Haft (1956), and Jouanna (1984: 41–43).

seen, the author of *On Ancient Medicine* significantly distorts the position of his opponents.

In *On the Nature of the Human Being*, Polybus similarly prefaces his own thesis with an attempt to situate himself in opposition to other thinkers. Yet again, we see a distinction between the doctor and the layman, as Polybus notably denies the term "doctors" (ἰητροί) to those thinkers who speculate about "air, fire, water, earth, or anything else not obviously present in human beings" (1.1, 6.32 L.). Like the authors of *On Breaths* and *On Ancient Medicine*, Polybus also focuses on the topics of "judgment" (γνώμη) and "experience" (πεῖρα). His opponents do not make correct judgments (οὐκ ὀρθῶς γινώσκειν, 1.2, 6.32 L.), whereas he does (cf. γνοίης δ' ἂν τοῖσδε, 5.3, 6.42 L.), while his arguments are all rooted in the privileged experience of the practicing doctor: what it feels like to touch specific humors (5.2, 6.42 L., 7.2, 6.46 L.), the existence of drugs that target one humor instead of another (5.3, 6.42 L.), the sequential nature of purges (6.2–3, 6.44–46 L.), and the prevalence of specific diseases in one season rather than another (7, 6.46–50 L.). Here again, the commitment to oppositional thinking leads the speaker to significantly exaggerate the differences between himself and his opponents. Contrary to what Polybus implies in his use of the term "doctors," there really were some doctors who speculated about substances like fire and water. Moreover, Polybus's own system, which associates four humors with four fundamental principles (the hot, the cold, the dry, and the wet), is not as different from the systems of his opponents as he would like us to believe.[8] Instead of writing off such exaggerations as the product of a careless mind, we should view them as reflections of the oppositional thinking that was encouraged by a culture of public performance. In all of these texts (*On Breaths, On Ancient Medicine*, and *On the Nature of the Human Being*), the authors seek to establish themselves as authorities on truth, and they do so by framing some rival group as diametrically opposed to the correct way of thinking about the body.[9]

Another way in which sound reinforces meaning in *On Breaths* can be seen in the author's opposition between the one and the many. This is an area where Heraclitus's use of language is especially relevant, since both

---

[8] On this point, see especially Lloyd (1979: 92–94).

[9] Further examples of this tactic can be found in *On Regimen in Acute Diseases, Prorrhetic II, On Fractures, On Joints, On the Sacred Disease*, and *On the Art*. An interesting variation occurs in *On Regimen*, where the author distinguishes himself from all previous writers on regimen, but he rejects "refutation" (ἔλεγχος) in favor of accepting the positive contributions of his predecessors. A similar sentiment can be found in the opening of *On Flesh* (quoted on p. 202).

authors argue for a hidden unity amidst apparent diversity. The main thesis of *On Breaths* is presented in the following terms (2, 6.92 L.):

> Of all diseases, the type is the same while the location differs [ὁ μὲν τρόπος ωὑτός, ὁ δὲ τόπος διαφέρει]. It is because of the diversity of their locations that diseases seem to bear no resemblance to each other [δοκεῖ μὲν οὖν οὐδὲν ἐοικέναι τὰ νοσήματα ἀλλήλοισιν διὰ τὴν ἀλλοιότητα τῶν τόπων], but of all diseases there is one and the same class and cause [μία πασέων νούσων καὶ ἰδέη καὶ αἰτίη ἡ αὐτή].

In the first sentence, the author's larger point is that diseases exhibit a coexistence of similarity and difference, reinforced by his placement of the words ωὑτός ("the same") and διαφέρει ("differs") at the ends of their respective clauses. To further emphasize this point, he pairs the terms *tropos* and *topos*, two words that are themselves both similar and different in respect to their sounds. This echoing effect continues in the second sentence, where two words that convey notions of *diversity* and *difference* (ἀλλήλοισιν ... ἀλλοιότητα) also share similar sounds. In this passage, the author is not just manipulating language to dazzle his listeners; he is reinforcing his central thesis that, amidst all the variation of individual diseases, there is also a sense of *sameness*. Heraclitus, for his part, makes similar use of sound in his own discussion of unity amidst diversity. Some well-known examples include his play on the words βίος ("life") and βιός ("bow," an instrument of death) (DK 22 B48) and his deployment of echoing pairs in referring to "wholes and not wholes; agreeing, disagreeing; consonant, dissonant; one from all and all from one" (DK 22 B10). It is possible that the author of *On Breaths* intentionally mimics Heraclitus when making his own claims about unity amidst diversity. The medical writer is obviously not following the doctrines of Heraclitus, but he may have been attracted to the persuasive power imbued by Heraclitus's use of language.[10]

We should also bear in mind that, for many Greek authors of the Classical period, a control of language was thought to imply a more general control of rationality itself. In *On Ancient Medicine*, the author employs a rhyming doublet at 2.2, 1.572 L. (ἐξηπάτηται καὶ ἐξαπατᾶται). Another jingle has been suggested for 13.3, 1.600 L. (πυρὶ <δέδοται> καὶ ὕδατι δέδευται). Far from suggesting a lack of seriousness, such echoing pairs present the speaker as a person who

---

[10] For what it is worth, *On Breaths*' reference to a cause and class that are "one and the same" (μία ... ἡ αὐτή, 2, 6.92 L.) bears some resemblance to Heraclit. DK 22 B60 (ὁδὸς ἄνω κάτω μία καὶ ωὑτή, "a road up, down, one and the same"). Similarly, the juxtaposition of *peira* and *apeiria* in chapter 1 (ἡ πεῖρα τῆς ἀπειρίης) can be compared with Heraclit. DK 22 B1 (ἀπείροισιν ἐοίκασι πειρώμενοι).

carefully attends to fine details, making note of minor differences and speaking with the same "precision" (ἀκρίβεια) that one expects from a rigorous thinker. Isocrates recounts in his *Panathenaicus* that he himself spent his youth writing speeches "in a style rich in many telling points, in contrasted and balanced phrases not a few, and in the other figures of speech which give brilliance to oratory and compel the approbation and applause of the audience" (12.1–2, trans. Norlin, modified). In the *Panegyricus*, Isocrates further contrasts the "precision" (ἀκρίβεια) of display speeches with the simplicity of speeches delivered in the courts (4.11), while both Alcidamas and Aristotle similarly suggest that "precision" (ἀκρίβεια) was a common feature of public *epideixeis* (Alcid. *Soph.* 13, 16, Arist. *Rh.* 1413b8–9, 1414a8–15; cf. Kurz 1970: 32–34). In his comedies, Aristophanes lampoons this tendency of contemporary thinkers to carefully compose their words. In the *Clouds*, Strepsiades asserts that, after receiving training from the sophists, "my soul has taken flight at the sound of their voice, and now seeks to split hairs, prattle narrowly about smoke, and meet argument with counterargument, puncturing a point with a pointlet" (319–321, trans. Henderson). Similarly, Aristophanes presents Euripides as a thinker whose words are "linchpin-shavings and chisel-parings" (*Ra.* 819) and whose tongue "will sort out utterances and parse clean away much labor of lungs" (*Ra.* 828–829, trans. Henderson; cf. *Ra.* 954–958), again suggesting that some thinkers used their rhetorical "precision" as a tool for establishing their status as careful thinkers. Although Aristophanes finds humor in the precise, controlled manner in which some of his contemporaries expressed their ideas, there is no denying that this was a legitimate, even respected, form of expression in the Classical period. Some modern readers might prefer to separate logic from style, but for at least a certain subset of Greek thinkers, language was a critical tool for both exploring ideas and establishing one's own authority.

In light of these observations, it would be hasty to presume that the style of *On Breaths* must necessarily indicate a lack of seriousness. To judge the true nature of this text, we need to look beyond the author's use of language to consider the intellectual context of this work. In particular, we must consider what the author is arguing in this text, how his system of medicine can be compared with other works in the Hippocratic Corpus, and whether his views about *pneuma* are as radical as some scholars have supposed. Before we tackle these questions, however, I would like to touch briefly on one more important conversation regarding the authorship of this text. For whereas some have denied·the possibility that this work was the product of a doctor, others have suggested that the author was none other than Hippocrates.

3.2   The Work of Hippocrates?

The argument for attributing *On Breaths* to Hippocrates depends on a well-known passage from the *Anonymus Londiniensis*. In this passage, the doxographer transmits the views of Hippocrates as recorded by his Peripatetic source (V.35–VI.43, trans. Jones, modified):

> Hippocrates says that breaths [φῦσαι] are causes of disease, as Aristotle has said in his account of him. For Hippocrates says that diseases are brought about in the following fashion. Either because of (a) the quantity of things taken [τὸ πλῆθος τῶν προσφερομένων], or (b) through their diversity [τὴν ποικιλίαν], or (c) because the things taken are strong and difficult of digestion [ἰσχυρὰ καὶ δυσκατέργαστα], residues are thereby produced.

(a)   When the things that have been taken are too many, the heat that produces coction is overpowered by the multitude of foods and does not effect coction, and because coction is hindered residues are formed.[11]

(b)   When the things that have been taken are of many kinds [ποικίλα], they quarrel with one another in the belly [στασιάζει ἐν τῇ κοιλίᾳ πρὸς ἑαυτά], and because of the quarrel [στασιασμόν] there is a change into residues.

(c)   When they are very thick [πάχιστα Diels: ἐλάχιστα papyr.][12] and hard to digest [δυσκατέργαστα], there occurs hindrance of coction because they are hard to digest, and so there is a change into residues.

From the residues rise breaths [φῦσαι], which having arisen bring on diseases.

---

[11]   Here, "coction" (πέψις) refers to a stage in digestion whereby nutriment is heated before leaving the belly (cf. LSJ s.v. πέσσω III). Just as with the discussion of "concocting" peccant humors, it was commonly assumed that the body needs to "gain the upper hand" over foods and drinks through "cooking" before they can be properly assimilated as nutriment.

[12]   In support of Diels's emendation of ἐλάχιστα to πάχιστα, see *Vict.* 46.1, 6.544 L. (δύσπεπτα τῇσι κοιλίῃσι, διότι παχύαιμον καὶ πολύαιμόν ἐστι τοῦτο τὸ ζῷον, "difficult for cavities to digest because this animal has thick and abundant blood"), Phylotim. fr. 11 Steckerl (τὰ μὴ κατεργαζόμενα παχυτέρους ἕξει τοὺς χυμούς, "whatever is undigested will have thicker humors"), Gal. *Bon. Mal. Suc.* 6.788 K. (παχεῖαι καὶ σκληραὶ καὶ διὰ τοῦτο δύσπεπτοι, "thick and hard and therefore difficult to digest"), and the combination of all three adjectives ("strong," "thick," and "difficult to digest") in *To Ptolemy on the Differences of Foods* (δυσκατεργαστότεροι ... καὶ παχέος χυμοῦ γεννητικοὶ καὶ διὰ τοῦτο ἰσχυροτέρας γαστρὸς δεόμενοι εἰς πέψιν, "more difficult to digest and productive of a thick humor and therefore needing a stronger belly for effecting coction," 2.486 Delatte = Aët. 2.143). Manetti (2011) retains ἐλάχιστα, but she cites a parallel (*Anon. Lond.* VI.36) that is irrelevant insofar as it refers to *breaths* rather than nutriment. For this doxographer's interest in "thickness," compare XI.40, XII.25, XVIII.33, and see pp. 96–97.

The man said these things being moved [κινηθείς] by a notion such as this. *Pneuma*, he holds, is the most necessary and the supreme component in us, since health is the result of its free, and disease of its impeded passage. We in fact present a likeness to plants. For as they are rooted in the earth, so we too are rooted to the air by our nostrils and by our whole body. At least we are like those plants that are called "soldiers" [στρατιῶται].[13] For just as they, rooted in the moisture, are carried now to this moisture and now to that, even so we also, being as it were plants, are rooted to the air, and are in motion, changing our position now hither now thither. If this be so, it is clear that *pneuma* is the supreme component.

On this theory, when residues occur, they give rise to breaths, which rising as vapor cause diseases. The variations in the breaths cause the various diseases [παρά τε τὴν διαφορὰν τῶν φυσῶν ἀποτελοῦνται αἱ νόσοι]. If the breaths are many, they produce disease, as they also do if they are very few. The changes too of breaths give rise to diseases. These changes take place in two directions, towards excessive heat or towards excessive cold. The nature of the change determines the character of the disease. This is Aristotle's view of Hippocrates.[14]

There are a number of similarities between this testimony and *On Breaths*. Both define "breaths" (φῦσαι) as a central cause of disease, both invoke food and drinks that are either excessive (V.43–VI.4; cf. *Flat.* 7.1, 6.98 L.) or diverse and struggle with each other (ποικίλα . . . στασιάζει, VI.4–5; cf. τὰ γὰρ ἀνόμοια στασιάζει, *Flat.* 7.1, 6.98 L.) as a source of such "breaths," both claim that *pneuma* is more "necessary" or "needed" than anything else (VI.14–16; cf. *Flat.* 4.2, 6.96 L.), both refer to ailments that are caused when *pneuma* is trapped or otherwise impeded in the body (VI.16–18; cf. *Flat.* 4.2, 6.96 L., 8.7, 6.104 L., 9.1, 6.104 L., 10.3, 6.106 L.), and both attribute different ailments to differences in the quantity and temperature of *pneuma* (VI.35–42; cf. *Flat.* 8.1, 6.100 L.). On the basis of these similarities, many readers have concluded that the doxographer's testimony *must* refer to *On Breaths*.[15] Others, however, have contended that the case is far from clear.

---

[13] LSJ s.v. στρατιώτης identifies this plant as water-lettuce. For a fuller discussion of its identity, see O'Brien (1970: 171n145).

[14] Celsus also reports that Hippocrates attributed all diseases to *pneuma* (*omne vitium est . . . in spiritu, pr.* 15), a report that may derive from the same Peripatetic source as the *Anonymus Londiniensis*; compare Mudry (1980, 1982: 91–92). As Edelstein (1931: 137) observes, the Stoics may have also claimed that Hippocrates attributed all diseases to *pneuma*. Compare Gal. *Hipp. Epid.* VI 17b.250–251 K.

[15] Spät (1897), Ducatillon (1983), Langholf (1986, 1990b), and Jouanna (1988: 39–49) are all receptive to the possibility that the author of *On Breaths* was Hippocrates. Manetti (1999a: 103–108), van der Eijk (2012), and Bartoš (2020: 29) also support reading the testimony as a reference to *On Breaths*. Diels (1893b: 424–434), Fredrich (1899: 52n5), Wilamowitz-Möllendorff (1901: 22), Nelson (1909: 104–107), Wellmann (1926: 329–334), and Lichtenthaeler (1991: 15) accept that the *Anonymus Londiniensis*

In the Hippocratic Corpus, "breaths" or "winds" are commonly said to arise when food is left to stagnate in the belly, and such stagnation is itself frequently attributed to the consumption of foods and drinks that are either excessive or in conflict with each other.[16] Furthermore, we are often told that the free flow of *pneuma* is essential to maintaining health, and that pains can arise when this *pneuma* gets stuck in one part or another.[17] These beliefs are attested for *many* Greek doctors of the Classical period, too many to establish an exclusive relationship between these doctrines and *On Breaths*. It has also been observed that the testimony of the *Anonymus Londiniensis* includes information that cannot be found in this text. Most notably, there is an analogy between humans and "those plants that are called soldiers" that is conspicuously absent from *On Breaths*. There is no explicit reference in *On Breaths* to food that is "strong" or "very thick" (V.41, VI.8), one of the three sources of breaths that the *Anonymus Londiniensis* attributes to Hippocrates. Finally, we may note that the *Anonymus Londiniensis* only refers to breaths that arise from "residues," whereas *On Breaths* describes many other scenarios in which *pneuma* is the cause of disease.[18]

　　To understand the relationship between *On Breaths* and the *Anonymus Londiniensis*, we need to look beyond mere questions of overlapping details to consider the process by which the doxographer may have constructed this account. By doing so, we will be better equipped to talk about any

　　refers to *On Breaths*, but they all assert that the attribution of this text to Hippocrates must spring from some mistake on the part of the doxographer. Prince (2016) seems to accept that the report in the *Anonymus Londiniensis* is a summary of *On Breaths*. However, her suggestion that the Peripatetic doxographer somehow conspired to suppress the real views of Hippocrates (viz. the four-humor theory of *On the Nature of the Human Being*) exemplifies the lingering discomfort among some scholars with assigning *On Breaths* to Hippocrates.

[16]　See pp. 105–106. On the verb στασιάζειν, compare *Aër.* 9.2, 2.38 L. and Pl. *Ti.* 82a, 85e, and note the references to foods and drinks in conflict with each other at *Vict.* 56.8, 6.570 L. and Arist. [*Pr.*] 1.15, 861a1–9.

[17]　Recall the testimony quoted earlier on Philistion, who is said to have claimed that "when the whole body breathes well and the breath passes through unhindered, health is the result" (p. 23). See also *VM* 22.7, 1.630–632 L., *Acut. App.* 4, 2.400–402 L., 7, 2.404–406 L., *Epid. II* 2.23, 5.94 L., 3.6, 5.108 L., *Epid. V* 20, 5.220 L., *Nat. Hom.* 21.1, 6.80–82 L., *Morb. Sacr.* 7, 6.372–374 L., Pl. *Ti.* 84c–e, and Praxag. fr. 27 Steckerl = fr. 6–8 Lewis.

[18]　Doubts that the *Anonymus Londiniensis* must refer to *On Breaths* have been expressed by Blass (1901: 405–410), Edelstein (1931: 140–142), Pohlenz (1938: 65–74), Steckerl (1945: 176, 1958: 39–40), Bourgey (1953: 84–88), Deichgräber (1971: 159–160), Harris (1973: 31n1), Lloyd (1975: 175), and Mudry (1980). Smith (1979: 44–60, 1999) prefers to see a reference to *On Regimen*, but he has been rebutted by Mansfeld (1980a) and Lloyd (1991a: 195–196). In his own discussion of the Hippocratic Question, Mansfeld (1980a) shelves any consideration of the *Anonymus Londiniensis* on the grounds that it is late and unreliable; in fact, *On Breaths* never even merits a mention.

discrepancies between these two texts, and we will also be able to speak with more authority about whether the common opinions about *pneuma* that we see in this testimony – opinions that are not, on their own, unique to *On Breaths* – are strung together in such a way as to make *On Breaths* the most likely source for this report. To begin, we may consider the limited scope of the doxographer's report. In the *Anonymus Londiniensis*, one of the doxographer's central questions pertains to the attribution of diseases to either (1) the "elements" or (2) digestive "residues." In *On Breaths*, the author never talks about the elements, although he does mention several ways in which improper digestion gives rise to disease. We should not be surprised, therefore, if the doxographer centers his entire report around the topic of digestion. Even though *On Breaths* describes many other ways in which diseases arise from *pneuma*, those aspects of the author's system do not pertain to the central dichotomy between "elements" and "residues" that the doxographer has already established as the framework for his inquiries.

If this testimony about Hippocrates does refer to *On Breaths*, I would suggest that the entire report, with only one exception, has been extracted from a single passage. Let me first quote the passage in full, after which we will consider the process by which the doxographer may have transformed this passage into his report about Hippocrates (7.1–8.1, 6.98–100 L.):

[7.1] The community-wide diseases have been described – through what, how, in what, and from what they arise. I will pass to the fever that arises through bad regimen. Bad regimen is of such a sort: on the one hand, whenever someone gives his body nutriment, either wet or dry, that is more than his body can bear and opposes the quantity of nutriment with no exercise, and on the other, whenever someone sends in nutriment that is diverse and dissimilar within itself [ποικίλας καὶ ἀνομοίους ἀλλήλῃσιν]. For things that are dissimilar engage in strife [στασιάζει], and some are digested more quickly, others more leisurely.

[7.2] It is necessary that much *pneuma* enter with much food. For with all things that are eaten and drunk, *pneuma* goes out from them and into the body in a greater or smaller quantity. This is clear from the following: belching arises in most after foods and drinks. For the pent-up air runs upwards whenever one breaks the bubbles in which it is concealed. Thus, whenever the body, filled with nutriment, is filled also with *pneuma*, as the foods remain for a long time – and foods remain because they cannot pass through on account of their quantity [πλῆθος] – and as the lower cavity is blocked off [ἐμφραχθείσης δὲ τῆς κάτω κοιλίης], the breaths run through all the body, and when they fall upon the bloodiest parts of the body, they cool them. Whenever these places are cooled, where the roots and sources of the blood are located, a shivering passes through all the body, and when all the blood is cooled, the entire body shivers.

[8.1] Shivering arises before fevers because of this, and however the breaths rush forth in respect to quantity and coldness, such is the shivering that arises, stronger from more abundant and colder breaths, less strong from less abundant and less cold breaths.

In the *Anonymus Londiniensis*, the report about Hippocrates says that breaths arise from three sources: (1) the "quantity" (πλῆθος) of what is consumed, (2) their "diversity" (ποικιλία), and (3) the fact that what is consumed is "strong" (ἰσχυρά), "very thick" (πάχιστα), and "difficult to digest" (δυσκατέργαστα). As we have already noted, none of these three sources are especially remarkable on their own. They are mentioned by many Greek authors of the Classical period and therefore cannot establish an exclusive connection between the doctrines reported in the *Anonymus Londiniensis* and what we find in *On Breaths*. However, what is remarkable about this report is how neatly these three sources can be mapped onto section 7.1. First, the author of *On Breaths* mentions the quantity of what is consumed ("more than his body can bear"), which is later picked up by the noun πλῆθος in section 7.2. This mirrors the same use of the term πλῆθος that appears in the *Anonymus Londiniensis* (παρὰ τὸ πλῆθος τῶν προσφερομένων, V.39–40). Then, the author mentions the diversity of the foods that are eaten ("diverse and dissimilar within itself"), using an adjective (ποικίλος) that again directly corresponds to language employed by the doxographer (παρὰ τὴν ποικιλίαν, V.40; ποικίλα, VI.4). The author follows up this second point by offering an explanation about how dissimilar foods "engage in strife" (στασιάζει). This provides a third verbal parallel between *On Breaths* and the *Anonymus Londiniensis*, whose author repeats the same verb in exactly the same context as the author of *On Breaths* (στασιάζει, VI.5–6).

As for the reference to food that is "strong" (ἰσχυρά), "very thick" (πάχιστα), and "difficult to digest" (δυσκατέργαστα), we have already noted that *On Breaths* does not establish a third category under this heading. However, it is not difficult to see how a third category of this sort may have been extracted from the text. There is already a reference to slow digestion at the end of section 7.1 ("and some are digested more quickly, others more leisurely"), which could have been misread as a third cause of disease. In section 7.2, we also encounter a reference to food that "cannot pass through" (οὐ δυνάμενα διελθεῖν) and obstructs the digestive tract (ἐμφραχθείσης δὲ τῆς κάτω κοιλίης), which might have suggested to our doxographer that this food is too "thick" to pass through the proper channels. In *Parts of Animals*, Aristotle refers to vessels that do not provide a "passage" (δίοδος) for blood because they are "smaller than the blood's thickness" (ἐλάσσους τῆς τοῦ αἵματος παχύτητος, 668b1–3). In the *Problemata*, humors that are acid, bitter, and salty are similarly said to become trapped under the skin because "being thick ... the residues cannot be excreted owing to their thickness" (883b28–32; cf. Arist. [*Pr.*] 3.14, 873a6–7, 24.4, 936a27–29, [*Aud.*] 801a12–16). The author of *Diseases IV* writes that only bile enters the reservoir on the liver because the other humors are too "thick" to pass through the narrow vessels that lead into it (40.1, 7.560 L.). In the *Anonymus Londiniensis*, the doxographer himself comments on the sluggishness of "thick" things (XVI.2–4; cf. Arist. [*Pr.*] 11.61, 905b38–40), and he cites the pathological nature of "thickened" humors in three other reports.[19] In *Generation of Animals*, Aristotle even proposes that one way in which fluids become "thicker" is when air is mixed with their watery components (735b8–37; cf. *Mete.* 383b20–384a2), an idea that the doxographer may have implicitly compared with the references to air in *On Breaths*. As for the association of a humor's thickness with its "strength," two notions that the doxographer seems to conflate between V.41 and VI.8, we may compare *On the Seed-Nature of the Child*'s assertion that males are born from sperm that is "thicker and stronger" (31.3, 7.540 L.) and *On Regimen*'s claim that beef is "strong" (ἰσχυρά) and "hard of digestion" (δύσπεπτα) because this animal is "thick-blooded" (παχύαιμον, 46.1, 6.544 L.), again equating a liquid's "thickness" with its "strength." Associations of thickness and strength also appear in Xenophon's observation that "stronger" soil is also "thicker" (*Oec.* 17.8), Aristotle's claim that "thicker" blood is more productive of strength (*PA* 648a2–3), and the association of strength with both thick gruels and thick blood in two passages from *On Affections* (40, 6.250 L., 47, 6.258 L.). All of these passages suggest that, even without an explicit reference to food that is "strong," "very thick," and "difficult to digest," the doxographer may have nevertheless inferred such a category from the language of *On Breaths*.

In Chapter 1, we observed that this doxographer tends to follow up his reports about the "starting points" of disease with information about their "differentiations" (διαφοραί). We see such a passage in the final portion of this report, where the doxographer says that "variations in the breaths cause the various diseases" (παρά τε τὴν διαφορὰν τῶν φυσῶν ἀποτελοῦνται αἱ

---

[19] *Anon. Lond.* XI.33–41 (Hippon of Croton), XII.25–26 (Thrasymachus of Sardis), XVIII.30–35 (Philolaus of Croton). Compare also the phlegm that cannot pass through the vessels "because of its thickness and quantity" at *Morb. Sacr.* 8.1, 6.374–376 L.

νόσοι, VI.33–34). The doxographer specifically defines such variations as
follows: "If the breaths are many, they produce disease, as they also do if
they are very few. The changes too of breaths give rise to diseases. These
changes take place in two directions, towards excessive heat or towards
excessive cold" (VI.35–40). This statement strongly recalls section 8.1 of *On
Breaths*, where the author writes that "however the breaths rush forth in
respect to quantity and coldness [πλήθει καὶ ψυχρότητι], such is the
shivering that arises, stronger from more abundant and colder breaths,
less strong from less abundant and less cold breaths." Here, there is a minor
distortion on the part of the doxographer, who takes a particularized
discussion about shivering and expands it to all diseases in general. There
is also a minor distortion in the expansion of the reference to "coldness" to
purported excesses in both heat and cold. Beyond these changes, however,
it is remarkable that the same two factors (i.e., quantity and temperature)
are mentioned in both texts. What is more, both factors are reported in the
same order that we see in *On Breaths*, just as the three "causes" of breaths in
the *Anonymus Londiniensis* closely follow the three references to quantity,
diversity, and digestion in section 7.1.

Both the section on "starting points" and the section on "differentiations" closely mirror what we find in a single passage from *On Breaths*.
A further parallel comes in the central portion of the report, where the
doxographer attempts to explain why Hippocrates put so much emphasis
on "breaths" in the first place. In this section, the doxographer begins by
suggesting that Hippocrates praised *pneuma* because it is "the most necessary and the most authoritative of the things in us, since health is the result
of its flowing well, and diseases of its flowing poorly" (VI.15–18). If this
passage is based on *On Breaths*, I would suggest that it was extracted from
the following section (4, 6.96 L.):

> That air is powerful in all things in general has been stated. In mortals,
> moreover, it is responsible for life, and in the diseased it is responsible for
> diseases. All bodies happen to have such a great need for air that a human
> being could abstain from everything else, both foods and drinks, and live for
> two, three, or more days. But if someone should check the wind's conduits
> into the body, he would die in a fraction of a day, so great is the body's need
> for air. In addition, while humans take breaks from everything else – for life
> is full of changes – this alone all mortal living things do continuously,
> sometimes inhaling and sometimes exhaling.

Again, it is not just the repetition of common notions but the combination
and sequencing of these common notions that support a close connection
between the *Anonymus Londiniensis* and *On Breaths*. Both texts report that

pneuma is simultaneously "necessary" and "all-powerful," and both follow up this claim by referring to the obstruction of the channels through which respiration occurs. As with the previous section, the doxographer's report is not without distortions. In *On Breaths*, the author says that an obstruction of *pneuma* leads to *death*, while the doxographer says an obstruction leads to *disease*. To be fair to the doxographer, other passages in *On Breaths* actually do attribute diseases to obstructed *pneuma*,[20] so the doxographer is not technically incorrect on this point. There is also an emphasis on "change" (μεταβολή, VI.37) that does not appear in *On Breaths*, although this may simply be a structuring principle introduced by the doxographer himself. We may compare, for example, the similar reference to "change" in the report on Philistion (quoted earlier, p. 23).

More problematic is the doxographer's subsequent assertion that "we are rooted to the air" in the same way that the plants known as "soldiers" are rooted in water. A similar analogy cannot be found in *On Breaths*. This detail presents the greatest challenge for drawing a connection between the *Anonymus Londiniensis* and *On Breaths*.[21] We must remember, however, that it is not unusual for doxographers – especially those writing in the Peripatetic tradition – to insert musings on the *sorts* of argument that a thinker *may* have used when formulating a belief. In *On Sensation*, Theophrastus lists the assumptions that, in his view, led some thinkers to attribute sensation to "similarity," while others attributed sensation to "contrast" (*Sens.* 2). Aristotle also famously mused about why Thales, who left nothing specific on the matter, identified water as the first principle of all things (*Metaph.* 983b20–27). The participle κινηθείς ("being moved") at *Anon. Lond.* VI.14 ("the man said these things being moved by a notion such as this") is similar to the participle προαχθέντες ("being led") at Thphr. fr. 225 (trans. Fortenbaugh et al.):

> Thales son of Examyes, from Miletus, and Hippon, who is thought to have been an atheist, said that the principle was water, being led [προαχθέντες] to this (conclusion) from appearances in accordance with perception. For what is hot lives by means of moisture, and dead bodies dry up, and the seeds of all things are moist, and the nourishment of all things is juicy; and each thing is naturally nourished by that from which it has its origin. And water is the principle of what is naturally moist and holds all things together. For this reason they supposed that water was the principle of all things and declared that the earth rests on water.

---

[20] *Flat.* 8.7, 6.102–104 L., 9.1, 6.104 L., 10.1–3, 6.104–106 L.
[21] Compare Craik (2015: 101), who cites only this discrepancy when noting why someone might doubt the association of this report with *On Breaths*.

The participle κινηθείς also appears in a doxographical context at Philol. DK 44 A25 ("moved by this [ἀπὸ δὴ τούτου κινηθέντες], some . . . called the interval 'excess,' as Aelian the Platonist and Philolaus") and S.E. *M.* 10.261 ("having been moved by this [ἔνθεν κινηθείς], Pythagoras said that the principle of the things that exist is the monad"). In both passages, the doxographer is suggesting his own explanation for an otherwise unexplained feature of a thinker's system. Thus, it would be reasonable to suppose that the similar appearance of the participle κινηθείς in the *Anonymus Londiniensis* likewise introduces an observation that originates with the doxographer himself. In Peripatetic doxography, it was generally assumed that the doxographer should not only report previous opinions but also critically reflect on the considerations that led to such opinions. Even if these considerations were not explicitly set forth by the doxographer's sources, the doxographer was still expected to surmise what they may have been, since having access to such views made it easier to subject these opinions to critical analysis.

For our purposes, an even more important observation pertains to the entry on Plato in the *Anonymus Londiniensis*. In this passage, the doxographer completely invents an analogy between the intestines and winding rivers (XVI.21–31, trans. Jones):

> Around it has been placed a long and winding intestine [μακρόν τε καὶ εἱλιγμένον ἔντερον], in order that the nutriment taken may not easily sink but remain for specified periods of time. For as the streams of rivers that flow straight are irresistible, but those of winding streams are more gentle because impeded, so if the intestine leading to the lower belly had been made short and straight, the nutriment also would move easily. But since it is winding and very long, the nutriment for that reason remains there for long periods of time.

For the sake of comparison, here is Plato's original text, where no such analogy can be found (*Ti.* 73a, trans. Bury, modified):

> And round about therein they wound [εἵλιξαν] the structure of the entrails, to prevent the food from passing through quickly and thereby compelling the body to require more food quickly, and causing insatiate appetite, whereby the whole kind by reason of its gluttony would be rendered devoid of philosophy and of culture, and disobedient to the most divine part we possess.

In this passage, the doxographer echoes Plato's use of the verb ἑλίσσειν ("to wind, coil"). This verb is commonly applied to rivers in Greek literature, and it may have therefore inspired the doxographer to include this intrusive analogy in his report.[22] A similar spark may have arisen from the text of *On Breaths*, where the author notes that the chills which accompany fevers penetrate the "roots" of the blood (αἱ ῥίζαι ... τοῦ αἵματος, 7.2, 6.100 L.). One of Aristotle's favorite analogies is between the roots of plants and the mouths of animals, since both structures are used for the intake of food.[23] Even more relevant in this context is a testimony from Sextus Empiricus, in which Heraclitus is said to have compared respiration to a "root" (DK 22 A16), as well as two Orphic fragments of unknown date, which claim that "the soul for humans is rooted in the *aither*" (ἀιι' αἰθέρος ἐρρίζωται, *OF* 436) and that "by drawing air we pluck a divine soul" just as someone might pluck a plant from the ground (*OF* 422).[24] Directly connecting these respiratory theories to *On Breaths*' passing reference to the "roots" of the blood, Democritus is said to have claimed that, even after a person breathes out their soul during death, some links with this soul remain "rooted" in the marrow and the heart, thereby enabling a person to re-inhale their soul and thus come back to life (DK 68 B1). All of these passages suggest that our doxographer would have been familiar with an analogy between respiration and a root even before reading *On Breaths*.[25] Having seen a reference to "roots" in chapter 7, the doxographer may have recalled these other examples of the respiration-root analogy and concluded that the author of *On Breaths* must hold a similar view.

As for the doxographer's citation of a particular species of plant called a "soldier," this level of taxonomic specificity would be surprising to find in any medical text from the Classical period. When the authors in the Hippocratic Corpus draw analogies between humans and plants, they tend to focus either on plants *in general* or on broad categories of plants rather than invoking particular species. A reference to a particular species of plant does not even occur in the long botanical excursus in *On the*

---

[22] Note Hes. *Th.* 790–791, A. *PV* 138–140, E. *Or.* 1377–1379, and A.R. 3.1277. Manetti (1999a: 123) also points out that an earlier reference to rivers can be found at *Ti.* 43a–b, which may have further contributed to this doxographical intrusion.

[23] Arist. *de An.* 412b3–4, *Juv.* 468a9–12, *PA* 682a21, 686b35–687a1, *IA* 705b6–8; compare *PA* 650a20–31. More generally, Aristotle also observes that the heads of animals are like the roots of plants at *de An.* 416a4 and *Long.* 467b2. For Aristotle's comparison of the umbilical cord to a root, see *GC* 493a17–18 and *GA* 739b36–37, 740a33–35, 740b8–11, 745b24–26.

[24] Compare also *OF* 116, where *aither* is called the "root of all things." This botanical metaphor was also applied to Empedocles's four elements (DK 31 B6) and the Pythagorean tetractys (DK 58 B15). Note also Aristotle's comment that Xenophanes claimed the earth is "rooted in the infinite" (DK 21 A47), even though no reference to a "root" appears in the fragment preserved by Achilles Tatius (DK 21 B28). Parmenides is likewise said to have claimed that the earth is "rooted in water" (DK 28 B15a).

[25] For Aristotle's familiarity with the theory, attributed to both "Orphics" and "Pythagoreans," that we inhale souls from the air, see *de An.* 404a16–20, 410b27–411a1. This "respiratory" theory of the soul was held by many thinkers from this era, including the author of *On Regimen*.

Seed-Nature of the Child (22–27, 7.514–528 L.). By citing a particular species by name, this analogy is strongly reminiscent of the meticulous botanical and zoological research that was being carried out in the Lyceum. Aristotle's zoological works contain numerous analogies between animals and specific types of plants.[26] Likewise, Theophrastus's botanical works contain many analogies between plants and specific types of animals.[27] In one passage, Aristotle even compares sea cucumbers to a species of plant that survives without being rooted in the ground (*PA* 681a17–25), indicating that there was already an interest among the Peripatetics in comparing animals to "free-floating" plants whose roots do not penetrate the earth. Thus, what many scholars have perceived to be the primary, or even the only, reason to doubt the connection between the *Anonymus Londiniensis* and *On Breaths* might better be understood as a doxographical intrusion, not unlike the intrusive analogy between the intestines and a river that we find in the report about Plato.

On balance, these observations provide a good case for supposing that the report about Hippocrates likely refers to *On Breaths*. It is of course impossible to draw a definitive conclusion on the matter, but the preponderance of evidence all points in the same direction. This then leads to an even thornier question – could Hippocrates *really* be the author of this text? The *Anonymus Londiniensis* is careful to note that this report originated with Aristotle (V.36–47, VI.42–43), primarily because the author disagrees with his Peripatetic source. Aristotle was the son of a doctor, deeply interested in medical science, and not far removed from the lifetime of Hippocrates, all of which would make him a good witness for what the

---

[26] For example, *PA* 668a21–25 (emaciated bodies leave only vessels to be seen, just like the dried-up leaves of figs and vines leave nothing but their vessels behind), *GA* 715b16–30 (*testacea* are reminiscent of fig trees and mistletoe), 725b34–726a3 (overnourished goats behave like overnourished vines), 755b7–10 (some say that sex differentiation in fish is like the differences between the fig and the caprifig, the olive and the oleaster).

[27] For example, Thphr. *HP* 1.1.4 (plants that shed their leaves are like animals that shed their horns, feathers, or hair), 1.4.2–3 (some plants, like some animals, can only live in aquatic habitats, others only live in dry habitats, and still others are amphibious), 2.4.4 (just like plants, some animals, like the hawk and hoopoe, change according to the seasons; some, like the water-snake, change according to the nature of the ground; and some, like the caterpillar, change at different stages of their lives), 3.2.1 (like animals, some plants resist domestication, while others do not), 4.3.5 (thyme grows abundantly in places without rainfall, just as snakes and lizards thrive without water), 7.14.3 (bedstraw keeps its flower within itself, just as weasels and sharks keep eggs within themselves). Note also Theophrastus's general remarks about the drawing of analogies between animals and plants at *HP* 1.1.7: "if in some cases analogy ought to be considered (for instance, an analogy presented by animals) . . . we must of course make the closest resemblances and the most perfectly developed examples our standard" (trans. Hort). This methodological emphasis on *specificity* is more typical of Peripatetic analogies than the less restrictive use of analogy in the Hippocratic Corpus.

real-life Hippocrates may have actually believed. Other evidence has been advanced to bolster the attribution of *On Breaths* to Hippocrates,[28] but none of these supporting arguments are as strong as the testimony provided by the *Anonymus Londiniensis* itself.

For my part, I have little interest in being so provocative as to call the author of *On Breaths* "Hippocrates" from this point forward. Although I think this text has the best claim to Hippocratic authorship out of all the works that have been transmitted under his name, I am less interested in the so-called Hippocratic Question than in challenging the still common assumption that it is somehow *inconceivable* for Hippocrates to have authored this work.[29] The strong reactions that some have displayed against this attribution are largely due, I would argue, to a continued tendency to separate the cosmological doctors from other medical writers from this period. Thus, whenever *On Breaths* is assigned to Hippocrates, it is still generally supposed that we are somehow seismically changing our views about what early Greek medicine is all about. I would argue, by contrast, that there is nothing preventing the author of *On Breaths* from fundamentally agreeing with the bulk of what is written elsewhere in the Hippocratic Corpus. In fact, we will soon see that there is nothing excluding this author from having participated in even the sort of careful research on display in the *Epidemics*.[30] As we have already observed over the past two chapters, the cosmological doctors were not the extreme caricatures that *On Ancient Medicine* would want us to believe. They had much more in common with other medical writers than has traditionally been

---

[28] Note especially Langholf (1986). The evidence from Plato's *Phaedrus*, in which Hippocrates is said to have claimed that one cannot study the body without considering "the whole" (268a–270d), is notoriously vague, and can be applied to so many texts in the Hippocratic Corpus that it cannot provide much definitive support. For my own reading of that passage, see pp. 160–163.

[29] Compare Jones (1947: 2), who claims that *On Breaths* is a work which "no modern scholar would dream of thinking either authentic or genuine." The persistence of this view is illustrated by Walshe (2016: 24), who calls *On Breaths* "a sophistic exercise with little to suggest a powerful medical presence expected from the hand of Hippocrates." Jouanna (1984: 40–41), by contrast, notes that the contents of *On Breaths* are "in accordance with the essence of Hippocratic medicine, and also with its spirit." Langholf (1986: 21–22) is even more emphatic: "The author was not a sophist but a doctor. In fact, the arrangement of the material is impressively clear, its content by no means one-sidedly doctrinaire or outsiderish: the opinion represented in it neither says (which of course has been assumed) that man consists of a primary substance of air nor (which has also been assumed) that air is the sole cause of disease. The author is not an extremist in his theory, but only makes air the root cause of illness."

[30] On this point, I agree with Langholf (1990b: 358–359). Aristotle provides a good example of a thinker who combined detailed comparative research with high-level inquiries into the first principles of all things.

supposed, and they are in fact key representatives of some of the most important trends in medical thinking that occurred in the Classical period.

3.3   The Common Cause of All Diseases

Whatever we conclude about this doxographical report, one thing we can say for certain is that Greek doctors were not averse to citing *pneuma* as an important factor in pathogenesis. We have already seen Polybus attribute epidemic diseases to the *pneuma* that we breathe (p. 80). Philistion is also reported to have expressed many ideas about *pneuma*, including the theories that respiration cools the body's innate heat (Gal. *Ut. Resp.* 4.471 K.), that we breathe through both the nostrils and the skin (*Anon. Lond.* XX.45–47), that different foods can either encourage or repress the production of *pneuma* in the body (Ath. 3.83), and that "when the whole body breathes well and the breath passes through unhindered, health is the result" (*Anon. Lond.* XX.43–45). The *Anonymus Londiniensis* goes on to say that Philistion described *multiple* ways in which diseases are caused by *pneuma*: "When the body does not breathe well, diseases occur, and in different ways" (XX.47–49). The text breaks off soon after this statement, but it seems to have originally listed several ways in which *pneuma* gives rise to disease. If this is the case, then this testimony would have closely resembled the structure of *On Breaths*, which is also organized around a list of affections that can ultimately be traced back to *pneuma*.

   In other texts, "winds and humors" are cited side by side as the principal agents of disease. In the *Republic*, Plato complains about people who live in such a way as to fill their bodies with "fluids and winds" (ῥευμάτων τε καὶ πνευμάτων), thereby forcing doctors to give names to such diseases as "breaths and catarrhs" (φύσας τε καὶ κατάρρους, 3.405c–d; cf. *Ti.* 84d–e). Mnesitheus of Athens, a physician and younger contemporary of Plato, states that diseases can arise from either an excess or a deficiency "in either winds or fluids" (ἢ ἐν πνεύμασιν ἢ ἐν ὑγροῖς, fr. 11 Bertier), while the author of *On the Eight Months' Child* claims that newborn infants are more susceptible to diseases because "instead of winds and humors that are akin [sc. to the infant] . . . newborns use winds and humors that are all foreign, rawer, drier, and less adapted to human beings" (12.2, 7.456 L.). In *On the Sacred Disease*, the author attributes seizures to a downward flux of phlegm from the head, which congeals the blood and causes the *pneuma* in the vessels to become trapped. Unable to complete its normal circuit, the *pneuma* violently jerks back and forth, producing the various symptoms of an epileptic attack: "the patient becomes speechless and chokes; froth flows from the mouth; he gnashes his teeth and twists his hands; the eyes roll and intelligence fails, and in some cases excrement is discharged" (7.1, 6.372 L., trans. Jones).[31]

Many other works in the Hippocratic Corpus also refer to the interactions between *pneuma* and humors. *Pneuma* is the most commonly cited source of tremors and spasms,[32] and it is also one of the primary means of explaining how sweat, semen, and other fluids are expelled from the body.[33] As a contributor to sensation, intelligence, consciousness, and speech, *pneuma* must continually circulate through the vessels. If it is blocked, weighed down, or otherwise hindered, the patient can suffer from a variety of ailments, including numbness, paralysis, lethargy, drowsiness, mania, despondency, forgetfulness, and loss of speech.[34] By far the most important relationship between *pneuma* and humors, however, is to be found in the gastrointestinal tract. According to a widely attested belief that is invoked throughout the Classical period,[35] whenever someone ingests food and drink that is excessive, heavy, compact, or contrary to one's habits, the nutriment cannot be quickly digested, resulting in a stagnation of moisture in the belly. This moisture, in turn, gives off exhalations as it is heated, in the same way that liquids give off steam when they are boiled.[36] As the *pneuma* produced

---

[31] After this sentence the author explains in detail how each of these symptoms is created, recalling *On Breaths'* detailed description of how the various symptoms of a fever can all be traced back to *pneuma*. Similar explanations of seizures can be found at *Acut. App.* 7.2, 2.406 L., *Flat.* 14, 6.110–114 L., and Praxag. fr. 70–71 Steckerl = fr. 25–26 Lewis.

[32] *VM* 22.7, 1.630–632 L., *Acut. App.* 7, 2.404–406 L., *Aph.* 4.68, 4.526 L., *Epid. II* 6.2, 5.132 L., *Nat. Hom.* 21.1, 6.80–82 L., Praxag. fr. 27 Steckerl = fr. 6–8 Lewis.

[33] *Aph.* 5.63, 4.556 L., *Prorrh. I* 98, 5.536–538 L., *Morb. I* 25, 6.190 L., *Vict.* 62.2, 6.576 L., 64.2, 6.580 L., 66.3, 6.584 L., 89.12, 6.652 L., *Oss.* 15, 9.188–190 L., Pl. *Ti.* 84d–e, 91a; cf. *Epid. II* 5.25, 5.132 L., *Epid. VI* 3.5, 5.294 L., 3.14, 5.300 L., Arist. *GA* 737b27–738a9. See also the texts cited in note 63 on p. 39.

[34] *VM* 22.7, 1.630–632 L., *Prog.* 11, 2.138 L., *Acut. App.* 6–7, 2.402–406 L., 10, 2.414–416 L., 23, 2.440–442 L., 68, 2.522 L., *Coac.* 485, 5.694 L., *Vict.* 35.5, 6.516 L., 35.7, 6.518 L., 36.2, 6.522–524 L., 71.1–2, 6.610 L., *Morb. III* 10, 7.128–130 L., Praxag. fr. 69, 72–75 Steckerl = fr. 23–24, 27–28 Lewis; cf. *Oct.* 9.8, 7.450 L., Diog. Apoll. DK 64 A19, Thphr. *Sens.* 44–45.

[35] *VM* 10.3, 1.592 L., *Acut.* 37.2–3, 2.298–302 L., *Acut. App.* 41–42, 2.476–478 L., *Epid. II* 3.17, 5.118 L., *Epid. VI* 5.1, 5.314 L., *Nat. Hom.* 21.1, 6.80–82 L., *Flat.* 7, 6.98–100 L., *Aff.* 47, 6.256–258 L., *Loc. Hom.* 45.3, 6.340 L., *Vict.* 40.2–4, 6.536–538 L., 42.3, 6.540 L., 46.3, 6.546 L., 50, 6.552–554 L., 52.1, 6.554 L., 54.1, 6.556 L., 56.8, 6.570 L., 74.1, 6.614–616 L., *Int.* 44, 7.274–276 L., *Morb. IV* 49, 7.578–580 L., *Prorrh. II* 4, 9.16 L., *Anon. Lond.* IV.31–40 (Euryphon of Cnidos), IV.40–V.34 (Herodicus of Cnidos), V.39–VI.43 (Hippocrates), VII.40–VIII.10 (Alcamenes of Abydos), VIII.10–34 (Timotheus of Metapontum), IX.37–44 (Ninyas of Egypt), XII.8–36 (Dexippus of Cos), XIII.21–XIV.2 (Aegimius of Elis), XX.1–24 (Petron of Aegina). Note also the many references in the Hippocratic Corpus to foods that are "flatulent" (φυσώδης), a quality that is usually associated with slow or difficult digestion.

[36] For the analogy, see *Flat.* 8.3, 6.102 L., and compare *Flat.* 8.6, 6.102 L., Arist. *PA* 652b33–653a8, and *Somn.* 457b31–458a5. *Genit.-Nat. Puer.* 12.2, 7.486 L. formulates the principle in

by these exhalations tries to find an exit either upwards or downwards, the patient suffers not only from belching, yawning, and flatulence but also from swelling, pain, thirst, and rumblings in the intestines. In many cases, the upward exhalation brings its evaporated moisture to the head, where it is cooled, condensed, and initiates fluxes to other parts of the body.[37]

The author of *On Breaths* assumes that his audience is familiar with these concepts when making his own claims about *pneuma*. His goal is to show that *pneuma*, which is already commonly cited as an important factor in *some* diseases, is actually the "starting point and source" (ἀρχὴ καὶ πηγή, 1.4, 6.92 L.) of all diseases in general. The author supports this thesis with an argument from induction, illustrating the supremacy of *pneuma* in every class, type, or "tribe" (ἔθνος, 6.1, 6.96 L.) of disease. After observing that *pneuma* exerts its influence over the universe as a whole, controlling the seasons, nourishing the sun, pervading the sea, and supporting the earth (ch. 3), he claims that *pneuma* is not only the most essential requirement for life (ch. 4) but is also responsible for all diseases in the body (ch. 5). In chapters 6–14, the author describes the agency of *pneuma* in fevers (chs. 6–8), intestinal disorders (ch. 9), catarrhs (ch. 10), lacerations (ch. 11), dropsy (ch. 12), apoplexy (ch. 13), and the so-called sacred disease (ch. 14). In each case, he explains how a different action of *pneuma* initiates a different set of affections, thereby "proving" that these diseases, which outwardly seem dissimilar, in fact have a common *arche*. In chapter 15, the author reiterates his thesis that *pneuma* is "the most active agent throughout all diseases" and that all other agents are but "accessory and contributing causes." Finally, he claims that he could have cited many other diseases in addition to the ones described: "I have carried my account down to the diseases and affections that are well known, in which cases my foundational principle [ὑπόθεσις] has been shown to be true. If I were to discuss all diseases, my account would be longer, but it would not be any more precise or more convincing" (15.2, 6.114 L.).[38]

---

general terms: "everything that is heated gives off *pneuma*." Compare also *Acut.* 28.3, 2.284 L., 49.1, 2.332 L., *Acut. App.* 51.1, 2.494 L., *Int.* 5, 7.178 L., 24, 7.228 L., 40, 7.264 L., 44, 7.274 L., *Anon. Lond.* XII.36–XIII.11 (Phasilas of Tenedos), Arist. [*Pr.*] 1.41, 864a12–13, and the general references to wind coming from water at *Od.* 4.568, Xenoph. DK 21 B30, and Heraclit. DK 22 B12, Emp. DK 31 B50, and *Genit.-Nat. Puer.* 25.1, 7.522 L.

[37] Compare *Epid. II* 3.17, 5.118 L., *Morb. I* 15, 6.168 L., *Morb. II* 11, 7.18 L., *Mul. I* 36, 8.84 L., *Gland.* 7.2, 8.560–562 L., *Anon. Lond.* IV.31–40 (Euryphon of Cnidos), V.22–34 (Herodicus of Cnidos), VII.40–VIII.10 (Alcamenes of Abydos), VIII.10–26 (Timotheus of Metapontum), Arist. *PA* 652b33–653a8, and *Somn.* 457b–458a.

[38] In this closing statement, the author plays on the ambiguous meaning of *hupothesis* as both a "foundational principle" and a "thesis" to be proved. For its relationship with the *hupotheseis* of *On Ancient Medicine*, see Schiefsky (2005: 122–123).

In my discussion of *On the Nature of the Human Being*, I argued that cosmological principles like the hot, the cold, the dry, and the wet were never intended to replace more traditional theories about the humors. Instead, these principles occupied a two-tiered framework of remote and proximate causes, wherein the hot, the cold, the dry, and the wet played the role of the remote, triggering cause, while the more familiar proximate cause could still be identified as the "separating out" of humors within the body. This two-tiered model of pathogenesis would have carried practical benefits for Greek doctors. First, it facilitated their interest in treating both diseases and their source, since the removal of an initiating cause was viewed as critical to restoring a patient's health. Second, this two-tiered model promised to open up new avenues in disease prevention. Equipped with an understanding of how diseases come to be, doctors could counteract remote causes before the patient falls ill, counterbalancing the hot with the cold, the cold with the hot, the dry with the wet, and the wet with the dry. As we saw in Chapter 2, Polybus was still deeply concerned with the differences between individual patients. In fact, we might speculate that one of the primary benefits of his system was that it intervened at the point in the causal chain before differentiation occurs. Far from denying the many variables that can change from one case to the next, Polybus may have formulated his entire system, in which the humors are said to be "always alike the same, whether the patient be young or old, or whether the season be cold or hot" (2.5, 6.36 L.), as a solution to the problem of individual variation.

I would now like to suggest that the author of *On Breaths* advances his thesis about *pneuma* with the same concerns for remote versus proximate causes and individual variation that we see in *On the Nature of the Human Being*. In fact, one could argue that *On Breaths* and *On the Nature of the Human Being* are both products of the same intellectual milieu. There are a number of similarities, some of them very close, between these two texts, both of which seem to have been written in a context where doctors were publicly debating the "starting point" of diseases.[39] Like Polybus, the author of *On Breaths* claims that the cause of a disease should be treated by applying its opposite (ἐκ τῶν ἐναντίων ἐπιστάμενος τῷ νοσήματι, 1.3, 6.92 L.; cf. ἐναντίον ἵστασθαι τοῖσι καθεστηκόσι, *Nat. Hom.* 9.2, 6.52 L.), and in a move that strongly reinforces the connection between these texts, he also gives the same examples of causes and cures that we find in *On the*

---

[39] For these and other parallels between *On Breaths* and *On the Nature of the Human Being*, see Jouanna (1988: 31–34).

Nature of the Human Being. The author of *On Breaths* notes that "evacuation cures repletion, repletion cures evacuation, rest cures exercise, and exercise cures rest" (1.4, 6.92 L.). Similarly, Polybus asserts that "diseases due to repletion are cured by evacuation, and those due to evacuation are cured by repletion; those due to exercise are cured by rest, and those due to idleness are cured by exercise" (9.1, 6.52 L., trans. Jones). Another parallel between these texts comes in the sixth chapter of *On Breaths*. In this chapter, the author describes two types of fevers: (1) those that arise from regimen and (2) those that are caused by respiration. The fevers that arise from regimen are particular to individuals (ἰδίη), while the fevers that arise from respiration are common to everyone (κοινὸς ἅπασιν, 6.1, 6.96 L.). Not only is this the same distinction that we find in *On the Nature of the Human Being*, but the author of *On Breaths* also frames it, like Polybus, in the language of commonality and difference (6.2, 6.98 L.):

> The fever that is common to many [πολύκοινος] is of such a sort because all people inhale the same *pneuma*, and when similar *pneuma* is mixed with the body in a similar way, the fevers that arise are also similar. But perhaps someone will say: why, then, do such diseases not befall all animals, but only a certain tribe of them? This is because, I'd say, body differs from body, nature from nature, nutriment from nutriment. For the same things are neither unfitting nor fitting for all tribes of animals, but some things are beneficial to some, while others are not beneficial to others. So whenever the air is steeped with such pollutions that are hostile to human nature, humans become diseased, and whenever the air becomes unfit for some other tribe of animals, those animals become diseased.

Just as Polybus divides patients into classes, distinguishing each class by its habits and underlying "nature," so too does the author of *On Breaths* plainly assert that the development of a disease is not determined by a single factor but it rather depends on a constellation of factors that can change from one case to the next. In the above-quoted passage, the author invokes the important concept of "fitness to the individual" (ἁρμονία). This language implies that differentiation is due as much to the individual patient as to the nature of the initiating cause. In fact, the author uses the same language that appears in *On Ancient Medicine*. The author of *On Ancient Medicine* writes that medicine has grown more effective as doctors have determined what is "fitting" (ἁρμόζων) for each class (3.4, 1.576 L., 5.1, 1.580 L.). Similarly, the author of *On Breaths* believes that a key aspect of medical thinking is to match causal factors to particular constitutions, noting that "the same things are neither unfitting nor fitting [οὔτ' ἀνάρμοστα οὔτ' εὐάρμοστα] for all tribes of animals, but some things are beneficial to some, while others are not beneficial to others" (6.2, 6.98 L.).

This emphasis on the *contingency* of disease is essential to understanding *On Breaths*. The author is very interested in the causes of disease, and especially in how a single cause can produce a wide range of effects. As it happens, the author's observation that "body differs from body, nature from nature, nutriment from nutriment" is the same argument that *On Ancient Medicine* uses to *oppose* the cosmological doctors. Both authors stress that "nature differs from nature" (διαφέρει . . . καὶ φύσις φύσιος, *Flat.* 6.2, 6.98 L.; cf. διαφέρουσιν οὖν τούτων αἱ φύσιες, *VM* 20.6, 1.624 L.), and both claim that an initiating cause – be it *pneuma* or cheese – will only bring about disease if it is "hostile" to one's *phusis* (φύσει πολέμια, *Flat.* 6.2, 6.98 L.; cf. πολέμιον, *VM* 20.6, 1.624 L.). The author of *On Ancient Medicine* presents this observation as a rebuttal to the theories of the cosmological doctors. Instead of contemplating universal *hupotheseis*, doctors should divide patients into classes and then focus on the effects of different foods on each class. The author of *On Breaths*, for his part, does not think that the recognition of individual differences should hinder his search for high-level commonalities. Instead, he asserts that there are secondary factors in addition to the common cause, factors that will ultimately determine how the ailment will be manifested from one case to the next.

It is important to stress that the author of *On Breaths* does not claim that *pneuma* is the *only* cause of a disease. Rather, he claims that *pneuma* is a *common* cause, and also, incidentally, the most important cause.[40] This is a critical point, as some readers have erroneously assumed that the author of *On Breaths* rejects humoral pathology in favor of a radically new system of medicine.[41] On closer examination, we can see that the author is not

---

[40] Compare the author's reference to "accessory and contributing causes" at 15.1, 6.114 L. This passage puts into perspective the author's bold assertion that "of all diseases there is one and the same class and cause" (2, 6.92 L.). I will come back to these passages later in my discussion.

[41] Compare Carrick (2001: 28–29): "the author of another treatise, *On Breaths*, drops the humoral model in favor of an explanation of diseases based on the presence or absence in the body of the correct amount and blend of air inhaled from one's environment and drawn into the interstices of various organs." Note also Brǎtescu (1980: 67), who claims that in the Hippocratic Corpus, "the treatises focus either *exclusively* on the principles of pneumatism or on those of pure humorism" (my emphasis). By contrast, Langholf (1990b: 340–341) correctly observes that "the modern terms 'humoral doctrine,' 'humoral pathology' (terms which are not found in the *Hippocratic Collection*) imply a simplification of complex theories: in the *Collection*, there is no theory which is confined to humors. The treatises *On Breaths* and *The Sacred Disease* perfectly demonstrate that the pneumatic doctrine is in principle and in practice compatible with humoral theories." Compare also Thivel (1981: 146): "The author of *On Breaths* is not seeking to create a new medicine, that would be an

rejecting the humors or even wandering very far from what *pneuma* was already deemed capable of doing within the body. Toward the end of *On Breaths*, the author claims to have discussed "well-known diseases" (τὰ γνώριμα τῶν ἀρρωστημάτων, 15.2, 6.114 L.). By calling these affections "well known," he suggests that his goal is not to introduce a whole new system of medicine but rather to supplement widely held views on the nature of disease. In several passages, the author emphasizes his reliance on opinions shared by "everyone." "I think it is clear to everyone," he writes, "that ileus, tormina, colic, and intestinal fixations are products of breaths" (9.1, 6.104 L.). In another passage, the author raises a potential objection: "Perhaps someone might say, 'How then do humoral fluxes arise on account of breaths? In what way is *pneuma* responsible for hemorrhages around the chest?'" (10.1, 6.104 L.). By raising this objection, the author implies that *everyone* believes in fluxes from the head, that *everyone* recognizes hemorrhages in the chest. His task is not to prove or disprove such widely held beliefs but rather to illustrate how *pneuma* can unite and govern them all.

To demonstrate that *pneuma* is the common cause of all diseases, including fevers, intestinal disorders, catarrhs, lacerations, dropsy, apoplexy, and the so-called sacred disease, the author starts with familiar narratives of how each of these diseases comes to be, reframing them only insofar as it is necessary to draw attention to preexisting, widely accepted views about what *pneuma* tends to do within the body. At this point, I would like to go through the author's various descriptions of disease, noting how his accounts can be paralleled elsewhere in the Hippocratic Corpus. By observing these parallels, I ultimately hope to illustrate the inherent conservatism of this text. Although the author's overarching thesis would have been a point of contention among his contemporaries, the observations he uses to argue his point do not significantly deviate from what we find in other works from the Hippocratic Corpus.

The author's first topic is fever, with which he claims to begin because it is "the most common malady" and because it "accompanies all other diseases" (6.1, 6.96 L.). In this section, he divides all fevers into two "tribes" (ἔθνεα), one of which is common to all and is caused by the *pneuma* that we breathe, while the other is particular to individuals and is caused by bad regimen. Since "common" diseases were already attributed to *pneuma* in

absurd claim, but he believes that the best way to preserve the ancient heritage is to cast it in the mold of a new theory."

this familiar division between "common" and "particular" diseases (cf. p. 80), the author does not find it necessary to make any adjustments on this front. When he comes to "particular" diseases, however, he argues that these, too, do not occur without the involvement of *pneuma* (7.1, 6.98 L.). The author begins by describing two ways in which a person can make use of "bad regimen." The first is the consumption of more food than is expended by exercise, while the second is the consumption of food that creates "conflict" in the belly. In both cases, the end result of such "bad regimen" is the stagnation of moisture in the belly, which in turn gives rise to "breaths." As we have already seen, "breaths" were commonly thought to arise from the stagnation of nutriment in the belly. Many Greek doctors would have therefore found parallels between this part of the author's treatise and popular notions about the generation of "breaths."

As for the particular symptoms of a fever (chills, trembling, yawning, debility, sweating, headaches, burning heat), the author explains each of these phenomena as a natural consequence of "breaths." Chills are attributed to the cooling of blood by the *pneuma* that falls upon it (7.2, 6.100 L.), echoing a commonly held belief that one purpose of respiration is to cool the body's innate heat.[42] In *Diseases I*, the author explicitly attributes chills to the cooling of the blood, noting that such cooling can arise "from external winds, water, clear air, and other such things, and also from ingested foods and drinks" (24, 6.188 L.). After explaining the cause of chills, the author of *On Breaths* then discusses other symptoms that attend a fever, at no point providing explanations that dramatically differ from what we find elsewhere in the Hippocratic Corpus. Trembling occurs when the blood, repelled by the cold *pneuma*, "darts" (διαΐσσει, 8.2, 6.100 L.) to the warm parts of the body. *Diseases IV* and *Diseases of Women I* also refer to chills "darting" through the body,[43] while the author of *Diseases of Unwed Girls* echoes the idea that blood is repelled by the cold when he writes that "the blood very rapidly moves upward [from the feet] whenever the patient stands in cold water up to the ankles" (2.2, 8.468 L.). Yawning is the next symptom to be explained in *On Breaths*. The author says that this symptom occurs when some of the *pneuma* rises from the belly and exits through the mouth (8.3, 6.102 L.), invoking what appears to have

---

[42] On the cooling power of *pneuma*, see *Genit.-Nat. Puer.* 24.2, 7.520 L., 25.5–6, 7.524–526 L., and the passages quoted in note 9 on p. 20.

[43] *Morb. IV* 46.4, 7.572 L., 57.2, 7.610 L.; *Mul. I* 35, 8.82 L.; compare *Epid. II* 4.1, 5.122 L. and *Morb. Sacr.* 7.10, 6.374 L.

been a common explanation for this phenomenon.[44] Debility is attributed to the warming and relaxation of the joints (8.4, 6.102 L.), while sweating occurs when some of the *pneuma* reaches the exterior of the body, where it condenses back into moisture like steam hitting the lid of a pot (8.6, 6.102 L.). Both of these explanations, together with the author's attribution of throbbing headaches to the trapping of *pneuma* in the vessels (8.7, 6.102–104 L.), are well within the limits of what we find in the Hippocratic Corpus.[45] As for the burning heat that is the hallmark of every fever, the author writes that the blood, fleeing the cold *pneuma*, gathers together in a mass, after which it stagnates, grows hot, and overpowers the *pneuma* in turn, transforming the once cold *pneuma* into a conveyor of heat. "Overpowered by the heat" (κρατηθεὶς ὑπὸ τῆς θέρμης, 8.5, 6.102 L.), the *pneuma* then distributes this heat to the rest of the body, thereby explaining how a concentrated humor in just one part of the body can end up passing its heat to every part. A similar mechanism accounts for the alternation between chills and fever in *Diseases I*, where it is not *pneuma* but rather bile and phlegm that first cool the blood and are then heated by this humor (24, 6.188–190 L.; cf. *Genit.-Nat. Puer.* 15.4, 7.494 L.). As the author of *Diseases I* also writes about blood "gaining the upper hand" over the substance that had cooled it and discusses many of the same attendant symptoms that appear in *On Breaths* (e.g., trembling and sweating), it seems likely that the author of *On Breaths* drew on an account very similar to this one, swapping out *pneuma* for noxious humors but nevertheless staying well within the limits of what *pneuma* was deemed capable of doing within the body.

From this description of fevers, we can see that the author of *On Breaths* has no intention of creating a whole new system of medicine. Instead, he simply shifts his audience's attention to the activity of *pneuma*, which was already thought to play an important role in many aspects of pathogenesis. The rest of the author's explanations are similarly constructed in such a way that they build on widely attested beliefs about the origin of disease. In many cases, the author's contemporaries were already attributing certain

---

[44] Compare *VM* 10.3, 1.592 L., *Epid. II* 3.1c, 5.102 L., 3.7, 5.110 L. (= *Epid. VI* 2.4, 5.278 L.), *Epid. IV* 2.11, 5.282 L., 5.1, 5.314 L., *Flat.* 13.2, 6.110 L., and Arist. [*Pr.*] 10.1, 886a24–28, 11.29, 902b9–15, 11.44, 904a16–22, 32.13, 961a37–b6.

[45] For the connection between debility and the loosening of the joints, see *Epid. VI* 1.9, 5.270 L., 1.15, 5.274 L. and Arist. [*Pr.*] 1.24, 862a30–33. On the throbbing caused by the trapping of *pneuma* in the vessels, see pp. 104–105. The author of *Epidemics II* specifically refers to the presence of "breaths" in the head (3.17, 5.118 L.).

affections to *pneuma*, as was the case for diseases where the free flow of *pneuma* was thought to be impeded in some way. In chapter 9, the author explicitly states that "everyone" believes that the twisting pains of intestinal disorders are caused by the blockage of *pneuma*, while his explanations of apoplexy in chapter 13 and of epileptic seizures in chapter 14 are fully in keeping with what we find in other texts (see note 63 on p. 39). Where the author is most original is when he talks about affections in which *pneuma* was not usually thought to play a major role. Since these are the passages in which we will best judge the nature of this text, I would like to look more closely at two passages in particular: (1) the author's discussion of humoral fluxes in chapter 10 and (2) his account of dropsy in chapter 12.

In chapter 10, the author acknowledges that fluxes from the head are not normally thought to be caused by *pneuma*. Raising a hypothetical objection of the sort one often finds in Greek rhetoric, he notes that "Perhaps someone might say, 'How then do humoral fluxes arise on account of breaths? In what way is *pneuma* responsible for hemorrhages around the chest?'" (10.1, 6.104 L.). A similar hypothetical objection appears in *On Ancient Medicine*, in which the author uses this tactic to show just how strong his own position is (17.1–2, 1.612 L.; cf. *Carn.* 6.4, 8.592 L., *Cord.* 2, 9.82 L.). In *On Breaths*, the author begins with an assumption that is commonly accepted in the Hippocratic Corpus, namely that *pneuma* travels through the vessels and that it shares these same pathways with the blood.[46] The author claims that fluxes from the head are initiated when a large amount of *pneuma* enters its vessels, which are narrower than the vessels in other parts of the body (10.1, 6.104 L.; cf. 8.7, 6.102–104 L.). Once the *pneuma* has entered these vessels, it "squeezes" the blood and exerts so much pressure that it eventually gives rise to an *apokrisis* (10.1–2, 6.104–106 L.):

> The thinnest part of the blood is pressed out [ἐκθλίβεται] through the vessels, and when this fluid collects in large quantity [ἀθροισθῇ πολλόν], it flows through the other passages, and in whatever part of the body it arrives in a mass, in that part of the body the disease becomes established.

The "fluid" in this case is a concentrated humor, which the author later identifies as phlegm (10.2–4, 6.106 L.). It had previously been mixed together with the blood, but as the *pneuma* exerts pressure on the blood, this blend of humors is disrupted and the thinnest part (i.e., the phlegm) is

---

[46] Praxagoras of Cos (late fourth century BCE) is traditionally said to have been the first Greek thinker to put *pneuma* in the arteries and humors in the veins. Before then, it was widely supposed that blood and *pneuma* simply flow together through the vessels.

"separated out." The author is careful to note that a flux does not immediately happen at this point. Rather, the concentrated humor must gradually build up until it reaches a critical mass (ἀθροισθῇ πολλόν, 10.2, 6.104 L.). Once enough phlegm has gathered together, it can then travel to other parts of the body, creating different affections depending on the place to which it flows. A similar delay between an *apokrisis* and flux can be found in *Prognostic*, in which the author observes that a headache that lasts for twenty days without a fever will be resolved in one of two ways: either (1) the patient will hemorrhage through the nostrils or (2) there will be a downward movement of humors from the head (21, 2.172 L.).[47] As for the assumption that different affections arise depending on the terminus of the flux, this was a common belief among the authors of the Hippocratic Corpus, one we have already encountered in our discussions of *On Ancient Medicine* (p. 52) and *On the Nature of the Human Being* (p. 82). There is only one detail in this description of humoral flux in which the author of *On Breaths* stands apart from other sources. This is his identification of *pneuma* as the root cause of an *apokrisis*, squeezing the blood and causing phlegm to be "pressed out." It is precisely on this point, however, that medical writers were primed to offer up new theories. Many texts in the Hippocratic Corpus presuppose the existence of *apokriseis*, but there were competing theories about what precisely caused the "separating out" of one humor from the rest. In *On Ancient Medicine*, the author says that *apokriseis* are caused by a "disturbance" (τάραχος, 14.6, 1.604 L.), which might occur when a patient consumes food and drink that is unblended and "strong." In works that emphasize the hot, the cold, the dry, and the wet (e.g., *On the Nature of the Human Being*, *On Affections*, *On Regimen*), an *apokrisis* can still arise from a "disturbance," but these authors more often attribute *apokriseis* to the heating, cooling, drying, or moistening of the humors themselves. In *On Breaths*, the author takes a mechanical approach, claiming that an *apokrisis* occurs when the blood, which contains a mixture of all the humors, is "squeezed" by the *pneuma* and a specific humor is "pressed out" (ἐκθλίβεται). The specific mechanism of "squeezing" is not unique to our author, and it is actually paralleled in other texts that talk about *apokriseis*. In *On Places in the Human Being*, the author notes that one cause of fluxes from the head is the squeezing of both the flesh and the vessels: "When the flesh shivers, contracts,

---

[47] For *On Regimen*'s presumption of a similar delay between an *apokrisis* and flux, see pp. 243–244.

and creates pressure, the vessels press out the moisture [ἐκφλίβουσι; cf. ἐκθλίβεται, *Flat.* 10.1, 6.104 L.] and the flesh simultaneously presses out its moisture in turn" (9.1, 6.292 L.). In the *Anonymus Londiniensis*, Philolaus is said to have attributed the thickening of the blood to the squeezing of the flesh (παραθλιβομένης τῆς σαρκός, XVIII.33–34). Similar references to "squeezing" can be found in *On Glands* ("The glands in the intestines press out [ἐκπιεζόμεναι] and distribute moisture," 5.2, 8.560 L.) and *Epidemics V* (sticky *ichor* is "pressed out" (ἐκθλίβεται) from a wound, 65, 5.242 L.; cf. *Epid. VII* 61, 5.426 L.), while Anaximenes is said to have claimed that rain arises when the clouds are condensed and their moisture is "pressed out" (ἐκθλίβεται, DK 13 A17).[48] In *On Breaths*, the author attributes this squeezing to the presence of *pneuma* in the vessels. He stands apart inasmuch as he identifies *pneuma* as the primary trigger of such an *apokrisis*, but neither the mechanism itself nor the fact that *pneuma* can be present in the vessels are conceptually out of place in the Hippocratic Corpus.

When the author explains "dropsy" (ὕδρωψ), he also draws on common notions of pathogenesis while arguing that *pneuma* is the root cause of this affection. Like other doctors from the Classical period, the author attributes dropsy to the collection of moisture in and around the flesh, where it stagnates, grows hot, and then causes the surrounding flesh to "melt" and flow to other parts.[49] The author claims that when the body's *pneuma* is loaded with moisture, it leaves some of this moisture behind as it travels through the flesh. The deposited moisture then does what stagnating moisture tends to do in this situation: it causes the surrounding flesh to melt and flow away (12.1, 6.108 L.). In this case, the only adjustment that the author makes to preexisting theories about dropsy is to claim that *pneuma* is the agent that initially deposited moisture around the flesh. Even on this point, however, the author is not without precedent. *On Regimen* also describes how *pneuma* travels around the flesh, consuming moisture from one part and depositing it somewhere else (see p. 234). In fact, medical writers often claim that *pneuma* transports moisture from one place to another. The most common example of this process is the conveying of moisture from the belly to the head. The author of *On*

---

[48] Compare Democritus's mechanistic explanation of how pressure differentials cause the body's soul to be "squeezed out" (ἐκθλίβεσθαι) and how respiration resists this squeezing by replenishing the *pneuma* within the body (DK 68 A106). At *Nat. Hom.* 14.1, 6.66 L., stones are said to be "squeezed out" into the bladder, although Jouanna (2002: 293) prefers to read λείβονται rather than θλίβονται. At *Ti.* 60c, Plato attributes the formation of stones to air "squeezing" and "pushing" the earth.

[49] Compare *Acut. App.* 52–53, 2.496–502 L., *Aff.* 22, 6.232–234 L., *Loc. Hom.* 21.1, 6.312–314 L., 24.1, 6.314–316 L., and *Int.* 23–26, 7.224–236 L.

Glands, for example, plainly states that "the body sends all kinds of vapors up to the head, which in turn the head transmits back" (7.2, 8.562 L., trans. Craik). At no point do we get the sense that the author of *On Breaths* is speaking tongue-in-cheek when making his own claims about *pneuma*. All of his explanations are far too reasonable and far too close to contemporary theories of pathogenesis for us to conclude that this work was not intended as a genuine contribution to medical knowledge.

3.4   Accessory and Contributing Causes

What allows the author of *On Breaths* to draw on preexisting disease narratives is the fact that he does not adopt the same definition of a "cause" that we find in *On Ancient Medicine*. He neither assumes that diseases are *necessarily* produced whenever *pneuma* is present, nor does he think that diseases are *always* cured whenever *pneuma* is taken away. In many cases *pneuma* is envisioned as a triggering, procatarctic cause, and it is also combined with accessory causes that determine the precise nature of its effects in different circumstances. In chapter 15, the author writes that *pneuma* is "the most active agent throughout all diseases" (διὰ πάντων τῶν νοσημάτων μάλιστα πολυπραγμονοῦσαι) and that all other agents are but "accessory and contributing causes" (συναίτια καὶ μεταίτια). In this passage, the author seems to restrict what deserves to be called a true "cause" to whatever bears the most responsibility in triggering an event.[50] In doing so, he recalls the legal debates we find illustrated in works such as Antiphon's *Tetralogies*, where the speakers seek to establish who bears the most responsibility for events involving multiple actors.[51] As for his reference to "accessory and contributing causes" (συναίτια καὶ μεταίτια), the author's downgrading of these factors should not distract us from the important role such causes still play in pathogenesis. The term *metaition* is not otherwise attested in the Hippocratic Corpus, but *sunaition* appears in four other passages, once in *Instruments of Reduction* and three times in *Epidemics VI*.[52] In *Instruments of Reduction*, the position in which

---

[50] For the idea, compare Cels. *pr.* 59: "Nothing is due to one cause alone, but that which is taken to be the cause is that which seems to have had the most influence (*contulisse plurimum*). Indeed it is possible that when one cause acts alone, it may not disturb, yet when acting in conjunction with other causes it may produce a very great disturbance" (trans. Spencer).

[51] See especially *Tet. II* 2.8, 3.10, 4.6, 4.10, *Tetr. III* 2.1, 3.2, 4.3–5, and *In Nov.* 20.

[52] See also the discussion of *aitia* and *sunaitia* at Pl. *Ti.* 46c–e and the reference to *sunerga* in the testimony on Philolaus (*Anon. Lond.* XVIII.47–XIX.1). We cannot presume, however, that the term *sunergon* originated with Philolaus himself, as this was also a technical term among the Stoics; compare Manetti (1990: 232–233, 1999b: 31). In tragedy, the adjectives *metaitios* and *sunaitios* typically imply a notion of "complicity" or "co-responsibility" (cf. Vegetti 1999: 288n17).

the patient sleeps is said to be a *sunaition* for the pathological curvature of the spine (37, 4.382 L.), while in *Epidemics VI*, a propensity for flatulence is said to be a *sunaition* for protruding shoulder blades (3.5, 5.294 L.), the hardness of the body is said to be a *sunaition* for the rupture of the vessels (3.6, 5.294 L.), and a winter cough in Perinthus is said to have been a *sunaition* for other diseases that afflicted the same patients during the spring (7.10, 5.342 L.). In all four passages, the *sunaition* specifically refers to something that distinguishes one group of patients from another. In the passage from *Instruments of Reduction*, it refers to a habitual activity (i.e., the patient's sleeping position), while in the three passages from *Epidemics VI*, it refers either to a permanent aspect of the patient's "nature" (i.e., a propensity for flatulence, a hardness of the body) or to a temporary state brought on by a disease (i.e., the physical condition that follows a winter cough). In all four passages, it is implied that the patients who possess these qualities will be more likely than others to experience certain effects. These *sunaitia* do not produce the effects on their own, but their presence will make them more likely to occur. In some cases, the *sunaitia* may even be *prerequisites* for the effects: the effects will not occur *unless* these conditions are met.[53] We have already seen another passage from *On Breaths* in which the author explicitly states that the same *pneuma* will not sicken all "tribes" of animals, since "body differs from body, nature from nature, nutriment from nutriment" (6.2, 6.98 L.). This assertion recalls the references to *sunaitia* that we see in *Instruments of Reduction* and *Epidemics VI*, and one assumes that this is at least partly what the author has in mind when he makes his own assertion about "accessory and contributing causes."

Of course, it is not *just* the characteristics of the individual patient that are responsible for variations in disease. When the author discusses the various diseases caused by *pneuma*, he also notes that different ailments are caused by differences in the parts with which the *pneuma* interacts, as well as differences in the quality, quantity, and source of the *pneuma* itself. In chapter 8, the author writes that "however the breaths rush forth in respect to quantity and coldness, such is the shivering that arises, stronger from more abundant and colder breaths, less strong from less abundant and less cold breaths." In chapter 2, the author invokes a similar set of notions while introducing his general thesis:

> Of all diseases, the type is the same while the location differs [ὁ μὲν τρόπος ωὑτός, ὁ δὲ τόπος διαφέρει]. It is because of the diversity of their locations

[53] Compare *Epid. VI* 7.1, 5.336 L.: "As I have written, these were the relationships of the affections. The first described occurred also without the later, but the later ones not without the former" (trans. Smith). A similar observation appears at *Epid. I* 10.1, 2.630 L.

that diseases seem to bear no resemblance to each other, but of all diseases there is one and the same class and cause.

In this passage, the author emphasizes that the location (τόπος) of a disease is responsible for its particular manifestation. This assertion should remind us of *On the Nature of the Human Being*, specifically the passage in which Polybus invokes the notion of humoral flux to illustrate how three diseases that appear to be very different in fact have a common *arche* (p. 82). Polybus describes an ailment that begins in the flesh and then flows to the intestines, the chest, and the bladder, creating different affections depending on the place to which it flows. In *On Breaths*, a similar discussion of humoral fluxes appears in chapter 10 (trans. Jones, modified):

> When the vessels about the head are loaded with air, at first the head becomes heavy through the breaths that press against it. Then the blood is compressed, the passages being unable, on account of their narrowness, to pour it through. The thinnest part of the blood is pressed out through the vessels, and when a great accumulation of this liquid has been formed, it flows through other channels. Any part of the body it reaches in a mass becomes the seat of a disease. If it go to the eyes, the pain is there; if it be to the ears, the disease is there. If it go to the chest, it is called sore throat; for phlegm, mixed with acrid humors, produces sores wherever it strikes locations [τόπους] unaccustomed to its presence, and the throat, being soft, is roughened when a flux strikes it.

In both *On the Nature of the Human Being* and *On Breaths*, fluxes are said to begin from a common source, but they give rise to different ailments depending on the place to which they flow. Neither author claims that all diseases are the same in their final manifestation, but they both emphasize that there is a single "starting point" (ἀρχή) that is the same in every case. When the author of *On Breaths* identifies *pneuma* as the "starting point and source" (ἀρχὴ καὶ πηγή) of all diseases in general, and when he says that the differences between diseases are due to differences in "location" (τόπος), he seems to be appropriating the language of humoral flux to frame his general thesis. All diseases belong to the same class because they all have a common cause. The differentiation that happens when we move beyond this common cause is like the differentiation that happens when a humor gathers in one place and then flows to other parts. As we see in the rest of this text, the location of an ailment is just one of many "accessory causes" that give rise to the variations between one patient and the next, but the familiarity of humoral flux to Classical Greek doctors enables the author to use this language as a shorthand for *any* differentiation that arises when you start from a common *arche*.[54]

3.5 A Single Class for All Diseases

In chapter 2, the author makes it clear that his goal is not simply to praise the unlimited power of *pneuma* but more specifically to identify a high-level commonality that transcends particular differences. This high-level commonality comes in the form of a "cause" (αἰτίη) and it places all diseases within one and the same "class" (ἰδέη). The author's specific assertion that all diseases belong to the same class is counterintuitive and clearly meant to be provocative. In the Classical period, Greek doctors frequently assert that there are many "types" or "classes" of disease – too many to catalog all conceivable permutations.[55] Polybus refers to four "types" (εἴδεα) of fevers, all of which originate from bile (15.1, 6.66 L.). He also asserts that "there are many forms of diseases and also many modes of treatment" (πολλαὶ μὲν ἰδέαι τῶν νοσημάτων, πολλὴ δὲ ἡ ἴησις, 2.3, 6.34–36 L.), apparently contradicting the assertion in *On Breaths* that "of all diseases there is one and the same class and cause" (μία πασέων νούσων καὶ ἰδέη καὶ αἰτίη ἡ αὐτή, 2, 6.92 L.). The contradiction is merely an illusion, however, as the author of *On Breaths* clearly accepts that diseases can take many forms.[56] Instead of postulating a single ailment with a single treatment, the author uses the term ἰδέη in its taxonomic sense, whereby the existence of a commonality establishes the existence of a "class," just as the so-called acute diseases (ardent fever, pneumonia, pleuritis, etc.) all belong to the same class because they all have certain traits in common. In *On Breaths*, the author divides diseases into classes and subclasses (cf. the reference to two "tribes" of fevers at 6.1, 6.98 L.), but his ultimate goal is to show that all these different classes have a common point of origin, a "source" from which they ultimately branch off. Whereas other doctors from this period looked for the "source" (ἀρχή) of humoral fluxes, our author looks for the source of all diseases, identifying an undifferentiated

---

[54] For another parallel with *Flat.* 2, 6.92 L., compare the universalizing statement at *Mul. II* 28, 8.308 L.: "For all diseases that are wont to arise from the uterus, I state the following: When the uterus moves out of its natural position, it moves sometimes in one direction and another time in another direction, and wherever it comes to rest it provokes violent pains" (trans. Potter).

[55] See pp. 137–168. On the use of the terms εἶδος and ἰδέη in the Hippocratic Corpus, see Gillespie (1912) and Diller (1971), both of whom observe that Greek doctors had a penchant for dividing patients, diseases, and treatments into "classes" and then considering the interactions between one class and another.

[56] Contrast Jouanna (1988: 31, 105n4), who claims that these two passages are "radically opposed."

arche in respect to which *all* diseases, despite their individual variations, can be said to belong to one and the same "class."

The obvious question that arises at this point is why the author of *On Breaths* would have wanted to advance such a thesis in the first place. Why would he want to identify a common cause of all diseases, and why does he take such pride in saying that all diseases belong to a single class? To start, we may observe that the author of *On Breaths* seems to relate his general thesis to the treatment of disease, observing that "if someone knows the cause of the disease, he will be able to administer what is beneficial to the body, opposing the disease by means of contraries" (1.4, 6.92 L.). The author then gives specific examples of what he means by the treatment of "opposites with opposites":

> Hunger is a disease. For whatever causes a person pain is called a disease. Now, what is the drug for hunger? It is what stops hunger, and this is eating. Accordingly, that malady must be cured with this remedy. Again, drinking stops thirst. Or again, evacuation cures repletion, repletion cures evacuation, rest cures exercise, and exercise cures rest. In a word, opposites are cures for opposites. For medicine is subtraction and addition: subtraction of what is in excess, addition of what is lacking. Whoever does this best is the best physician, while whoever most falls short of this most falls short of the art.

We have already noted the parallel between this passage and *On the Nature of the Human Being*, where the claim that "opposites are cures for opposites" conceals a more complex model of pathogenesis. Polybus holds that repletion, evacuation, exercise, and rest give rise to diseases by heating, cooling, drying, and moistening the humors. This action encourages the heat, cold, dryness, and moisture that is present in the humors themselves, with the humor that gains the most "strength" in this process being the one that separates off from the rest. In this framework, the hot, the cold, the dry, and the wet may be called the common cause of all diseases. They link the external, triggering cause (e.g., repletion, evacuation, exercise, and rest) with the "separating out" of one humor from the rest, and they bring a level of simplicity to medicine without entailing the extreme causal and therapeutic reductionism that is attacked in *On Ancient Medicine*. In *On Breaths*, *pneuma* takes the place of the hot, the cold, the dry, and the wet within this causal framework. There are many different triggers of disease and many different forms that diseases can take, but in between these two stages there is a common cause (i.e., *pneuma*) that is the same in every case. For both Polybus and the author of *On Breaths*, the identification of this common cause is directly relevant to treatment. In cases where a disease has already arisen, the doctor needs to remove the remote cause so that the patient's body can "gain the upper hand." In cases where the patient is still healthy, a knowledge of how diseases come to be enables the doctor to keep the patient from falling ill, heading off diseases at their source by treating any imbalance with its opposite.

On the one hand, then, the author of *On Breaths* seems to be promoting an idea that is directly relevant to treatment. So many diseases are caused by *pneuma* that the best way to ward off an illness is to remove anything that introduces noxious *pneuma* into the body. At the same time, we must admit that by claiming that *pneuma* is the common cause of *all* diseases, and by asserting that *pneuma* is the most powerful force in the universe as a whole, the author of *On Breaths* goes well beyond what is needed to make this otherwise practical point. We have already seen that the author of *On Breaths* is not creating a whole new system of medicine. He recognizes the many differences between individual cases, and he presumably prescribed all the same treatments that his contemporaries employed, strengthening the healthy parts and identifying concentrated humors with the ultimate goal of removing these humors from the body. His assertion that all diseases have a common cause and belong to a single "class" does not change the ultimate forms that diseases can take. There is no clear medical benefit in the author's claim that *pneuma* plays a *universal* role in pathogenesis, and there is also no therapeutic relevance in saying that in addition to being the strongest power in the body, *pneuma* also governs the sun, moon, and stars. Such observations provide the strongest possible support for claiming that *On Breaths* advances a thesis that is not meant to be taken seriously. Another explanation can be offered, however, one that fits better with the equally important observation that the author of *On Breaths* appears to be well versed in the concerns of Greek doctors, and that none of his explanations wander very far from what we find elsewhere in the Hippocratic Corpus.

By claiming that *pneuma* is not only the common cause of all diseases but also the most powerful force in the universe as a whole, the author of *On Breaths* manifests what might be called a "cosmological impulse"; that is, a belief that whatever their applicability, high-level generalizations are inherently desirable and directly relevant to the medical art. We have already noted that Eryximachus claims to have gained his insight about the universal power of *eros* "from medicine, our art" (186a), as if to imply that the search for first principles is a natural pursuit for the practicing doctor. We have also seen an intense interest in commonality and difference in *On the Nature of the Human Being*, in which Polybus not only claims that different affections, located in different parts, can all be traced back to one and the same "source" but also that the constituents of human beings are "always alike the same, whether the patient be young or old, or whether the season be cold or hot" (2.5, 6.36 L.). In the next chapter, I would like to move beyond the narrow limits of *On Breaths* to argue that Greek doctors were actually training themselves to look for commonalities that transcend particular differences. They divided patients, diseases, and treatments into groups, and they looked for general principles that were common to each. This search for commonalities became so closely associated with medical thinking that we should hardly be surprised if a handful of Greek doctors took this mode of inquiry to what, to them, seemed its logical extreme. Because medical research was predicated on the belief that the most valuable generalizations apply to the widest range of cases, some doctors looked for principles that were common to all patients, to all diseases, and to all things in general, genuinely believing that, by considering the first principles of the cosmos, they were making a direct contribution to the advancement of the medical art.

CHAPTER 4

The Cosmological Impulse

4.1 The Problem of Individual Variation

I would like to begin this chapter by digging into an especially striking phrase from *On Breaths*. This is the assertion that different animals will react to *pneuma* in different ways because "body differs from body, nature from nature, nutriment from nutriment" (διαφέρει ... καὶ σῶμα σώματος καὶ φύσις φύσιος καὶ τροφὴ τροφῆς, 6.2, 6.98 L.). This phrase, which combines the verb διαφέρει with nominative-genitive doublets, can be paralleled in other texts from the Hippocratic Corpus. Very often, this formulaic phrase is deployed when an author wishes to assert that certain prognoses and treatments cannot be generalized with "precision" (ἀκρίβεια) because there are simply too many variables to put these prescriptions in writing. In *On Fractures*, the author writes that "it takes about thirty days altogether as a rule (τὸ ἐπίπαν) for the bone of the forearm to unite, but there is nothing exact about it (ἀτρεκὲς δὲ οὐδέν), for constitution differs greatly from constitution and age from age" (μάλα γὰρ καὶ φύσις φύσιος καὶ ἡλικίη ἡλικίης διαφέρει, 7, 3.440 L.). Elsewhere, the same author observes that "one cannot make a single statement as to when the bones will come away, for some separate sooner owing to their small size, others because they come at the end of the fracture, while others do not come away as wholes but are exfoliated after desiccation and corruption. Besides this, treatment differs from treatment" (διαφέρει τι καὶ ἰητρείη ἰητρείης, 33, 3.532–534 L., trans. Withington, modified). In *Diseases I*, the author says in reference to patients suffering from internal suppuration, "It is impossible to know precisely [τὸ ἀκριβὲς εἰδέναι] and to hit the mark when stating [τυχεῖν εἴπαντα] the period within which these patients die, not even whether it will be long or short. For the period of time that some people give is not precise [ἀκριβής] in most cases, nor does this information, of itself, suffice; for year differs from year and season from season" (διαφέρει γὰρ καὶ ἔτος ἔτεος καὶ ὥρη ὥρης, 16, 6.170 L., trans. Potter, modified). Similarly, the author of *On Regimen* compiles a long list of

factors that can change from one case to the next, all in order to demonstrate
that it is impossible to write with "precision" (ἀκρίβεια) regarding the proper
balance between eating and exercise (67.1–2, 6.592 L.):

> Regarding human regimen, as I have already said, it is impossible to write
> with such precision [ἀκριβείην] as to produce a due proportion of exercises
> with respect to the quantity of foods. For there are many things that stand in
> the way. First, the constitutions of human beings differ from one another
> [φύσιες ... διάφοροι]. Dry constitutions taken as a class are more or less dry
> in comparison with themselves and in comparison with each other, and the
> same goes for wet constitutions and all the rest. Then the various times of
> life do not have the same needs, nor the situations of regions, the changes in
> the winds, the shiftings of the seasons, or the constitutions of the year.
> Within foods as a class there is abundant difference [διαφορή]. Wheats are
> different from wheats, wine from wine [πυροί τε γὰρ πυρῶν καὶ οἶνος
> οἴνου], and all the other things that we use in our regimens differ among
> themselves, ultimately standing in the way of our being able to write with
> precision [ἀκριβείην].[1]

The main point in all of these passages is that certain prognoses and
treatments cannot be generalized in such a way that they hold good on
all occasions – there are simply too many variables to put these prescriptions in writing. Regarding some of these details, we may say what is true
"as a rule" (τὸ ἐπίπαν), but anything more specific would depend on the
circumstances. Regarding others, there is not even a general tendency in
one direction or the other: if we want to achieve precision in any of these
areas, we will have to approach the question from an entirely different
angle.

The above-quoted passage from *On Regimen* is especially striking as it
presents the art of medicine as a source of seemingly infinite variation.
There are so many factors that can influence disease, so many *differences*
between one case and the next, that it is impossible to write with precision
when describing even the most basic medical procedures. A similar observation appears in *On Places in the Human Being*, whose author claims that
medicine cannot be learned quickly because it has no "fixed technique" (41,
6.330–332 L., trans. Craik, modified):

> It is not possible to learn medicine quickly because of this: it is impossible
> for any fixed technique [καθεστηκὸς σόφισμα] to come about in it, such as
> when a person who has learned how to write in the one way by which it is

---

[1] For more examples of this formulaic phrase, see *Fract.* 35, 3.536–538 L., *Art.* 8, 4.94 L., *Morb. I* 22,
6.182–184 L., *Aff.* 60, 6.268 L., and *Genit.-Nat. Puer.* 15.3, 7.494 L.

taught knows everything. And all who have knowledge how to write have the same knowledge because of this: the same thing, done in the same way, now and at other times, would never become the opposite, but is always steadfastly the same and does not require *kairos*. But medicine now and at other times does not do the same thing; and does opposite things to the same individual; and the same things are opposites to one another.

Two general points should be made about this passage. The first concerns the emphasis it gives to "the same thing, done in the same way, now and at other times" (τὸ αὐτὸ καὶ ὁμοίως ποιεύμενον, νῦν τε καὶ οὐ νῦν). This phrase seems to explain what the author means by a "fixed technique": it is a procedure that, when performed in the same way, always has the same effect. When we learn how to write the alphabet, for example, we find that the same strokes of the pen always produce the same letters, no matter when we write. In medicine, by contrast, the same treatment, administered in the same way, might have one effect at one time and an entirely different effect at another. There is no single result that always comes from the same procedure, and hence no single procedure that the doctor should always perform. The second point regards the central position this passage gives to the *kairos*, the "due measure" or "right proportion" that is uniquely suited to each occasion.[2] It is in this respect, the author writes, that medicine differs from writing: medicine requires attention to the *kairos*, while writing does not; medicine must be adapted to changing circumstances, while writing involves an action that is "always steadfastly the same." Closely related to this emphasis on the *kairos* is the author's assertion that whoever learns how to write does so "in one way" and then "knows everything," the implication being that while doctors must adapt to changing circumstances, everything a person needs to know when writing is inherent in the skill itself. Aristotle makes a similar comparison between medicine and writing in the *Nicomachean Ethics*, where he notes that medicine, navigation, and gymnastics all require "deliberation" (βουλή) when they are put into practice. Writing, on the other hand, needs no such deliberation: it belongs to a class of arts that are "precise" (ἀκριβεῖς) and "sufficient in themselves" (αὐτάρκεις), arts in which the practitioner can learn one procedure and then apply it in every case (1112a34–b9).[3]

---

[2] On the history of this concept, see Trédé (1992).

[3] Elsewhere, Aristotle observes that good conduct, like medicine, requires constant attention to the *kairos* because it has "nothing fixed" (οὐδὲν ἐστηκός, *EN* 1104a3–10), echoing the claim in *On Places in the Human Being* that medicine has no "fixed technique." For still more parallels with this passage, see Isoc. 3.12–13, where the comparison is between writing and rhetoric, and *Morb. I* 9, 6.156 L., where the author observes that "there is no demonstrated starting point of healing" (trans. Potter). Note also Th. 2.51.2, where no "fixed" treatment produced the same result for all sufferers from the plague, and

When aiming for the *kairos*, it was generally believed that doctors should begin by carefully assessing the situation, determining what is needed after considering many variables. These variables are the same factors we find listed in the above-quoted passages, the factors that make it impossible to write with "precision" about some topics because "constitution differs from constitution, age from age, season from season," and so on. In *Diseases of Women I*, the precision that cannot be committed to writing is transferred to the judgment of the practitioner (11, 8.42 L., trans. Hanson, modified):

> Looking at these things, and testing them with precise judgment [γνώμη σκεθρῇ βασανίσας], one must examine the entire body to see whether or not it seems to need frequent purgation, while one takes into consideration the patient's coloring, her age, her strength, the season of the year, and what kind of a regimen she follows.

A similar idea can be seen in *On Fractures* in a passage that explicitly connects the existence of many variables with the doctor's need to consider the *kairos* (35, 3.536–538 L., trans. Withington, modified):

> Treatments differ greatly from treatments and bodily constitutions from bodily constitutions as to power of endurance [μελέται γὰρ μελετέων μέγα διαφέρουσι, καὶ φύσιες φυσίων τῶν σωμάτων ἐς εὐφορίην]. It also makes a great difference whether the bone protrudes on the inner or outer side of the arm or thigh, for many critical vessels stretch along the inner side, and some of them are fatal when wounded; there are also some on the outside, but fewer. In such injuries, then, one must not overlook their dangers, what sort they are, but foretell them with a view to the *kairoi*.

The central idea in these passages is that some factors do not just differ among themselves; they also *contribute* to the final prognosis.[4] In the same way that a rhetorician might claim that the place, the time, and the audience all have a "power" (δύναμις) to determine whether a speech will be effective, Greek doctors viewed such variables as the age, sex, habits, and constitution of the patient as contributing causes, each of which has a "power" to influence the course of a disease.

On Fractures' criticism of "wisdom-mongering doctors" for presuming that a fixed technique can be applied to the setting of broken bones (quoted earlier, pp. 63–64).

[4] Compare *Aff.* 60, 6.268 L.: "Cereals and wines differ among themselves in their nature with regard to strength and weakness, and to lightness and heaviness; also, the places where they grow differ [διαφέρει δὲ καὶ χώρη χώρης], one place being well-watered and another unwatered, one sunny and another thickly shaded, one good and another bad; thus it follows that all these things contribute [συμβάλλεται] to each kind of food's being stronger or weaker" (trans. Potter, modified).

The existence of these many variables made *akribeia* ("precision") a prime target for medical thinking. Whereas other crafts could be extremely precise, mastering the triad of "measure, number, and weight," Greek doctors did not always enjoy success when treating their patients.[5] In Plato's *Philebus* (55e–58a), the various *technai* are sorted into tiers according to their level of *akribeia*. In this arrangement, the mathematical *technai* are the most precise, followed by carpentry. As for medicine, it is placed in the lowest category, alongside music, farming, navigation, and generalship.[6] As we saw in the above-quoted passage from *On Places in the Human Being*, the same act, performed in the same way, could produce one effect in one situation and a completely different effect in another, a variability that, to some observers, suggested that the "art" of medicine did not actually exist. Instead of *techne* ("know-how"), doctors were dependent on *tuche* ("chance"). Multiple references to this charge can be found in the Hippocratic Corpus, which suggests that it was not just an idle accusation but a source of genuine discomfort among some Greek doctors in the fifth and fourth centuries BCE.[7]

One of the defining characteristics of Classical Greek medicine was a growing concern for individual differences.[8] Von Staden (2002: 43) calls Greek medicine "a *techne* constantly ambushed by

---

[5] For the centrality of "measure, number, and weight" in defining a *techne* that exercises "precision," see Schiefsky (2005: 13–18). These qualities are specifically denied to medicine at *VM* 9.3, 1.588–590 L. and *Vict.* 2.3, 6.470–472 L.

[6] For the connection of *akribeia* to medicine's limitations as a "craft," see *Morb. I* 5, 6.148 L., 16, 6.170 L., and *Prorrh. II* 1–4, 9.6–20 L. Solon provides an early reference to such limitations at fr. 13.57–62 West.

[7] Compare especially *VM* 1, 1.570–572 L., 9–12, 1.588–598 L., *Acut.* 8.1, 2.240 L., *De arte* 4, 6.6 L., and *Loc. Hom.* 46, 6.342 L. Note also the contrast between *techne* and *tuche* in the epigram allegedly inscribed on Hippocrates's tomb (*AP* 7.135). On the possible identity of the critics who denied medicine's status as a *techne*, see Lloyd (1991b: 252–253). Dean-Jones (2003: 102–103) suggests that these critics "may well have been composed more of straw than of flesh," although the charge is repeated so often in medical literature that it was, at the very least, part of the discourse on medicine's limitations as an "art." For a general discussion of *techne* versus *tuche* in Classical Greek medicine, see Schiefsky (2005: 5–18), who observes that "by the end of the fifth century BC there had developed a widespread conception of what might be called an exact τέχνη: an art that could achieve full ἀκρίβεια by using precision tools to make exact quantitative measurements. These τέχναι could attain an ideal of detailed, finished workmanship with a high degree of reliability, and they set a standard that other disciplines claiming the status of τέχνη were sometimes required to meet" (p. 17).

[8] On the "problem" of individualization in Classical Greek medicine, see Müri (1936: 41–47), Temkin (1953: 219–222), Kudlien (1967: 140–145), von Staden (2002), and Lloyd (2007). On the heightened concern for "precision" in the fifth and fourth centuries BCE, see Kurz (1970: 62–87) and Schiefsky (2005: 13–18).

particularity and individuality," in which even reliable generalizations must be accompanied with qualifiers such as "for the most
part" or "as a rule." In the above-quoted passages, we see that Greek
doctors were profoundly aware that individual variation constituted
a significant impediment to their art. Even more critically, these
authors repeatedly assert that such differences hinder what they
themselves can reliably put into writing. For the remainder of this
chapter, I will argue that the problem of individualization was felt so
deeply in the Classical period that some Greek doctors actually
rejected older forms of medical writing in favor of new strategies
for organizing medical knowledge. By reorienting their thinking
around a search for commonality, these doctors developed new
modes of medical inquiry, ultimately paving the way for some
medical writers to base the art of healing on the first principles of
the universe as a whole.

In making this argument, I will draw on a wide range of texts from
the Hippocratic Corpus, most of which are traditionally dated to the
fifth or fourth century BCE. More precise dates for these texts are
difficult to establish, although it should be stressed that my arguments
will not presuppose that any one text necessarily predates another.
Instead, I will be examining more general strategies for organizing
medical knowledge in the Classical period. Some of these strategies
responded to earlier methods, while others could have developed
concurrently with other techniques. In general, I have tried to keep
any forays into relative chronology to a minimum, with the only
exceptions being (1) my acceptance of the scholarly consensus that
the "diagnostic handbook" represents one of the earliest forms of
medical writing in the ancient Mediterranean and (2) my contention
that the cosmological doctors apply a series of organizational strategies
that developed at least partly in response to perceived weaknesses in
this format. Most of the specific developments that I discuss in this
chapter could be presented in whatever order one pleases. What
I intend to argue is not that the works in the Hippocratic Corpus
should all be laid end to end in some neat chronological order.
Instead, I will show that the *aggregate* of changes that occurred in
this period – changes that were primarily motivated by a desire to
attain greater "precision" in the art – are both detectable in the works
of the cosmological doctors and can in fact explain why these doctors
thought that cosmological principles were a legitimate, even desirable,
endpoint for medical thinking.

4.2 The Shortcomings of Diagnostic Handbooks

It is now generally agreed that the earliest stratum in the Hippocratic Corpus is represented by chapters 12–75 of *Diseases II.*[9] This text, whose precise date of composition is unknown, but which likely acquired its final form by the fifth century BCE, belongs to a genre of medical writing that I will hereafter call a "diagnostic handbook." What defines a text as a diagnostic handbook is its strategy for organizing medical knowledge. This form of medical writing comprises lists of symptoms, their prognoses, and their treatments, wherein each set of symptoms is presented as a separate disease. As a compositional technique, the diagnostic handbook has a long and well-documented history. It can be illustrated by Egyptian medical papyri of the second millennium BCE, including the Kahun gynecological papyrus (ca. 1800 BCE), the Edwin Smith papyrus (ca. 1600 BCE), and large portions of the Ebers papyrus (ca. 1550 BCE), as well as numerous tablets from ancient Mesopotamia, including the UGU therapeutic series and the *Sakikkū*/SA.GIG diagnostic-prognostic series (ca. 1050 BCE).[10] As practical works, diagnostic handbooks tend to be arranged in a systematic manner, with each entry following a formulaic scheme. The scheme usually contains three elements: (1) a title that identifies the ailment, (2) a description of its symptoms, and (3) a prognosis and treatment. For a representative entry, we may cite the following passage from *Diseases II* (49, 7.74–76 L., trans. Potter, modified):

> Another consumption: there is coughing, the sputum is copious and moist, and sometimes the patient without difficulty coughs up pus that resembles hail stones which, on being rubbed between the fingers, are hard

[9] On the relative antiquity of this text, see Bourgey (1953: 37n3), Jouanna (1974, 1983), Grensemann (1975), Mansfeld (1980b: 381), Langholf (1990a: 3–4, 25, 52–53), and Roselli (2018: 188). Of similar antiquity are some passages in the gynecological treatises, for which see Grensemann (1987) and Roselli (2016).

[10] On the Egyptian medical papyri, the standard reference is Grapow (1954–73). See also Nunn (1996) for English summaries and analyses of these texts, as well as the general discussions of Bardinet (1995) and Westendorf (1999). Heeßel (2004, 2010), Geller (2004, 2018), and Arbøll (2021) give good introductions to the diagnostic literature of ancient Mesopotamia. For comparisons between the earliest Greek medical texts and the medical literature of Egypt and Mesopotamia, see the essays collected in Horstmanshoff and Stol (2004). Some scholars have argued for direct lines of influence between these neighboring traditions, noting their geographical proximity, the tendency of healers to travel long distances, and some close parallels in their prescriptions, while others have advocated a more cautious approach to the study of such affinities. For our purposes, what is most important is how the medical literature of Egypt and Mesopotamia reflects a specific *mode* of medical thinking that is also attested for the Greeks. Although I am not opposed to suggesting that Greek doctors drew on the ideas and practices of their Egyptian and Mesopotamian counterparts, for the purpose of this study, I will treat any similarities as parallel modes of thinking rather than presupposing direct lines of influence from one culture to the next.

and evil-smelling. The voice is clear, the patient is free of pain, and there are no fevers, although sometimes fever heat; the patient is especially weak. You must make this patient drink hellebore and a decoction of lentils, and feed him as well as possible, while avoiding sharp vegetables, beef, pork and mutton; have him do a few exercises, take walks, vomit after meals, and refrain from sex. This disease lasts for seven or nine years; if the patient is treated from the beginning, he recovers.

In some diagnostic handbooks, the diagnosis, prognosis, and treatment are all combined in a single entry, as we see in the above-quoted passage from *Diseases II.* In others, this information is split into parts, with one document correlating symptoms with specific diagnoses and/or prognoses, while another correlates diagnoses with lists of possible treatments. In some traditions, a different professional might even be tasked with different steps in this movement from diagnosis to treatment. In Mesopotamia, for example, it has been suggested that the act of diagnosis was primarily the task of a professional called the *āšipu*, while another healing professional, the *asû*, was an expert in pharmacology.[11]

Since diseases do show reliable patterns, it is not surprising that the diagnostic handbook remained the dominant form of medical writing until the fifth century BCE. These handbooks not only identify the most common patterns of disease but they also draw authority from the fact that their treatments have been "tested" over a long period of time. The Egyptian papyri cite cures so effective they have worked "a million times" (e.g., *P. Ebers* 123, 131, 251, *P. Kahun* case 33, and *P. Edwin Smith* v. 4.8–5.10). In Mesopotamia, recipes are often marked *bulṭu latku* ("a proven treatment"),[12] while one tablet is impressively labeled, "Proven and tested salves and poultices, fit for use, from the mouth of ancient antediluvian sages from Šuruppak [= the home of Ubara-Tutu, the last king before the flood], which Enlil-muballiṭ, sage of Nippur, left to posterity in the second year of Enlil-bani, king of Isin [= ca. 1860 BCE]."[13] This final passage is especially significant as it suggests that diagnostic handbooks

---

[11] Scurlock (1999).

[12] For example, *BAM* 168 70–81: "If a man's groin hurts him at an inappropriate time, and his shins cause him a stinging pain, he is weak in his thighs and his knees gnaw at him with pain, that man suffers in the rectum [already] during his youth. To cure him . . . you dry out Dilmun dates, horned alkali, fat of the kidney of a male sheep, *kukru*, juniper, *ṣumlalû*, *baluhhu*-resin, *abukkatu*-resin – 8 drugs – insert a suppository into his anus to stop flatulence; a proven remedy [*bulṭu latku*]" (trans. Geller 2010: 103). For other examples, see *BAM* 152:7, 159 iv 2′–7′, 16′–22′, 168:12, 503 i 17′–18′, *BM* 78963:16, *SpTU* 2.50:1–4, 10–14, 25–26, and *STT* 95:7–12, 35–40. The practice is discussed by Leichty (1988) and Stol (1991–2: 60–61).

[13] *AMT* 105 (trans. Geller 2010: 17). On this tablet, which is to be dated no earlier than the eighth century BCE, see Elman (1975: 31) and Rochberg (2004: 215). Compare also *STT* 30:6 ("proven [*latkutum*]

were originally composed by "the ancients" and could thereby tap into a cultural preference for traditional, inherited wisdom.[14] By the late sixth century BCE, however, this cultural preference was starting to change, as inherited wisdom was being supplanted by a self-conscious turn toward "inquiry" (ἱστορία).[15] We have already encountered this emphasis on inquiry in *On Ancient Medicine*. In this text, the author claims that humans have advanced from primitive beginnings, and that medicine continues to be refined as doctors identify more and more distinctions between different classes of patients. Putting aside the dubious historicity of this account, the specific narrative that the author constructs is one of increasing "precision." For this author, medicine is constantly improving on what has come before, and the primary means by which this improvement has occurred is by more carefully distinguishing one patient from the next.

Before we consider how a growing concern for individual differences inspired new strategies for organizing medical knowledge, some general remarks are in order. First, it is important to stress that a concern for "precision" was already a feature of medical thinking well before the Classical period. In a fragment from the *Iliupersis*, an epic poem from the seventh century BCE, it is said that the god Poseidon placed "all that was precise" (ἀκριβέα πάντα) in the heart of Podalirius, a legendary healer (fr. 5 Allen, trans. West):

> Their father the Earth-shaker himself gave them both [sc. the brothers Machaon and Podalirius] the healing gift; but he made one higher in prestige than the other. To the one he gave defter hands, to remove missiles from flesh and cut and heal all wounds, but in the other's heart he placed all that was precise [ἀκριβέα πάντα], to diagnose what is hidden and to cure

poultices originating in Eridu [= the first city in the world and home of the first kings in the Sumerian king list]") and *BAM* 159 iv 16'–22' ("proven [*latku*] eye-salve from Hammurabi [= a famous king of the eighteenth century BCE]"; cf. *SpTU* 2.50:10–14). Similar pedigrees can be cited from Egyptian medical literature; the London medical papyrus, for example, refers to a prescription that was "good during the time of the Majesty of the Dual King Nebmaatre [= Amenhotep III]."

[14] On the preclassical emphasis on inherited wisdom, see Clifford (2007). For inherited wisdom in the Greek tradition, see Kleingünther (1933: 5–11).

[15] On the shifting emphasis from inherited wisdom to personal inquiry, see Edelstein (1967) and Dodds (1973: 1–25). For the "humanizing" of knowledge that once belonged to the gods, see Lesher (2008). Geller (2010: 123–126) observes that Mesopotamian medicine also shows an interest in personal inquiry in the fifth century BCE. It is much less pronounced than what we find in Greece, however, and it does not involve as dramatic a break with the authority of ancestral knowledge. An emphasis on personal inquiry does not, of course, have to invalidate all reverence for inherited wisdom (cf. Eryximachus's proud reference to the invention of medicine by Asclepius at Pl. *Smp.* 186e), but the inherited wisdom that we see venerated in these contexts is presented as a foundation on which new advances have been made, not a ready-made system that needs no further improvements.

what does not get better. He it was who first recognized the raging Ajax's flashing eyes and burdened spirit.

This passage contains the first attested use of the adjective ἀκριβής in Greek literature. In this case, "precision" is defined as an ability to take visible symptoms that usually go unnoticed (e.g., Ajax's "flashing eyes") and then align those external symptoms with both a cause and a treatment. A similar approach to precision can be seen in the medical literature of ancient Mesopotamia. In the *Sakikkū*/SA.GIG diagnostic-prognostic series, we find an impressively detailed catalog of medical inferences, many of which hinge on slight differences between one symptom and the next. In some Mesopotamian texts, we even see entire syndromes described in minute detail, such as the following entry from the Nineveh recension of the UGU therapeutic series (*BAM* 578 i 27–32, trans. Scurlock 2014: 519):

> If, (despite) his not having eaten, a person's stomach continually rises up to vomit, he continually produces a lot of phlegm, liquid continuously flows from his mouth, his face continually (feels like it) is spinning, his insides are continually bloated, his hips (and) his shins continually hurt him intensely, he is hot and then cold, he continually has sweat, his appetite for bread and beer is diminished, he drinks a great deal of cold water (and then) vomits, he pours yellow/green (matter) from his anus (and) his penis, his appearance continually changes (for the worse), his flesh is tense (and) whatever he eats does not agree with him, the gall bladder has turned over on that person.[16] To cure him, you take these three plants while still fresh: *kukru*, *burāšu*-juniper (and) *ṣumlalû*. You dry (and) grind (them). [You have him drink (it)] on an empty stomach (mixed) with undiluted wine. He should have a bowel movement and then you bandage his epigastrium (and) his abdomen. You have him eat hot things [. . .] three days [. . .][17]

This passage is a good reminder of the sophistication of medical thinking well before the fifth century BCE. Here, we see a healer carefully examining the symptoms of his patient, identifying the internal cause of the disease, and then applying a multistage treatment that begins with a purge of the bowels, followed by an external manipulation of the patient's body, and concluding with a generalized diet of "hot things" until the patient recovers. Egyptian medical literature also presents the doctor as a careful examiner of his patients. In the Edwin Smith papyrus, an Egyptian diagnostic handbook that is primarily concerned with the

---

[16] For a discussion of this condition, with parallel texts, see Scurlock and Andersen (2005: 136–138).

[17] The missing final portion of this entry would have included a prognosis. Compare the ending of *BAM* 77 30′–32′: "If you have him eat (it) for three days on an empty stomach and then if he drinks water, he should recover" (trans. Scurlock 2014: 534).

treatment of wounds, fractures, and dislocations, the healer is regularly instructed to "probe the wound" in order to distinguish one affection from another. Most of the entries in this papyrus come with one of three prognoses: (1) "an ailment I will handle," (2) "an ailment I will fight with," or (3) "an ailment for which nothing is done." In this framework, "an ailment I will handle" is a case in which recovery is likely, while "an ailment I will fight with" is a case in which recovery is uncertain. Finally, "an ailment for which nothing is done" is a case in which recovery is either unlikely or simply cannot be influenced by the doctor's interventions. In the cases where recovery is either uncertain or unlikely, the papyrus often instructs the healer to apply some initial treatment and then wait until the disease has reached a "turning point." Like the Greek concept of a "crisis," these "turning points" are moments of uncertainty in which a case could develop in one direction or another, leading to either recovery or death.

In the Hippocratic Corpus, we find similar references to cases that are either uncertain or beyond the doctor's abilities to intervene. What is different among the Greeks is a growing interest in examining the limits of this uncertainty and, if possible, in removing such uncertainty altogether. As I mentioned earlier, this new perspective on "precision" seems to have arisen from the direct comparison of medicine with other crafts. Alongside his assertion that anyone who intends to discuss medicine correctly must consider "what is said and done with precision in the art," the author of *Diseases I* notes that one should also contemplate "to which of the other arts medicine has similarities, and to which it has none" (1, 6.142 L., trans. Potter). By choosing *akribeia* as their point of focus, these doctors were not seeking to completely overturn their traditional understanding of health and disease. "Precision" implies the refinement of a preexisting system, not the replacement of one system with a completely new worldview. When the author of *On Ancient Medicine* writes about the historical development of his art, he assumes that doctors have always been on the right track, and that the best way to proceed is simply to build upon what has come before. At no point in this text does the author suggest that his understanding of disease is a relatively new development. In fact, he attacks his opponents for allegedly replacing time-tested definitions of health and disease with a radically different set of "foundational principles." As we have already noted, even the cosmological doctors viewed the body as a setting where fluids cause disease by becoming concentrated and/or by moving from one location to another. There is no evidence that this understanding of disease was ever seriously challenged in the Classical period, and there are in fact good reasons to suppose that the basic principles of humoral pathology are very old, if not prehistoric.[18] Thus, in the absence of a revolutionary new way of either defining disease or restoring a patient's health, "precision" became the central focus of these early attempts to improve the medical art.

For our purposes, the most important outcome of these conversations about "precision" is the challenge they brought to the diagnostic handbooks that had purported to catalog all diseases and their treatments. The primary complaint against these texts was that they failed to account for all the variables that can change from one case to the next. In a fragment from Euripides, we are told that the doctor must attempt cures "after looking to the illness [πρὸς τὴν νόσον ... ἰδόντ'], not by giving pre-ordained remedies, unless these remedies befit the disease [μὴ ἐπίτακτα φάρμακα διδόντ', ἐὰν μὴ ταῦτα τῇ νόσῳ πρέπῃ]" (fr. 286b.1–3 K.). In other words, the doctor must adapt his remedies to the situation. He cannot just follow some written instructions but must take an active role in determining what is needed. In the *Statesman*, Plato distinguishes doctors who administer cures "in accordance with writings" (κατὰ γράμματα) from those who treat patients "without writings" (χωρὶς γραμμάτων, 293a–b). He also notes that lawgivers should follow the example of doctors by departing from written instructions when the situation demands it (294e–300a; cf. *Phdr.* 268c, *Chrm.* 156b–c). In Aristotle's *Politics*, we learn that some Greek thinkers criticized Egyptian medicine for its overreliance on written laws: "The advocates of kingship maintain that the laws speak only in general terms, and cannot provide for circumstances; and that for any science [τέχνη] to abide by written rules is absurd. In Egypt the physician is allowed to alter his treatment after the fourth day, but if sooner, he takes the risk" (1286a9–14, trans. Jowett *apud* Barnes). For a similar criticism of Egyptian medicine for

---

[18] Compare Temkin (1953: 219–220), Parker (1983: 213–216), and Laskaris (2002: 2n5). An association between bile and the liver can already be found in the seventh century BCE (Archil. fr. 234 West; cf. Hippon. fr. 73 West). On the history of phlegm, which seems to be derived from the verb *phlegein* ("to inflame"), see Fredrich (1899: 36–43), Jouanna (1974: 92–108), and Lonie (1981: 277–279). For Mesopotamian ideas about bile, phlegm, and "wind," see Geller (2007), Böck (2014: 122–128, 142–145, 152), and Arbøll (2021: 56, 79–83, 93, 192). As Lonie (1977: 245n44) observes, the attribution of various ideas to "the ancients" in *On Regimen in Acute Diseases* – ideas that the author himself simply takes for granted and does not feel compelled to explain to his audience – "indicate[s] the existence of a relatively complex rational medicine which is already well established by or before the end of the fifth century."

doctoring "by the book," we may compare the following passage from the historian Diodorus (1.82.3, trans. Oldfather):

> On their military campaigns and their journeys in the country [the Egyptians] all receive treatment without the payment of any private fee; for the physicians draw their support from public funds and administer their treatments in accordance with a written law which was composed in ancient times by many famous physicians. If they follow the rules of this law as they read them in the sacred book and yet are unable to save their patient, they are absolved from any charge and go unpunished; but if they go contrary to the law's prescriptions in any respect, they must submit to a trial with death as the penalty, the lawgiver holding that but few physicians would ever show themselves wiser than the mode of treatment which had been closely followed for a long period and had been originally prescribed by the ablest practitioners.

Perhaps the most famous complaint against diagnostic handbooks can be found in *On Regimen in Acute Diseases*, an early medical text that directly critiques a diagnostic handbook entitled *Cnidian Signs*.[19] Using language very similar to what we see in these other passages, the author of *On Regimen in Acute Diseases* complains that *Cnidian Signs* prescribes remedies that are too simple and not "suited" (ἁρμόζοντα, 3.1, 2.226 L.) to the diseases for which they are recommended. Later on, the same author contrasts the method of *Cnidian Signs* with his own preference to "apply my mind in all the art" (ἐν πάσῃ τῇ τέχνῃ προσέχειν τὸν νοῦν, 4.1, 2.230 L.), a statement that recalls the claim in Euripides that it is only "after looking to the illness" (πρὸς τὴν νόσον ... ἰδόντ') that a doctor can select a fitting treatment.[20]

In all of these texts, we find a similar objection to diagnostic handbooks: their rigid prescriptions leave little room for the doctor to adapt to changing circumstances. Whereas diagnostic handbooks might divide the same disease into two or more forms (cf. "Another consumption" in *Diseases II*), some Greek doctors claimed that these minor divisions are not enough: there is an infinite variety in human disease, a manifold

---

[19] On the translation of Κνίδιαι γνῶμαι as *Cnidian Signs*, see Langholf (1990a: 13n9). A parallel use of γνώμη in the sense of "sign" can be found at Thgn. 60. Other potential translations of this title include *Cnidian Judgments, Cnidian Opinions, Cnidian Sentences*, or even *Cnidian Maxims*. However we translate it, the title seems to imply that the work is intended to assist the practitioner in making "judgments" (γνῶμαι) about diseases, which would have been assisted by identifying particular "signs" (γνῶμαι) that point to one diagnosis over another.

[20] For the use of προσέχειν τὸν νοῦν in the sense of "adapt to the situation," see *Prog.* 19, 2.164 L., 22, 2.174 L., *Epid. I* 26.3, 2.680 L., *VC* 12.4, 3.228 L., 18.2, 3.250 L., *Fract.* 30, 3.516 L., *Art.* 30, 4.144 L., *Epist.* 24, 9.400 L., and Isoc. *Ant.* 184. Note also the use of προσέχειν at *Acut. App.* 21.1, 2.434–436 L., 23.2, 2.440–442 L.

division for which simple lists of affections and their treatments will not suffice. The point is made most explicitly in the following passage from *On Regimen in Acute Diseases* (1–3, 2.224–228 L.):

> Those who composed the work entitled *Cnidian Signs* have correctly written the sorts of things that patients undergo in each of the diseases, as well as how some of them turn out. And up to this point even a non-doctor could write correctly if he made good inquiries from each of the patients into the sorts of things they undergo. But as to what the physician should grasp in addition [προσκαταμαθεῖν], without the patient's telling him, they have omitted many of these things, things which are different in different circumstances, and some of which are critical for the drawing of inferences [ἐπίκαιρα . . . ἐς τέκμαρσιν]. . . . Some of them [sc. the compilers of *Cnidian Signs*] were not unaware of the varieties [πολυτροπίας] in each of the diseases and of their manifold division [πολυσχιδίην], but in wishing to indicate distinctly [σάφα] the number of diseases, they did not write correctly [ὀρθῶς]. For the enumeration would not be easy if one identifies the disease of each patient on the basis of how one disease differs from the other [τῷ ἕτερον ἑτέρου διαφέρειν τι], and on the assumption that no two diseases are the same unless they have the same name.

According to this author, the key problem with *Cnidian Signs* is not its attempt to identify disease patterns but its choice to look for such patterns exclusively at the level of aggregate diseases. Like other diagnostic handbooks, *Cnidian Signs* seems to have presented each set of symptoms as a separate entity, to which prognoses and treatments were then attached. The author admits that the compilers of this handbook made room for some degree of variation, but he implies that their method of enumerating diseases "on the basis of how one disease differs from the other" (τῷ ἕτερον ἑτέρου διαφέρειν τι) is both impractical and insufficient. This method is impractical, on the one hand, because there are simply too many variables to make a separate entry for every conceivable permutation. If such factors as the patient's age, sex, habits, and constitution all have a power to influence a disease, then doctors would need to make a separate entry for every human on earth – at which point it is no longer possible to generalize disease patterns. Diagnostic handbooks are insufficient, moreover, because there is much that the doctor should "grasp in addition" to these patterns, "things which are different in different circumstances, and some of which are critical for the drawing of inferences." Later on, the author clarifies what he means by this phrase (7–9, 2.238–244 L.):

> I think it is worth writing all the things that have not been grasped by physicians, although they are critical [ἐπίκαιρα] to know, and things that

bring great benefits and great harms. Now, the following have not been grasped [ἀκαταμάθητα]: why do some physicians, in acute diseases, administer unstrained gruels through the whole duration of the illness and believe that they are treating the patient correctly, while others think it all important that the patient not ingest any barley – for they deem it a source of great harm – but administer the juice after straining it through linen cloth, while still others would give neither thick gruel nor juice, some not until the seventh day, and others not until the disease reaches a crisis? Very many physicians are not accustomed even to propose such inquiries. ... But I affirm that this investigation is wholly fine and akin to the most, and the most critical [ἐπικαιροτάτοισι], components of the art. For it has great power to bring about health in all who are sick, the preservation of health in those who are well, good condition in those in training, and whatever each person desires.

In this passage, the author complains about the lack of individualization in medical treatment: some doctors always give barley gruel at the beginning of a disease, others administer only the juice, while still others make the patient fast until the seventh day or until the disease has reached a crisis. What we should be doing, the author implies, is not simply to employ the same treatment in all cases, but to make sure that whatever treatment we do select coincides with the needs of the situation.

4.3 A Search for Commonality

But how, exactly, are doctors supposed to approach clinical decision-making when no two cases are the same? How are they to find the *kairos* amidst so many different variables? To put it simply, Greek doctors responded to the growing emphasis on individual differences by reorienting their inquiries around a search for commonality. They decided that if no two cases are exactly alike, then doctors must focus on what is unaffected by changing circumstances. In *On Regimen in Acute Diseases*, we see a clear example of this new mode of inquiry in the author's attempts to formulate general principles regarding the proper administration of treatment. Instead of moving from one disease to the next, the author moves from one treatment to the next, developing general rules for administering each treatment that are independent of any particular diagnosis. As the author discusses the application of these general rules to particular cases, he uses the same language he had previously employed to criticize *Cnidian Signs*. The doctor should give either melicrat or wine, he writes, "whichever is suited [ἁρμόζῃ]," adding that he will later describe "what is suited in each of the types [of ailments]" (τὸ δ᾽ ἁρμόζον ἐφ᾽

ἑκάστοισι τῶν τρόπων, 12.1, 2.250 L.; cf. 3.1, 2.226 L.).²¹ The author frequently describes his rules of thumb as *epikairos* ("critical"),²² just as he had rebuked *Cnidian Signs* for omitting much that is "critical for the drawing of inferences" (ἐπίκαιρα ἐς τέκμαρσιν, 1, 2.224 L.), and he generally envisions the primary job of the doctor as paying precise attention (ἀκριβέως θεωρέων, 20.2, 2.268 L.) and thereby figuring out what is "needed" (δεῖ, χρή) in any given set of circumstances. At various points within this text, the author observes that certain principles hold good "always,"²³ "in all diseases,"²⁴ "both at the beginning and throughout the disease,"²⁵ and for all classes of patients.²⁶ In chapter 48, he notes that one such principle is useful in all circumstances (ἐς πάντα ... εὔχρηστον), while he elsewhere formulates principles that are not quite universal, but merely hold true "as a general rule" or "for the most part" (τὸ ἐπίπαν, τὸ πάμπαν, ὡς ἐπὶ τὸ πολύ, κτλ). In chapter 11, the author writes that "all who use gruel in these diseases [i.e., acute diseases] must not fast, generally speaking [ὡς ἔπος εἰπεῖν], on any day, but they must use it and not intermit – unless there is some need to intermit because of a purge or clyster." In this case, the author cites a general principle that holds true in most cases, but he notes that the physician should be ready to break this rule if the circumstances demand it. Similar attempts to generalize within the constraints of contingent factors can be seen in the author's descriptions of how one class of patients should be treated in one way, another in another,²⁷ in his recording of incidental symptoms that only some patients manifest,²⁸ in his reference to the need to adjust the quantity, quality, and timing of prescriptions to particular situations,²⁹ and in his noting of

---

[21] The author returns to this topic in chapter 19. For other references to what is "fitting" or "suited" in *On Regimen in Acute Diseases* (τὸ ἁρμόζον, τὸ ἐπιτήδειον, τὸ πρέπον, κτλ), see also 21.3, 2.270 L., 50.1, 2.332 L., 52.1, 2.336 L., 53.1, 2.336 L., and 66.2, 2.368 L. Jones (1923b: 91) and Joly (1972: 50) both translate the phrase οἷόν τε at 35, 2.296 L., as "it is possible." A better translation, however, is "it is fitting" (cf. LSJ s.v. οἷος III). Note also the author's use of the phrase πρός τι ("in relation to something") at 21.2, 2.270 L. This is the same language that we see in *On Ancient Medicine* when the author asserts that foods and drinks should be adapted to individual constitutions (20.3, 1.622 L.).

[22] *Acut.* 7.1, 2.238 L., 9, 2.244 L., 13, 2.250 L., 39.1, 2.304 L.

[23] *Acut.* 46.2, 2.324 L., 51.1, 2.334 L.   [24] *Acut.* 20.2, 2.268 L.

[25] *Acut.* 20.1, 2.266 L.; compare 21.1, 2.268 L.

[26] *Acut.* 28.2, 2.282 L., 35, 2.296 L., 46.2, 2.324 L.

[27] *Acut.* 11.1–2, 2.246 L., 19.1–2, 2.264–266 L., 22.1–2, 2.272 L., 23.1, 2.274 L., 53.1, 2.336 L. The author also observes that different classes of patients respond to the same factors in different ways: 29.2, 2.286–288 L., 34.1, 2.296 L., 37.1–3, 2.298–302 L., 50.1–2, 2.332–334 L., 53.2, 2.340–342 L.

[28] *Acut.* 17.1, 2.260 L., 19.1, 2.264 L., 22.2, 2.272–274 L., 28.3, 2.284 L., 30.2, 2.288–290 L., 42.1–3, 2.312–314 L., 53.2, 2.340–342 L.

[29] *Acut.* 11, 2.246–248 L., 12.2, 2.250 L., 13, 2.250 L., 19–20, 2.264–268 L., 22, 2.272–274 L., 24–25, 2.276–278 L., 29.1, 2.286 L., 33, 2.294 L., 48.2, 2.330 L., 50.1, 2.332 L., 52.2, 2.336 L.

additional procedures that may be required at one time or another.[30] His overall purpose is to determine, regarding each mode of treatment, "to whom it should be administered and to whom it should not be administered, as well as the reason why it should not be administered" (55, 2.342 L.). The author believes that by formulating such general principles, doctors will be able to individualize their treatments and thereby hit the *kairos* in each case.

Unlike the prognoses and treatments in diagnostic handbooks, the general principles in *On Regimen in Acute Diseases* are not tied to any particular disease. As long as the patient falls within the specified parameters, then the doctor should provide the corresponding treatment, an approach to clinical decision-making that seems to lie behind the author's criticism of *Cnidian Signs* for assuming that "no two diseases are the same unless they have the same name" (3.2, 2.228 L.). A similar approach to medicine can be seen in *Prognostic*, which attempts to do for prognosis what *On Regimen in Acute Diseases* does for treatment. In this text, the author moves from symptom to symptom, developing general guidelines about what each symptom indicates "in all diseases," "for the most part," or for a particular class of patients.[31] In the final chapter of this work, the author makes an important statement regarding his approach to general principles (25.3–5, 2.188–190 L.):

> Concerning indications and other signs, one must be well aware that in every year and in every season bad signs indicate something bad and good signs indicate something good, since the signs recorded above prove to hold true in Libya, in Delos, and in Scythia. Accordingly, one must know that it would not be strange if, in the same places, one should very often hit the mark if one has thoroughly grasped these things and knows how to distinguish and reckon them correctly. One must also not regret the omission from the present account of the name of any disease. For it is by the same signs in all cases that you will recognize what comes to a crisis in the aforementioned times.

---

[30] *Acut.* 10, 2.246 L., 11.1, 2.246 L., 12.1, 2.248–250 L., 16, 2.256–260 L., 19, 2.264–266 L., 21.1, 2.268 L., 22, 2.272 L., 28.3, 2.284 L.

[31] Note in particular the author's penchant for universalizing language: *Prog.* 3.6, 2.120 L. (ἐν πᾶσι τοῖσιν ὀξέσι νοσήμασι), 5.2, 2.122 L. (ἐν πᾶσι τοῖσιν ὀξέσιν νοσήμασιν), 6.1, 2.122–124 L. (ἐν πᾶσι τοῖσιν ὀξέσι νοσήμασιν), 7.1, 2.130 L. (ἁπάντων . . . τῶν οἰδημάτων χρονιζόντων), 8.1, 2.130 L. (οἱ δὲ ὕδρωπες οἱ ἐκ τῶν ὀξέων νοσημάτων πάντες), 13.3, 2.144 L. (πᾶσαι δὲ αἱ ὑπόσαπροι καὶ δυσώδεες ὀδμαὶ . . . ἐπὶ πᾶσι τοῖσιν ἐμεομένοισι), 14.1, 2.144 L. (ἐπὶ πᾶσι τοῖσιν ἀλγήμασι τοῖσι περὶ τὸν πλεύμονά τε καὶ τὰς πλευράς), 14.5, 2.146 L. (ἐπὶ πᾶσι τοῖσι περὶ τὸν πλεύμονα νοσήμασι), 14.7, 2.146 L. (πάντα δὲ τὰ πτύελα), 17.1, 2.152 L. (τοὺς δὲ ξύμπαντας ἐμπύους), 18.4, 2.160 L. (αἱ δὲ ἀποστάσιες αἱ ἐς τὰ σκέλεα . . . πᾶσαι).

In these concluding remarks, the author asserts that his generalizations hold true in the extreme south (Libya), the extreme north (Scythia), and the center of the world (Delos) – a metonym for all geographical and climatic variations.[32] He also stresses that these generalizations remain valid "in every year and in every season" and "in all cases," regardless of the diagnosis, clearly illustrating how a concern for variation has inspired this author to seek out high-level commonalities that transcend individual differences.

As Greek doctors started to reorient their thinking around a search for commonalities, they developed new modes of inquiry specifically designed to uncover new generalizations. We see this most clearly in the seven books of *Epidemics*, where individual cases are compared with one another in the hope of finding generalizable truths. In these texts, the authors record how different diseases, occurring in different seasons, were experienced by different classes of patients (men vs. women, the young vs. the old, the bilious vs. the phlegmatic, and so on). They also provide detailed, day-by-day descriptions of individual cases, all in the hope of finding common elements that can then be applied in future cases.[33] In *Epidemics III*, the author prefaces a series of case histories by noting that "it is necessary to grasp precisely [καταμανθάνειν . . . ἀκριβῶς] the constitution of the seasons and the disease, [observing] what common element [κοινόν] in the constitution or in the disease is good, and what common element in the constitution or in the disease is bad" (16.2, 3.102 L., trans. Jones, modified).[34] Elsewhere, we are told that doctors should make note of what is "either similar or dissimilar" (ἢ ὅμοια ἢ ἀνόμοια, *Epid. I* 20.2, 2.660 L.; cf. *Off.* 1, 3.272 L. and *Epid. VI* 8.26, 5.352 L.) and that one should "do nothing at random, overlook nothing" (*Epid. VI* 2.12, 5.284 L.) since even the smallest deviation from the *kairos* can dramatically change a patient's outcome. In many passages, the authors compare specific patients by name, noting the similarities and differences between their

---

[32] For this use of Libya and Scythia to illustrate climatic extremes, compare *Aër.* 12–24, 2.52–92 L. and *Vict.* 37.1, 6.528 L.

[33] On the methodology of the *Epidemics*, see Diller (1964), Nikitas (1968), Deichgräber (1971), Manetti and Roselli (1982), Langholf (1990a), Jouanna (2000, 2016), and the essays collected in Baader and Winau (1989), especially Langholf (1989), Licciardi (1989), and Smith (1989). For the limitations of these attempts to formulate reliable generalizations, see Lloyd (2007).

[34] Note the parallels with *On Regimen in Acute Diseases*, which similarly stresses the importance of observing cases with "precision" (ἀκριβέως θεωρέων, 20.2, 2.268 L.) and "grasping" (καταμανθάνειν) general principles that can later be applied to particular cases. Note also the inclusion of "the constitutions of the year" (τοῦ ἐνιαυτοῦ αἱ καταστάσιες) in *On Regimen*'s list of variables that can change from one case to the next (quoted earlier, p. 124).

cases.[35] They also compile lists of factors that can distinguish one case from the next,[36] using their implicit understanding of human physiology to guide their clinical observations.

In *Epidemics VI*, the author describes this mode of inquiry in general terms (3.12, 5.298 L., trans. Smith, modified):

> The summary conclusion [κεφάλαιον] comes from the coming to be and the point of departure,[37] and from very many accounts and things learned little by little, when one gathers them together [συνάγοντα] and grasps [καταμανθάνοντα] whether the things are like one another, and in turn, whether the dissimilarities in them are like each other, so that from the dissimilarities there arises one similarity [ὡς ἐκ τῶν ἀνομοιοτήτων ὁμοιότης γένηται μία]. This would be the road [ὁδός; i.e., method]. In this way develop verification of correct accounts and refutation of what is incorrect.

In this passage, the author uses the phrase ὁμοιότης μία ("one similarity") in the same way that *Epidemics III* refers to a "common element" (κοινόν, 16.2, 3.102 L.), while his statement that one must gather together multiple accounts and compare those accounts with one another "so that from the dissimilarities there arises one similarity" recalls the assertion in *Epidemics I* that doctors should make note of what is "either similar or dissimilar," presumably in order to gain proper insights from the comparison of individual cases.[38] Another interesting term is κεφάλαιον, which usually denotes a "chief point" or "summary conclusion" that picks out whatever is essential from some longer account. In this context, the term may refer to

---

[35] For example, *Epid. I* 14–17, 2.642–650 L., 20–21, 2.660–666 L., *Epid. II* 1.12, 5.82 L., 2.1, 5.84 L., 2.9, 5.88 L., 3.11, 5.114 L., *Epid. IV* 1–4, 5.144–146 L., 20d–f, 5.158–160 L., 25, 5.164–168 L., 29, 5.172 L., 31, 5.174–176 L., 33, 5.176–178 L., 36, 5.178 L., 40–41, 5.182 L., 45, 5.188 L., 50, 5.190 L., 55, 5.194 L., 57, 5.196 L., *Epid. V* 4, 5.204–206 L., 8, 5.208 L., 30, 5.228 L., 65, 5.242–244 L., 87, 5.252 L., 96–99, 5.256 L., *Epid. VI* 3.5, 5.294 L., 3.14, 5.300 L., 8.18, 5.350 L., and *Epid. VII* 5, 5.376 L., 9, 5.380 L., 27, 5.398 L., 30, 5.400 L., 34–35, 5.402–404 L., 45, 5.412 L., 52, 5.422 L., 61, 5.426 L., 112, 5.460 L.

[36] For example, *Epid. I* 23, 2.668–670 L., *Epid. II* 1.6, 5.76 L., 3.2, 5.106 L., *Epid. IV* 43, 5.184 L., 46, 5.188 L., and *Epid. VI* 2.14, 5.284 L., 6.14, 5.330 L., 8.7–15, 5.344–348 L.

[37] That is, from considering everything that led up to the disease. This information is important because it helps the doctor distinguish conditions with similar symptoms but different causes, each of which must be treated in a different way (cf. *Acut. App.* 22, 2.436–438 L., *Epid. II* 1.11, 5.82 L., and *Epid. VI* 3.20, 5.302 L.). It is also important because knowing the day on which a disease begins allows the doctor to predict its crises and exacerbations, a central consideration for determining the *kairos* (cf. *Epid. II* 1.6, 5.74 L. and *Epid. IV* 20b, 5.158 L.).

[38] In the *Timaeus*, Plato echoes this language when he observes that multiple humors were given the common designation of bile "either by certain physicians or by someone who was capable of surveying a number of dissimilar cases [ἀνόμοια] and discerning amongst them one single type [ἓν γένος] worthy to give its name to them all" (83c, trans. Bury). The interest of Greek doctors in discussing "similars" and "dissimilars" is also reflected in Eryximachus's speech, especially his assertion that "what is healthy in the body is different and dissimilar from what is sick, and what is dissimilar longs for and desires dissimilar things" (186b).

either the "chief point" of the author's methodology or the "essential generalization" that comes from a series of particular observations. The word may have even been chosen specifically to recall the phrase ὡς ἐν κεφαλαίῳ εἰρῆσθαι ("to speak in summary"), which introduces generalizations in *On Regimen in Acute Diseases, Epidemics III, On Fractures,* and *On Joints.*[39]

In the *Metaphysics*, Aristotle describes a similar process of moving from the particular to the general (981a7–12, trans. Ross *apud* Barnes, modified):

> To have a judgment that when Callias was suffering from this or that disease this or that benefited him, and similarly with Socrates and various other individuals, is a matter of experience; but to judge that it benefits all persons of a certain type, marked off as one class, who suffer from this or that disease (e.g. the phlegmatic or bilious when suffering from ardent fever) is a matter of art.

Just as the author of *Epidemics VI* refers to the "gathering together" of individual accounts, so too does Aristotle begin by describing the collection of particular observations. When Callias was suffering from a certain illness, he was benefited by a certain treatment. The same data has been collected for Socrates, and so on for other individuals. What moves these observations from "experience" (ἐμπειρία) to "art" (τέχνη) is an act of generalization.[40] The medical researcher classifies patients according to their shared characteristics (e.g., "the phlegmatic or bilious when suffering from ardent fever") and identifies some other trait (e.g., a positive reaction to a specific form of treatment) that is common to all members of this class.

When Greek doctors followed this method for formulating general principles, they often codified them in the form of aphorisms. As its name implies, an aphorism (from ἀφορίζειν, "to mark off by boundaries") is a generalization that holds good for all members of a specified class.[41]

---

[39] *Acut.* 12.2, 2.250 L., 61, 2.356–358 L., *Epid. III* 8.3, 3.88 L., *Fract.* 26, 3.500 L., 31, 3.524–526 L., 43, 3.554 L., 45, 3.556 L., and *Art.* 40, 4.174 L., 48, 4.216 L., 58, 4.254 L., 61, 4.260 L.

[40] Compare Arist. *Rh.* 1356b28–32: "But none of the arts theorizes about individual cases. Medicine, for instance, does not theorize about what will help to cure Socrates or Callias, but only about what will help to cure any or all of a given class of patients [τῷ τοιῷδε ἢ τοῖς τοιοῖσδε]: this alone is subject to art [ἔντεχνον] – individual cases are so infinitely various that no knowledge of them is possible" (trans. Roberts *apud* Barnes). A similar point is made at *EN* 1180b7–28.

[41] Note Aristotle's use of the verb ἀφορίζειν in the above-quoted passage: "all persons of a certain type, marked off as one class" (πᾶσι τοῖς τοιοῖσδε κατ' εἶδος ἓν ἀφορισθεῖσι), with which compare *APo.* 97b7–28: "To reach the definition [ὁρισμός] of something, we must first examine a set of individuals that belong to the same species, identifying what they have in common. Then we must examine individuals that belong to another species, then another and another, all of which belong to the same

The Hippocratic Corpus contains many collections of aphorisms, including not only the seven books of *Aphorisms* but also *Prognostic, Prorrhetic I, Coan Prognoses*, and certain sections of the *Epidemics*. The aphorisms in these collections are relatively brief (most are only a single sentence), and they often contain qualifiers to note that they hold good "in all diseases," "for the most part," or for a particular class of patients. Despite the authoritative ring of these high-level generalizations, the production of aphorisms usually required a significant smoothing out of contradictory observations. As Lloyd (2007: 349) observes, "The price the practitioners were always paying for their generalizations (whether this was recognized or not) was the elision of some of the possibly relevant information in the original data." On some occasions, medical writers had great faith in their generalizations, stressing the "precision" (ἀκρίβεια), "stability" (βεβαιότης), and universal applicability of their aphorisms,[42] while other passages suggest that some doctors were aware of the methodological difficulty with picking out one significant detail from a sea of contradictory information. In *Epidemics VI*, the same text that describes the "method" (ὁδός) for arriving at "one similarity" (ὁμοιότης μία) that rises above dissimilars, we are told that

---

genus as the first. When we have identified the common elements for each of these species, the elements that are shared across *all* species provide the definition of the genus. Every definition is always universal [αἰεὶ δ᾽ ἐστὶ πᾶς ὅρος καθόλου]. For example, the physician does not say what is healthy for an individual eye (e.g., the eye of Socrates). He declares what is healthy for *every* eye, or for a *species* of eye, which he marks off from the rest [οὐ γάρ τινι ὀφθαλμῷ λέγει τὸ ὑγιεινὸν ὁ ἰατρός, ἀλλ᾽ ἢ παντὶ ἢ εἴδει ἀφορίσας]" (trans. Barnes). Outside the title of the *Aphorisms*, neither the noun ἀφορισμός nor the verb ἀφορίζειν appear in the Hippocratic Corpus. The specific term ἀφορισμός seems to have first been applied to general principles in the fourth century BCE (e.g., Thphr. *HP* 9.2.1, with which cf. Pl. *Chrm.* 173e, Epicr. fr. 10.13 K–A), although the concept of an aphorism is already developing in the Hippocratic Corpus (note especially the use of the term ὅρος at *Epid. VI* 2.21, 5.288 L. and ὅριον at *Epid. VI* 6.6, 5.326 L.; cf. also *De arte* 5.6, 6.8 L.).

[42] Note especially the universalizing language at *Epid. II* 1.6, 5.74 L. and *Epid. VI* 3.16, 5.300 L. and the questions about whether general principles apply universally at *Epid. V* 77, 5.248 L., *Epid. VI* 2.5, 5.278 L., and *Epid. VII* 57, 5.424 L. On the stability of aphorisms, note also the references to a "precise sign" (σημεῖον ἀκριβές) at *Epid. VII* 112, 5.460 L., to the "surest [literally, 'most stable'] relapses" (βεβαιόταται ὑποστροφαί) at *Epid. II* 1.11, 5.82 L. (= *Epid. VI* 3.21, 5.302 L.), to events that will occur "surely" (βεβαίως) at *Art.* 63, 4.270 L., to a "sure crisis" (βεβαίαν κρίσιν) at *Coac.* 147, 5.614 L., to a treatment that removes thirst "surely" (βεβαίως) at *Morb. III* 17, 7.160 L., and to "uncertain remedies" (ἄκεά τ᾽ οὐ βέβαια) at A. *Eum.* 506. The implicit contrast between "stability" (βεβαιότης) and depending on other factors informs the assertion in *On Places in the Human Being* that "medicine as a whole is firmly established [βέβηκε], and the finest of the techniques collected in it clearly have the least dependence on chance" (46.1, 6.342 L.). *Pace* Craik (1998: 85), the perfect tense of βαίνειν does not suggest the "advancement" of medicine over a period of time but rather its ability to "hold steady" and "stand in place" for doctors who know how to use it (cf. LSJ s.v. βαίνω I.2 and note the similar claims at *De arte* 4–6, 6.6–10 L.).

for good physicians similarities cause wanderings and uncertainty, but so do the opposite. It has to be considered what kind of cause [πρόφασις] there is, and that reasoning is difficult even if one knows the ways. For example, if a man has a pointed head and flat nose, is sharp-nosed, bilious, vomits with difficulty, full of black bile, young and has lived at random: it is hard for all these to be in concord with one another. (8.26, 5.352–354 L., trans. Smith, modified)

As we see in this final passage from *Epidemics VI*, the search for commonalities led some Greek doctors to become interested in different modes of classification. Just as the author of *On Ancient Medicine* associates the advancement of the healer's art with the division and subdivision of patients into "classes" (εἴδη), each of which shares a common nature (φύσις), mode of life (δίαιτα), or physical state (διάθεσις), so the compilers of the *Epidemics* divided patients into groups, attributing their common experiences to the shared characteristics of each group. The most important "groups" in the *Epidemics* pertain to the patients' *diathesis* (i.e., their symptoms in a given disease).[43] Other important divisions involve the patients' sex and age,[44] as well as their complexion,[45] weight,[46] exercise habits,[47] fertility,[48] and (in the case of women) marital status,[49] along with the color and straightness of their hair (or the lack thereof),[50] the color and size of their eyes,[51] the shape of their nose,[52] the shape of their heads,[53] the size of their spleen,[54] the nature of their voice,[55] their habits of work and travel,[56] their propensity to certain emotions,[57] their tendency to suffer

[43] Compare especially the highly generalized attempts to classify pains around the head and neck at *Epid. I* 12, 2.636–638 L. and the different "modes" (τρόποι) of fevers at *Epid. I* 24–26, 2.670–682 L.

[44] Note, for example, the following passage from *Epidemics VI*: "Women did not suffer similarly from the cough, but few of them had fever, and of those very few went into pneumonia, and those the older. All survived. I attributed this to their not going out as the men did and because they were not otherwise susceptible like the men" (7.1, 5.334 L., trans. Smith).

[45] *Epid. I* 19.1, 2.656 L., *Epid. II* 5.1, 5.128 L., and *Epid. VI* 2.6, 5.280 L., 2.19, 5.286 L., 3.13, 5.298 L.

[46] *Epid. II* 1.8, 5.80 L.   [47] *Epid. I* 1.6, 2.602 L.   [48] *Epid. VI* 7.8, 5.342 L.

[49] *Epid. I* 16.2, 2.646–648 L. Note also the distinction between free women and slave women at *Epid. VI* 7.1, 5.334 L.

[50] *Epid. I* 19.1, 2.656 L., *Epid. III* 17.5, 3.118 L., and *Epid. II* 5.1, 5.128 L., 5.23, 5.132 L., 6.1, 5.132 L.; compare *Epid. VI* 3.1, 5.292 L., 7.1, 5.334 L.

[51] *Epid. I* 19.1, 2.656 L., *Epid. II* 5.1, 5.128 L., 6.1, 5.132 L., and *Epid. VI* 7.1, 5.334 L.; compare *Epid. II* 6.14, 5.136 L. and *Epid. VI* 7.6, 5.340 L.

[52] *Epid. II* 5.1, 5.128 L., 6.1, 5.132 L. and *Epid. VI* 8.26, 5.352–354 L.

[53] *Epid. VI* 1.2, 5.266 L., 8.26, 5.352–354 L.   [54] *Epid. VI* 3.2, 5.292–294 L.

[55] *Epid. I* 19.1, 2.656 L., *Epid. II* 1.8, 5.80 L., 5.1, 5.128 L., 6.1, 5.132 L., 6.22b, 5.136 L., and *Epid. VI* 4.19, 5.312 L., 7.1, 5.334 L., 7.6, 5.340 L.

[56] *Epid. I* 19.1, 2.656 L., *Epid. IV* 50, 5.190 L., and *Epid. VI* 7.1, 5.332 L., 8.26, 5.352–354 L.

[57] *Epid. I* 19.1, 2.656 L., *Epid. III* 17.11, 3.134 L., *Epid. II* 6.1, 5.132 L., and *Epid. VI* 2.20, 5.288 L., 4.19, 5.312 L.

apokriseis of blood, phlegm, bile, or black bile,[58] their propensity to gener-
ate "breaths" (φῦσαι) in the body,[59] their innate susceptibility to specific
diseases,[60] and the inclination of their "natures" (φύσεις) to the hot, the
cold, the dry, or the wet.[61] This final criterion is especially significant as it
recalls the emphasis on the hot, the cold, the dry, and the wet that we see
among the cosmological doctors. In *Epidemics I*, older men are said to be in
the period of their lives when "the hot is now being dominated [sc. by the
cold]" (ἤδη τὸ θερμὸν κρατεῖται, 12.3, 2.638 L.), while in *Epidemics VI*, the
author notes that "sedimentation after urination is more frequent in
children," following this with the question, "Is it because they are warmer?"
(3.7, 5.296 L., trans. Smith). Such transitions from external symptoms to
internal causes were not discouraged by the compilers of the *Epidemics*. In
fact, some doctors seem to have been attracted to such explanations largely
because they provided yet another means of overcoming the many variables
that can change from one case to the next.

4.4   The Stability of Causal Explanations

In the Hippocratic Corpus, many authors incorporate causal explanations
into their broader search for high-level commonalities. Like the aphorisms
that correlate symptoms with prognoses or treatments, causal explanations
imply the existence of stable, highly generalized principles that guarantee
a certain result under a given set of circumstances.[62] One advantage of this
mode of inquiry is that causal explanations less often require qualifying
statements that would blunt their universal application. An obvious problem, however, is that causal explanations are also far more difficult to
determine with any certainty, especially when both the causes and their
effects are hidden within the body.[63] As we observed in Chapter 1, the

---

[58]   *Epid. III* 14, 3.96–98 L., *Epid. II* 1f, 5.104 L., 5.1, 5.128 L., 6.1, 5.132 L., *Epid. IV* 20f, 5.160 L., *Epid. V* 22, 5.222 L., and *Epid. VI* 8.20, 5.352 L., 8.26, 5.352–354 L., 8.31, 5.354–356 L. See also *Epid. VI* 2.20, 5.288 L., 5.8, 5.318 L., 6.5, 5.324–326 L.

[59]   *Epid. VI* 3.5, 5.294 L.

[60]   Note especially *Hum.* 8, 5.488 L. ("As to the body generally, know to what disease the *phusis* most inclines," trans. Jones, modified). See also *Epid. I* 2.1, 2.604–606 L., 3.3, 2.614 L., *Epid. III* 1.6, 3.52 L., *Epid. II* 5.1, 5.128 L., 6.1, 5.132 L., and *Epid. VI* 6.5, 5.324–326 L., 7.6, 5.340 L., 7.8–9, 5.342 L., 8.12, 5.348 L., 8.31, 5.354–356 L.

[61]   *Epid. I* 12.3, 2.638 L. and *Epid. VI* 1.6, 5.268 L., 3.7, 5.296 L., 4.13, 5.310 L., 4.18–19, 5.312 L., 5.15, 5.322 L., 6.2, 5.324 L., 6.8, 5.328 L.

[62]   In many passages, medical writers use the term ἀνάγκη and its cognates ("it is necessary, necessar-
ily") when constructing causal explanations: for example, *VM* 19.3, 1.616–618 L., 22.7, 1.632 L., *Aër.* 4.2–3, 2.18–20 L., 7, 2.26–30 L., *Acut. App.* 14.1, 2.422 L., and *Morb. Sacr.* 5.3, 6.370 L., 8.2, 6.376 L.

[63]   For the strategies that medical writers used to uncover hidden causes, including the common
assertion that one should investigate "the invisible from the visible," see p. 164.

author of *On Ancient Medicine* believes it is crucially important to identify the internal cause of a disease, since it is only by removing that internal cause that the patient will get well. In *On the Art*, the author similarly observes that "the same intelligence is required to know the causes of diseases as to understand how to treat them" (11.4, 6.20 L., trans. Jones), again suggesting that the primary motivation for seeking causal explanations is to enable the doctor to provide a fitting treatment. In Chapter 2, we encountered multiple passages that stress the importance of treating both an ailment and its "source." In Chapter 3, we also saw that the author of *On Breaths* frames his entire investigation as an inquiry that is directly relevant to treatment, noting that "if someone knows the cause of the disease, he will be able to administer what is beneficial to the body, opposing the disease with the use of contraries" (1.4, 6.92 L.).

While attempting to identify the cause of a disease, many Greek doctors organized their thinking around the same principles of classification and commonality that we find in the *Epidemics*. These doctors divided and subdivided patients into groups, and they used the similarities and differences between those groups to guide their search for causal factors. In *Diseases of Unwed Girls*, the author leans heavily on such acts of classification when he seeks his own explanation of

> the so-called "sacred disease," apoplexies, and all the terrors that make human beings sorely afraid, so that they lose their mind, see malevolent spirits, sometimes by night, sometimes by day, and sometimes at both times, and then, from such a vision, many hang themselves, more women than men, for the nature of women [ἡ φύσις ἡ γυναικείη] is more prone to despondency and depression than that of men. (1.2, 8.466 L.)

Already in this opening statement, we can see how the author is carefully navigating the language of both commonality and difference. He begins with a general category of "human beings" (ἄνθρωποι), after which he immediately subdivides humans into two subclasses, noting that the above-mentioned diseases occur more often in women than in men (πλέονες δὲ γυναῖκες ἢ ἄνδρες).[64] The reason for this tendency, he claims, can be found in the common *phusis* of all women. Here, the word *phusis* is closely associated with the act of classification. It indicates some feature that is common to all women, and which explains why they suffer these

---

[64] This phrase echoes many comparisons between men and women in the *Epidemics*. Compare, for example, *Epid. I* 16.1, 2.646 L. ("women fell sick in large numbers, but in smaller numbers than men").

affections more often than men. However, the division into groups is not yet complete, as the author then observes that, within the class of women, "unwed girls of marriageable age suffer this more [μᾶλλον] when the menses descend, and not very much [οὐ μάλα] before this point" (2.1, 8.466 L.). As he divides and subdivides patients into groups, the author relies on general tendencies (πλέονες, μᾶλλον, μάλα) that point to the underlying cause of this condition, which he finally attributes to the flooding of the heart and diaphragm with excess blood. After describing the etiology of this condition, the author then concludes with yet another act of classification, noting that "within the class of married women, barren women suffer the same things" (3.6, 8.470 L.). This final statement is especially noteworthy as it implies an analogical relationship between unwed girls and barren women. These two classes of women suffer the same condition more often than others because both groups experience the same underlying cause: menstruation without pregnancy.[65] In other words, classification not only distinguishes one group from another but it also encourages the drawing of connections across otherwise dissimilar groups.

As we see in the introduction to *Diseases of Unwed Girls*, where the author groups together "the so-called 'sacred disease,' apoplexies, and all the terrors that make human beings sorely afraid," patients were not the only factors that Greek doctors classified in their search for causal agents. Diseases were also sorted into groups, with conditions that outwardly seem dissimilar nevertheless grouped together because they all share the same "starting point" (ἀρχή) and "nature" (φύσις). We have already seen this process of disease classification in *On the Nature of the Human Being*, where Polybus invokes the notion of humoral flux to observe that conditions that appear very different can in fact have a common *arche*. We also saw this process in *On Breaths*, whose author gathers together the various classes of disease, notes a common cause shared by them all, and then uses this derivation of all diseases from a single "starting point and source" (ἀρχὴ καὶ πηγή, 1.4, 6.92 L.) to conclude that "of all diseases there is one and the

---

[65] As we see in this example (whose association of unwed girls with barren women recurs at *Mul. II* 18, 8.272–274 L.), preconceived notions and social expectations factored into the creation of classes and even the "observed" propensities of each class. These doctors were not strict empiricists: what they saw was influenced by what they *expected* to see. This is especially clear in their discussions of women, where the Greek male perspective is emphatically on display (cf. Dean-Jones 1994; King 1998). For the inseparability of observation from theory, see Mansfeld (1980b: 382n3), Craik (2001a), and Kuriyama (2002: 111–151). Langholf (1990a) has persuasively shown that the compilers of the *Epidemics*, once praised as "empiricists" untainted by "theory," in fact rely on implicit assumptions about humoral pathology to guide their clinical observations.

same class and cause" (μία πασέων νούσων καὶ ἰδέη καὶ αἰτίη ἡ αὐτή, 2, 6.92 L.). Many texts in the Hippocratic Corpus are organized in a similar manner, placing diseases into classes, comparing those classes with each other, and striving to find a common "starting point" that will allow the different classes to be subsumed under something higher. A partial list of texts that illustrate this approach includes *On Affections, Diseases of Women I–III, Diseases I, Diseases IV*, the first eleven chapters of *Diseases II*, and chapters 9–40 of *On Places in the Human Being*. This format can also be found in many of the so-called surgical texts, including *On Fractures, On Joints, On Wounds, On Head Wounds, On Fistulas*, and *On Hemorrhoids*.

In these works, the authors usually follow the traditional format of a diagnostic handbook, giving each disease a name and providing a summary of its symptoms and treatments.[66] However, they accompany each entry with an important addition – an *explanation* of the internal processes that give rise to that condition. In all of these texts, the authors show a deep concern for the many variables that can change from one case to the next. They observe that "body differs from body, age from age, season from season,"[67] that diseases are manifested differently in men versus women, the young versus the old, and the bilious versus the phlegmatic,[68] that doctors need to adjust their treatments to fit the age, constitution, and personal habits of the patient,[69] and that the same treatments can have different effects on different patients.[70] At the same time, there is a strong desire to generalize and to arrange diseases hierarchically, where each condition is said to spring from something higher. In *On Places in the Human Being*, the author lists seven fluxes from the head, each of which gives rise to a different class of ailments (10–23, 6.294–314 L.). In *Diseases IV*, the author similarly traces the various classes of disease back to a limited number of "reservoirs" (πηγαί), assigning phlegm to the head, blood to the heart, bile to the gallbladder, and water to the spleen. In the sixth chapter of *On Affections*, the author describes a general category of

---

[66] On some occasions, it appears that these authors are *directly* revising a diagnostic handbook, the clearest example of which is *Diseases II*, chapters 1–11, which represents a partial rewriting of the same handbook that gave rise to *Diseases II*, chapters 12–75. For the compositional history of these revised diagnostic handbooks (which scholars once hastily attributed to a "Cnidian school" of medicine), Jouanna (1974) remains an indispensable starting point.

[67] For example, *Morb. I* 16, 6.168–170 L., 22, 6.182–184 L., *VC* 2.6, 3.192 L., *Fract.* 7, 3.440 L., 33, 3.532–534 L., 35, 3.536–538 L., and *Art.* 8, 4.94 L.; compare *Acut. App.* 21, 2.434–436 L.

[68] For example, *Morb. I* 22, 6.182–188 L., 29, 6.198 L., *Aff.* 28, 6.240 L., 30, 6.242 L., *Acut. App.* 29.1, 2.450 L., and *VC* 19.3, 3.254 L.

[69] For example, *Acut. App.* 20, 2.434 L., 31.2, 2.458–460 L., 40.2, 2.476 L., *VC* 20.2, 3.256 L., *Fract.* 8, 3.446–448 L., and *Haem.* 9, 6.444 L.; compare *Acut. App.* 24, 2.442–444 L.

[70] For example, *Aff.* 40, 6.250 L., 61, 6.268–270 L.

"acute" diseases that includes pleurisy, pneumonia, ardent fever, and phrenitis (6, 6.214 L.), but he then places this category under a larger umbrella of "fevers of winter" (12, 6.220 L.), whose differences are merely attributable to how bile or phlegm fall upon different parts. After discussing this major class of "winter fevers," the author then turns to a second class of diseases: those that occur during the summer (14, 6.220–222 L.). The author provides a general cause of these summer diseases (i.e., a moistening of the body when it is heated by the sun), and he urges his readers to treat these diseases "at the beginning" (ἀρχόμενα, 17, 6.224–226 L.), before they have a chance to become ingrained. By stressing the need to treat diseases at their *arche*, this author recalls the system of disease prevention that we find in *On the Nature of the Human Being*. In both texts, it is stressed that one should strive to identify the starting point of a disease and counteract that cause with speedy treatment, which can be greatly simplified when applied at this point in the causal chain. After concluding his discussion of summer diseases, the author of *On Affections* observes that tertian and quartan fevers have a *phusis* that arises from the same things (ἐκ τῶν αὐτῶν γίνεσθαι πεφύκασιν, 18, 6.226 L.). He then proceeds to a more general discussion of "supervening" conditions such as white phlegm, splenomegaly, and dropsy, all of which arise in consequence to the diseases that have already been described.[71] In this section, the author engages in some important pivots toward high-level generalization, noting that "In general, you must investigate the other diseases too in the same way, looking to see whence the *phusis* arises for each; by investigating in this way and seizing upon the starting point of diseases [τὴν ἀρχὴν τῶν νοσημάτων], you will err the least" (25, 6.236 L., trans. Potter, modified). With this statement, the author implies that the various classes of disease are best understood by tracing them back to a limited number of "starting points" (ἀρχαί). Just as the major diseases have their various "modes" (τρόποι), each with a particular "nature" (φύσις), so too can entire disease classes be subsumed under something higher.[72] In fact, the author prefaces his entire exposition with the assertion that "all diseases arise in human beings from bile and phlegm" (νοσήματα τοῖσιν ἀνθρώποις ἅπαντα

---

[71] On the changing of one disease into another, see the general discussion at *Morb. I* 3, 6.144–146 L.

[72] Compare *Aff.* 28, 6.240 L., where the author observes that strangury has many different "modes" (τρόποι). Sometimes, this method of organizing diseases according to their *arche* reveals that diseases with the same name actually arise from different sources. Note, for example, *Aff.* 22, 6.232 L., where dropsy is said to arise from six different ailments. The push for a higher *arche* is also emphasized at *Morb. I* 26, 6.194 L., where the author notes that some people do not go far enough when identifying the "cause and starting point" (αἴτιον . . . καὶ ἀρχήν) of a particular illness.

γίνεται ὑπὸ χολῆς καὶ φλέγματος, 1, 6.208 L.). This universal starting point applies to all diseases in general, and it therefore suggests that all known ailments can be sorted into one and the same class. The author takes so much pride in his overarching principle that he concludes his disease catalog with a full-throated endorsement of this principle's reliability (37, 6.246 L., trans. Potter):

> When you come to a patient, you must question him thoroughly about what he is suffering, in consequence of what, for how many days, whether his cavity has passed anything, and what regimen he is following. Consider first [ἐνθυμεῖσθαι πρῶτον] whether the disease has arisen from bile or from phlegm or from both, and have full confidence that it must be because of these, either one or both of them.

Like the author of *On Breaths*, the author of *On Affections* shows profound confidence in the universality of his first principle. By comparing various diseases with each other and identifying their common elements, he traces all diseases back to a single *arche* that rises above the many variables that can change from one case to the next.

As we saw in Chapter 1, the author of *Diseases I* also identifies bile and phlegm as the common source of all diseases. In his discussion of these humors, the author claims that "bile and phlegm come into being together with [people] coming into being, and are always present in the body in greater or lesser amounts" (2, 6.142 L., trans. Potter, modified). With this reference to "coming into being," the author recalls the interest in embryology and anthropogony that we find in both *On Flesh* and *On Regimen*, as well as Polybus's description of the humors as innate from birth (5.3–4, 6.42–44 L.) and "always alike the same, whether the patient be young or old, or whether the season be cold or hot" (2.5, 6.36 L.). Another text that connects human *phusis* with human origins is *Diseases IV*. In this text, the author claims that all diseases arise from "four forms of moisture" (ὑγροῦ τέσσαρα εἴδεα, 32.1, 7.542 L.), namely phlegm, blood, bile, and water, which are all present in human beings from the point of conception. Since a patient's *phusis* is largely determined at birth (note the connection with the verb *phuesthai*, "to grow" or "be born"), these doctors conclude that the best way to understand human *phusis* is to go back to the *arche* of a human being. Although the author of *On Ancient Medicine* associates this type of thinking with the narratives of Empedocles and other cosmologists,[73] it is important to stress that an emphasis on origins was also well suited to

---

[73] Compare especially *VM* 20.1, 1.620 L. with the comments of Schiefsky (2005: 19–25, 294–295).

medical thinking in this era. All of these authors approach human *phusis* in the same manner that they approach the *phusis* of disease. In both instances, they identify certain principles that hold true in all circumstances, and they justify the stability of these principles by tracing them back to a common source. When the author of *Diseases IV* traces human *phusis* back to the womb, he is mirroring his attempt to trace each humor back to a specific reservoir within the body. Similarly, when both Polybus and the author of *Diseases I* claim that specific humors are innate from birth, they justify the universality of these disease agents by making them a universal feature of human nature. Whether they are discussing the *phusis* of human beings or the *phusis* of disease, these authors seek out the permanence, simplicity, and precision that exists at the origin of things. Such an interest in origins is not merely some trickle-down effect from the inquiry into nature, but an extension of Greek doctors' thinking about how the best way to rise above individual differences is to go back to a common *arche*.

4.5 From the Common to the Particular

One reason why Greek doctors were so keen to seek out causal explanations was that such information would not leave doctors in the lurch when confronted with a wholly new set of circumstances. Even when a doctor had never experienced a particular situation, he could nevertheless analyze the "nature" (φύσις) and "power" (δύναμις) of each factor that influences a patient's health, using this information to determine what is likely to occur under a given set of conditions. This "adaptability" advantage of causal explanations is well illustrated by *Airs Waters Places*. In this text, the author addresses itinerant doctors who regularly travel from one community to the next. Toward the end of his preface, the author reflects on what a doctor can do if he studies all the "powers" of the various factors that can influence human health (2.1–2, 2.14 L.):

> Starting from these things, one should contemplate the particular cases [καὶ ἀπὸ τούτων χρὴ ἐνθυμεῖσθαι ἕκαστα]. For if someone knows these things well – especially all of them, but if not, at least most – neither the local diseases nor the nature [φύσις] of the peoples' bellies will escape his notice when he arrives at a city with which he is unfamiliar. Accordingly, he will not be at a loss or miss the mark in his treatment of diseases – things which are likely to occur unless one knows these things beforehand when reflecting on each case in advance. As the time and the year progresses, he

can say both what diseases, being common to all [πάγκοινα], will seize the city in the summer or winter and what diseases, being particular to individuals [ἴδια ἑκάστῳ], may arise from a change in regimen. For by knowing the changes of the seasons and both the risings and settings of the stars, how each of these things occurs, he can know in advance how the year will turn out. By thinking in this way and predicting the *kairoi*, he can attain the best knowledge about each case, most often hit the mark when aiming at health, and achieve not inconsiderable successes in the art.

In this passage, we see the same distinction between diseases that are "common to all" and diseases that are "particular to individuals" that appears in both *On Breaths* and *On the Nature of the Human Being*. Yet again, "common" diseases are attributed to environmental factors that are shared by an entire community, while "particular" diseases are attributed to a person's regimen (δίαιτα), a factor that can change from one patient to the next. In this text, the author claims that doctors can master both "common" and "particular" diseases if they "contemplate" (ἐνθυμεῖσθαι) the causal factors that give rise to a disease.[74] At the beginning of *Airs Waters Places*, the author specifically asserts that the most important activity for the medical researcher is to consider how causal factors can differ from one case to the next (1.1–2, 2.12 L.):

Whoever intends to investigate medicine correctly should do the following. First, he should contemplate [ἐνθυμεῖσθαι] the seasons of the year, considering what each season has the power to bring about. For the seasons are not at all similar to one another, but are very different both in themselves and in the changes from one to the next. Next, he should contemplate the winds, both the hot and the cold, especially those that are common to all human beings, and then also those that are native to each locale. He should also contemplate the powers of waters, for just as they differ in taste and in weight, so too is the power of each very different.

In this passage, every factor that influences human health is given a particular "power" (δύναμις). This "power" determines what effects that factor will have on the body, and it is the primary consideration for doctors who want to adjust their treatments to fit the needs of

---

[74] Compare the assertion in *On Affections* that one must "contemplate first" (ἐνθυμεῖσθαι πρῶτον) the common origin of all diseases from bile and phlegm (37, 6.246 L.). The verb ἐνθυμεῖσθαι elsewhere refers to the "contemplation" of causal factors at *Aër.* 2.1, 2.14 L., 10.1, 2.42 L., 13.4, 2.58 L., 24.10, 2.92 L., *Prog.* 20.5, 2.170 L., 25.2, 2.188 L., *Aff.* 6, 6.214 L., 37, 6.246 L., and *Prorrh. II* 4, 9.14 L., 18, 9.44 L., 21, 9.50 L.; compare *Morb. I* 1, 6.140–142 L.

particular situations. In *On Breaths*, the author recalls this emphasis on "powers" when he refers to *pneuma* as the greatest "potentate" (δυνάστης) in the universe as a whole (3.2, 6.94 L.; cf. 4.1, 6.96 L., 15.1, 6.114 L.). Eryximachus similarly asserts that "the undivided *eros*, taken as a whole, has a wide, a strong, nay an absolute power" (πολλὴν καὶ μεγάλην, μᾶλλον δὲ πᾶσαν δύναμιν ἔχει, 188d), again suggesting that what makes a causal factor especially important is its "power" to influence the outcome of an event.

Since the most useful commonalities apply to the widest range of cases, there was an incentive to arrange these generalizations into hierarchical systems, with some principles receiving more attention than others. When the author of *Airs Waters Places* describes the powers of winds, he notes that one should pay the most attention to the winds that are "common to all human beings" (μάλιστα μὲν τὰ κοινὰ πᾶσιν ἀνθρώποισιν) and only after that consider the winds that are particular to local communities (ἔπειτα δὲ καὶ τὰ ἐν ἑκάστῃ χώρῃ ἐπιχώρια ἐόντα, 1.2, 2.12 L.). In *Epidemics I*, we are similarly told that medical reasoning should take its origin "from the common nature of all and the particular nature of each" (ἐκ τῆς κοινῆς φύσιος ἁπάντων καὶ τῆς ἰδίης ἑκάστου, 23.1, 2.668–670 L.), and many texts in the Hippocratic Corpus are arranged in accordance with this principle, beginning with what is "common to all" before moving to particular cases. In *On Affections*, we have already seen how the author prefaces his discussion of specific diseases with the assertion that "all diseases arise in human beings from bile and phlegm" (1, 6.208 L.). By doing so, he presents a general principle that is remarkably close to the thesis of *On Breaths*, simply replacing *pneuma* with the two humors of bile and phlegm. *On Wounds* begins with a discussion of "all wounds in general" (ἕλκεα ξύμπαντα, 1.1, 6.400 L.), noting that wounds, considered as a group, should not be moistened with anything except for wine. The author then justifies this rule with a highly generalized principle about the "dry" and the "wet," observing that "the dry is nearer to health, and the wet to unhealthiness, since a wound is wet, but healthy flesh dry" (1.1, 6.400 L., trans. Potter, modified). The author of *On Wounds* follows up this general principle with more instructions that are arranged from the common to the particular, including what should be done for "all old wounds" (1.2, 6.400 L.), for "all fresh wounds" (1.3, 6.400 L.), for "every fresh wound *except* in the cavity" (2.1, 6.402 L.), and finally for various subcategories of wounds. Another transition from the common to the particular can be found in the beginning of *Prorrhetic II* (5, 9.20 L., trans. Potter, modified):

> About dropsies, consumptions and gouty conditions as well as persons taken by what is called the sacred disease, I say that, concerning all of them, they have something in common [κατὰ μέν τι περὶ πάντων τὸ αὐτό], namely that in whomever these diseases are to a degree hereditary, you can be sure that they are hard to get rid of. Their other features I shall describe disease by disease [τὰ δὲ ἄλλα καθ᾽ ἕκαστον γράψω].

Sometimes, medical writers begin their texts by observing that a certain commonality does not exist. In *On Head Wounds*, the author opens with the observation that "the heads of human beings are in no way like one another [οὐδὲν ὁμοίως σφίσιν αὐταῖς], nor do the sutures of the head have a *phusis* that is the same in all cases" (οὐδὲ αἱ ῥαφαὶ τῆς κεφαλῆς πάντων κατὰ ταὐτὰ πεφύκασιν, 1.1, 3.182 L.). The author then goes on to say that instead of having a common *phusis*, human skulls are divided into four types, with the first type having a prominence in the front of the head, the second in the back of the head, the third at each end, and the fourth at neither end. When this same author describes various injuries of the skull, he also divides them into "types" (τρόποι), each of which consists of several "forms" (ἰδέαι). In chapter 7, he writes that "the *hedra* taken by itself is long or short, rather bent, or straighter, or rounded; and there are many other forms of this mode [καὶ πολλαὶ ἄλλαι ἰδέαι τοῦ τοιούτου τρόπου], according to the shape of the weapon" (7.4, 3.208 L., trans. Withington). In *On Places in the Human Being*, an initial commonality is similarly rejected just to prop up many others. In this text, the author opens with the statement that "in my opinion, there is no starting point of the body, but all parts are alike the starting point and all the end point" (1.1, 6.276 L.). The author then goes on to describe the common anatomy of human beings, emphasizing that diseases that begin in one part of the body can eventually make their way to other parts. At one point, the author observes that he has only written about the joints and vessels that are "identical in all people" (πᾶσιν ὁμοίως). As for the joints and vessels that are "different in different persons" (ἄλλα ἄλλοισι), they are "unworthy of discussion" (οὐκ ἄξια λόγου) and have accordingly been omitted from his account (6.10, 6.290 L.). Yet another example of this movement from the common to the particular can be found in *On Glands*. In this text, the author opens his discussion "about glands as a whole" (περὶ δὲ ἀδένων οὐλομελίης, 1.1, 8.556 L.) by describing the common *phusis* of all glands. He then moves to specific glands in chapters 5–10, at one point interrupting his discussion to remark that "there are other really small glands in the body, but I do not wish to digress in my account; for my treatise is directed towards the glands that are critical [τὰς ἐπικαίρους]" (7.1, 8.560 L., trans. Craik, modified). In other texts that are arranged from the common to the particular, minor details are not omitted because they are assumed to be unimportant but because they can be derived from the principles already established. In *Airs Waters Places*, the author remarks that he cannot list every difference that exists between the communities in which people live. Instead, he focuses on the most extreme differences, concluding that "by drawing inferences from these things, you should contemplate the rest, and you will not miss the mark [when aiming at health]" (24.10, 2.92 L.).[75]

This privileging of the common over the particular became so integral to medical thinking that medical research came to be defined, very broadly, as a search for commonality. We have already mentioned the assertion in *Epidemics III* that doctors should look for what is "common" (κοινόν, 16.2, 3.102 L.) and the claim in *Epidemics VI* that researchers should note the similarities and differences between individual cases in order to identify "one similarity" (ὁμοιότης μία, 3.12, 5.298 L.) that unites and governs them all. In *Diseases I*, the author provides a list of topics to be considered by anyone who intends to engage in debates about medicine. The first entry in this list is "whence *all* diseases arise in human beings" (ἀφ' ὧν αἱ νοῦσοι γίνονται τοῖσιν ἀνθρώποισι πᾶσαι, 1, 6.140 L.), and he later observes that one must consider "what 'all' is in the art, being one and everything, and what 'one'" (ὅ τι ἅπαν ἐστὶν ἐν αὐτῇ, ἓν καὶ πάντα, καὶ ὅ τι ἕν, 1, 6.140 L.). This riddling statement is difficult to parse, but it seems to be related to an emphasis on the common and the particular. We may note, for example, that to be "one" and "everything" is a good way to describe a universal principle that encompasses all particulars.[76] In *On Places in the Human Being*, the author follows up his initial observation that medicine, unlike writing, has no "fixed technique" by claiming that medicine does in fact have a stable basis (βέβηκε

---

[75] Compare the final chapter of *On Breaths*, in which the author writes, "I have carried my account down to the diseases and affections that are well known, in which cases my foundational principle [ὑπόθεσις] has been shown to be true. If I were to discuss all diseases, my account would be longer, but it would not be any more precise or more convincing" (15.2, 6.114 L.). For the promise that contemplating general principles will prevent doctors from "missing the mark" (a term related to aiming for the *kairos*), compare *Aër.* 1.1–2.2, 2.12–14 L., *Acut. App.* 13.1–2, 2.420 L., *Prog.* 25, 2.188–190 L., and *Aff.* 25, 6.236 L.

[76] At *Nat. Hom.* 1.2, 6.32 L., Polybus notes that some thinkers identify a single element as "both the one and the all" (τὸ ἕν τε καὶ τὸ πᾶν). Compare also Heraclitus's description of the universal order as "one from all and all from one" (ἐκ πάντων ἓν καὶ ἐξ ἑνὸς πάντα, DK 22 B10).

γὰρ ἰητρικὴ πᾶσα, 46.1, 6.342 L.). This stable basis comes from the fact that medicine establishes "classes and non-classes" (τὰ εἴδεα καὶ τὰ μὴ εἴδεα, 44.1, 6.338 L.), where each genuine "class" is defined by the existence of some universal principle. The author is so confident about this method of sorting topics into classes that he banishes from medicine any dependence on chance. In chapter 46, he observes that "in my opinion, medicine has been discovered as a whole [ὅλη], medicine of the sort that teaches both the tendencies[77] and the *kairoi* in each case. Whoever has such a knowledge of medicine least depends on chance, but achieves successful outcomes both with and without chance."[78]

Another emphasis on the stability of universal principles can be found in *On the Seed-Nature of the Child*. In this text, the author begins with the sweeping assertion that "law governs all things" (νόμος μὲν πάντα κρατύνει, 1.1, 7.470 L.). This prelude has been belittled by modern

---

[77] Many editors have emended the author's reference to "tendencies" (ἔθεα), replacing it with either εἴδεα ("classes"; cf. *Loc. Hom.* 44.1, 6.338 L.) or ἤθεα ("characters"; cf. *Gland.* 12.2, 8.569 L. and *Prorrh. II* 3, 9.12 L., and note A. *Ag.* 727–728, where most editors replace ἔθος with ἦθος). Both emendations make good sense, but it is possible to read ἔθεα as a reference to the "habits" of disease (i.e., what "tends" to happen in a given set of circumstances). Compare the use of the verb εἴωθα (< ἔθω) to denote what "usually" happens in the course of a disease at *Aph.* 2.12, 4.472 L., 2.27, 4.478 L., 2.50, 4.484 L., 3.28, 4.500 L., 4.61, 4.524 L., *Epid. VI* 8.31, 5.354 L., *Coac.* 133, 5.610 L., *Aff.* 17, 6.224 L., 30, 6.242 L., 44, 6.254 L., and *Dent.* 19, 8.546 L. On the notions of tendency and probability, see also di Benedetto (1966, 1986: 126–142), Licciardi (1989), and von Staden (2002). On "chance" (τύχη), see p. 127.

[78] In *Diseases of Women III*, the author similarly observes that medicine lacks a "fixed standard" (σταθμός) for prescribing treatments (18.10, 8.442–444 L.). To overcome this difficulty, the author stresses that the doctor should consider the available treatments in relation to the patient's "body as a whole" (ὅλου τοῦ σώματος), looking to the patient's "physical state" (ἕξις) and "strength" (ἰσχύς) when determining what ought to be done. As an additional guide, the author immediately follows this statement with a universal principle: "whichever of these things you do, always employ fumigations: for this is what softens and leads down the humors." Interestingly, the author refers to this process of contemplating a patient's *phusis* as becoming an "inquirer into nature" (φυσικός). Additionally, he calls the specific factors that the doctor should consider his "elements" (στοιχεῖα). In the immediate context, the author does not seem to use the word *phusikos* to denote someone who contemplates the "nature" of the cosmos, but rather a doctor who thinks about the various categories of human *phusis*. Similarly, *stoicheia* are not here defined as the material "elements" from which the universe is composed but rather the "building blocks" that the doctor should use for making therapeutic calculations. It is possible that the author is intentionally appropriating the language of cosmology in this passage, just as the author of *On Ancient Medicine* seeks to reassert what it means to be a student of "nature" (20, 1.620–624 L.). However, it is also possible that the author is here relating the term *stoicheia* to its original sense of "letters of the alphabet," essentially replying to the observation in *On Places in the Human Being* that medicine, unlike writing, has no "fixed technique." Here, the author would be saying that medicine *does* have something like the letters that are constantly rearranged to create an infinite variety of words and statements, but these "letters" are the factors that the doctor should consider when calculating the *kairos* in each case. The "letters" of medicine are constantly reshuffled, but they are just as stable as the letters of the alphabet, the reason being that they are rooted in a knowledge of classes and the general principles that are inherent in each class.

commentators,[79] but it would have been felt more powerfully by a medical writer of the fifth or fourth century BCE. In this period, doctors were just starting to associate the isolation of universal laws with the advancement of the medical art. They would have therefore viewed the assertion that "law governs all things" as a good motto for medical research, just as the author of *On Fractures* introduces the phrase *nomos dikaios* to denote an "exact rule" where an unexpected outcome does not indicate an exception to the rule but rather an error on the part of the practitioner (7, 3.442 L.; cf. Pl. [*Min.*] 316c–317d).

Perhaps the most striking expression of this emphasis on high-level commonalities is the opening of *Diseases of Unwed Girls* (1.1, 8.466 L.):

> The beginning of my compilation of what is eternal in medicine (for it is impossible to understand the nature of diseases – which is the business of the art to discover – unless one knows the nature of diseases in the highest order, according to the starting point [κατὰ τὴν ἀρχήν] from which they were first divided).

The precise syntax of the first seven words in this passage (ἀρχή μοι τῆς ξυνθέσιος τῶν αἰειγενέων ἰητρικῆς) has been the source of some confusion. Previous translators have usually treated the genitive τῆς ξυνθέσιος as if it were nominative (e.g., Littré 1853, vol. 8: 526–529: "Le commencement de la médecine est pour moi la constitution des choses éternelles"), inserted a second ἀρχή before ἰητρικῆς (e.g., Bonnet-Cadilhac 1993: 147: "Le principe de la synthèse des phénomènes constants est à mes yeux le principe de la médecin"),[80] or else followed Ermerins (1862 [1859–64]: 903) by inserting the preposition ἀπό before the words τῶν αἰειγενέων (e.g., Potter 2010: 359: "The beginning point of my composition is from what is eternal in medicine").[81] The key to understanding this statement is to

---

[79] For example, Heidel (1941: 23): "Occasionally one is amused by an author's evident desire to show his speculative temper by solemnly declaiming a banal cliche that at the moment was current in philosophical circles, such as 'Law governs all things.' One could readily match such expressions with similar utterances of physicians today"; Lonie (1981: 103): "The phrase was frequently echoed and quoted in the fifth and early fourth centuries, and it was used to convey varying ideas. Here it is no more than a piece of hackneyed literary embellishment, a *captatio* placed at the beginning of the work and comparable to the pompous (and irrelevant) introductions to Virg. and Nat. Mul." Contrast the praise of this opening by Ilberg (1925: 10).

[80] Compare Schiefsky (2005: 147): "The beginning of medicine is in my opinion the principle of the ever-existing."

[81] Compare Lami (2007: 23): "Il principio che io do al componimento medico è a partire dagli elementi sempiterni." Flemming and Hanson (1988: 250) translate the phrase as if the preposition ἐκ appeared before τῆς ξυνθέσιος: "My beginning comes out of the totality of medicine's eternal aspects." Lami (2007: 27) is wary of the three genitives, but sequences of three genitives, one governing another, are not that unusual. Compare Cooper and Krüger (1998: 192 = 47.9.7).

observe that these first seven words do not form a complete sentence. Instead, they simply mark the physical "beginning" of the author's work, performing the same function as a similar formula that we see throughout the Ebers papyrus: "The beginning of a compilation of remedies" (*P. Ebers* 4); "The beginning of a compilation on the eyes" (*P. Ebers* 336); "The beginning of the book on the wandering of *wekhedu* in all parts of a man's body" (*P. Ebers* 856a). Closer in date to *Diseases of Unwed Girls*, Ion of Chios opens a work with the phrase, "The beginning of my discourse" (ἀρχὴ δέ μοι τοῦ λόγου, DK 36 B1), while similar phrases can be found in Euripides (ἀρχὴ δ' ἥδε μοι προοιμίου, *El.* 1060) and Plato (ἡ μέν μοι ἀρχὴ τοῦ λόγου, *Smp.* 177a; ἡ αὐτή μοι ἀρχή, *Prt.* 318a).[82] Here, the author calls his work a "compilation of medicine's eternal things," or, to render it more idiomatically, a "compilation of what is eternal in medicine." It has often been assumed that "what is eternal" (τῶν αἰειγενέων) refers to cosmology,[83] but it is important to emphasize the limiting function of ἰητρικῆς in this context, which here restricts the author's focus to "what is eternal *in medicine*." By adding this qualifier, the author does not refer to cosmology per se but simply to a set of general principles that retain their validity even when all other variables change. "What is eternal in medicine" are principles that hold true no matter the season of the year, the identity of the patient, or even the identity of the disease, much like Polybus's assertion that the basic constituents of human beings are "always alike the same [αἰεὶ ταὐτὰ ἐόντα ὁμοίως], whether the patient be young or old, or whether the season be cold or hot" (2.5, 6.36 L.).[84] The current work is a "compilation" (ξύνθεσις) of such principles insofar as the author brings them together to explain how diseases come to be.[85] The author may also be anticipating the Platonic notion of "collection" and "division," as he justifies his inquiry

---

[82] Note also the very next "sentence" in *Diseases of Unwed Girls*, which lacks a main verb and similarly acts as a title (1.2, 8.466 L.): "Concerning the so-called 'sacred disease,' apoplexies, and all the terrors that make human beings sorely afraid, so that they lose their mind, see malevolent spirits, sometimes by night, sometimes by day, and sometimes at both times, and then, from such a vision, many hang themselves, more women than men, for the nature of women is more prone to despondency and depression than that of men."

[83] For example, Littré (1853 [1839–61], vol. 8: 529–530), Heidel (1941: 22), Lami (2007: 28–29), and Bourbon (2017: 194–195).

[84] Compare also Heraclitus's description of his "account" (λόγος) as "always existing" (ἐόντος ἀεί, DK 22 B1). Most scholars who think that *Diseases of Unwed Girls* is referring to cosmology either make ἰητρικῆς depend on ἀρχή or treat it as an adjective modifying ξυνθέσιος. Lami (2007: 27) claims that, in order to be a substantive, ἰητρικῆς requires an article. Note, however, the many openings of Hippocratic treatises where ἰητρική (without the article) is clearly used as a noun: *VM* 1.1, 1.570 L., *Aër.* 1.1, 2.12 L., *Lex* 1, 4.638 L., *Nat. Hom.* 1.1, 6.32 L., and *Loc. Hom.* 2.1, 6.278 L.

[85] Compare the use of the verb συντίθεσθαι at *Carn.* 1.1, 8.584 L. and συγκεῖσθαι at *Loc. Hom.* 46.1, 6.342 L.

into "what is eternal" by observing that "it is impossible to understand the nature of diseases – which is the business of the art to discover – unless one knows the nature of diseases in the highest order [ἐν τῷ ἀμερεῖ, literally 'in the partless'], according to the starting point [κατὰ τὴν ἀρχήν] from which they were first divided [διεκρίθη]."[86]

With these words, the author implies that doctors should focus on both the common and the particular. They should consider the common "nature" of diseases ("the nature of diseases in the highest order," "the starting point from which they were first divided") at the same time that they investigate the peculiar "nature" of each affection. In this context, the word "nature" (φύσις) is closely associated with the act of classification. In fact, one could define the term *phusis* as the sum total of general principles that are inherent to all members of a class.[87] Whether one is discussing the "nature" of all diseases, the "nature" of a certain subset of diseases (e.g., the assortment of diseases that some Greek doctors called "acute"), or the "nature" of particular diseases such as pneumonia, pleuritis, tenesmus, or apoplexy, every division has a *phusis* that is specific to that group. From this passage, it is unclear whether the author is asserting that one should begin with the common nature of all diseases *in general* (e.g., something similar to the claim in *On Breaths* that all diseases are caused by *pneuma*) or simply with the common nature of all diseases that belong to a particular class (e.g., starting with the common nature of all pneumonias before considering specific manifestations of this ailment). The rest of this text only supports the second interpretation,[88] but we should not discount the possibility that this author had more general ideas about the shared *phusis* of all diseases. After all, these two interpretations are not mutually exclusive, as doctors could start with the common nature of all ailments before considering what is common to each subset. However we choose to interpret this passage, it is clear that the author of *Diseases of Unwed Girls* places the same emphasis on

---

[86] For the application of the terms σύνθεσις and διάκρισις to collection and division, see Gal. *PHP* 5.775 K. Flemming and Hanson (1988: 245) rightly observe that this section from *Diseases of Unwed Girls* "speaks of reaching to grasp universals, categories without parts (*ameres*), from which divisions are then made," comparing Arist. *APo.* 100b2 (τὰ ἀμερῆ . . . καὶ τὰ καθόλου, "the partless and the universal"). *Pace* Bonnet-Cadilhac (1993: 150), this reference to the "partless" does not presuppose the influence of Aristotle. Compare Parmenides's description of "what is" as "whole" and "consisting of only one part" at DK 28 B8.4.

[87] Compare *Acut. App.* 52.1, 2.496 L., where the author uses the term *phusis* to refer to a "form" of dropsy (ὑδρώπων δύο μὲν φύσιες).

[88] Note, for example, how the author sets as his topic "the so-called 'sacred disease,' apoplexies, and all the terrors that make human beings sorely afraid," establishing a class of diseases that all happen to share a common *phusis*.

high-level commonalities that we see in *On Breaths*. Both authors assume that there are many different "types" of disease, but they also assert that one must consider the shared "nature" (φύσις) and "starting point" (ἀρχή) that places these diseases within one and the same class.

4.6 The Cosmological Turn

Of course, Greek doctors did not have to refer to the entire cosmos when engaging in investigations of "the whole" (τὸ ὅλον). They could take any topic and break it down into its constituent parts, using a process of collection and division very similar to what we find in Plato's dialogues. In *Prognostic*, the author observes that "one ought to know the whole character of sweats [τὸ ξύνολον τῶν ἱδρώτων], for some are connected with prostration of strength in the body, and some with intensity of the inflammation" (6, 2.124 L., trans. Jones). By referring to "the whole character of sweats," the author simply means that the doctor must consider what is common to all sweats, and he must also consider the various categories into which sweating can be divided.

This observation is critical to understanding a notorious crux in Plato's *Phaedrus*, in which Socrates similarly associates medical inquiry with investigations into "the whole."[89] In this dialogue, Socrates argues that for rhetoric to be considered a genuine *techne*, it should be organized along the same lines as medicine. Socrates begins by distinguishing what it is necessary to learn as "preliminaries to the *techne*" (τὰ πρὸ τῆς τέχνης ἀναγκαῖα μαθήματα, 269b) from the *techne* itself. In medicine, such preliminaries would include knowledge of how to make a patient vomit, move their bowels, heat or cool their bodies, and other such things (268a–b), while to master the *techne* and become a true "doctor" (ἰατρός) one must also know "to whom he should apply such treatments, when, and to what extent" (268b). This passage recalls the assertion in *On Regimen in Acute Diseases* that doctors cannot simply apply the same treatment in every case, but they should also know "to whom [a treatment] should be administered and to whom it should not be administered, as well as the reason why it should not be administered" (55, 2.342 L.). This passage is also reminiscent of Eryximachus's assertion in the *Symposium* that whoever can differentiate good and bad *eros* is a "master of the healer's art," while whoever knows how to implant *eros* when it is absent and take it away when

---

[89] Over the next few pages, all translations from the *Phaedrus* will be adapted from Nehamas and Woodruff's translation in Cooper (1997).

it is present is a "good workman" (186c–d). For Eryximachus, the "work-man" (δημιουργός) would be the person who has learned what Socrates calls the "preliminaries to the *techne*," while the "master of the healer's art" (ἰατρικώτατος) resembles Socrates's true doctor who knows "to whom he should apply such treatments, when, and to what extent."[90]

In the *Phaedrus*, Socrates continues his argument by comparing medicine with two other arts: tragedy and music. First, he notes that tragedians cannot just know a few simple tricks to create pity and fear; they must also put these techniques together into a "composition" (σύστασις) wherein the various techniques "fit one with the other and with the whole work" (πρέπουσαν ἀλλήλοις τε καὶ τῷ ὅλῳ, 268d). Turning then to music, Socrates asserts that one must also differentiate those who know how to produce high or low notes from those who can produce a "harmony" (ἁρμονία, 268e), again distinguishing the preliminaries of an art from an understanding of the art itself. To fully acquire a *techne*, one must bring the pieces together in such a way that they are "fitting" (ἁρμόζων) for both each other and for the "whole" (τὸ ὅλον). After providing these examples, Socrates criticizes the so-called teachers of rhetoric because they merely give instruction in matters such as "speaking concisely" or "speaking in images" and presume that, after providing such lessons, they have educated their students "completely" (τελέως, 269c). In reality, these students need to learn more than just rhetorical devices. They also need to learn how to "put together the whole" (τὸ ὅλον συνίστασθαι, 269c), for this is what differentiates the *technai* from other knowledge. At this point in the dialogue, there is no indication that Socrates is thinking about cosmology when referring to "the whole." Instead, he seems to be associating this term with the notions of "composition" (σύστασις) and "harmony" (ἁρμονία), whereby the various components of an art must all be assembled in such a way as to complement each other and thereby achieve what is fitting in each case.

After setting forth these criticisms of rhetorical handbooks, Socrates provides his own advice for how to organize rhetoric as a *techne*. He begins by noting that "all the great arts require endless talk and ethereal speculation about nature" (πᾶσαι ὅσαι μεγάλαι τῶν τεχνῶν προσδέονται ἀδολεσχίας καὶ μετεωρολογίας φύσεως πέρι, 269e–270a). He then observes that, in both medicine and rhetoric, "we need to determine the

---

[90] Similar claims can be found at Arist. *EN* 1137a9–26 and [*MM*] 1199a29–b3. Compare also the distinction between knowing the methods (τρόποι) of reducing dislocations and knowing the best occasions on which to use them at *Art.* 1, 4.80 L.

nature [φύσις] of something – of the body in medicine, of the soul in
rhetoric," for we otherwise "won't be able to supply, on the basis of an art,
a body with the medicine and diet that will make it healthy and strong, or
a soul with the reasons and customary rules for conduct that will impart to
it the convictions and virtues we want" (270b). In one of the most widely
discussed portions of the *Phaedrus*, Socrates asserts that would-be teachers
of rhetoric should follow the example of Hippocrates, who claims that one
cannot understand the nature of the body without understanding "the
nature of the whole" (τῆς τοῦ ὅλου φύσεως, 270c). As Socrates elaborates
just after this statement (270d):

> Concerning the nature of anything must we not contemplate in the follow-
> ing way: first, whether the thing concerning which we want ourselves to be
> proficient in a craft and able to make someone else proficient is simple or
> multiform, then, if it is simple, to investigate its power [δύναμιν], viz. what
> power it naturally [πέφυκεν] has to act and in relation to what [πρὸς τί] it
> has that power, or what power it naturally has to be acted upon and by what,
> and if it has multiple forms [εἴδη], to enumerate them, and then to see in the
> case of each form, just as in the case of one [i.e., the simple nature], what it
> naturally [πέφυκεν] does and how it performs that action, or what it
> naturally has done to it, how it is acted upon, and by what?

As with the reference to "what is eternal" in *Diseases of Unwed Girls*, Plato's
references to "the whole" (τὸ ὅλον) and to "ethereal speculation about
nature" (μετεωρολογίας φύσεως πέρι) have occasionally been misread as
a nod to cosmology. Almost always, scholars have jumped to this conclusion while attempting to answer the so-called Hippocratic Question,
arguing that Hippocrates was the author of some text that currently
bears his name. As we see in the above-quoted passage, however, Plato's
discussion is more taxonomic than cosmological.[91] Socrates is not claiming
that doctors and rhetoricians should investigate the universe as a whole.
Instead, he speaks about the division of both bodies and souls into groups
and the consideration of what "powers" each group has to act and be acted
upon. Plato's use of the verb πέφυκεν ("is by nature") suggests that even
when a topic is "multiform" (πολυειδές), each division has a *phusis* that

---

[91] On this point, I agree with Steckerl (1945), Jouanna (1977), and Schiefsky (2005: 69–70). Note also
Edelstein (1931: 132–134), who correctly observes (*pace* Mansfeld 1980a: 346n16) that Plato tends to
associate the terms *adoleschia* ("endless talk") and *meteorologia* ("ethereal speculation") not with
discussions of the cosmos as a whole but with any form of speculation that involves high-level
generalizations. Compare *Phd.* 70c, *Prm.* 135d, *Tht.* 175d, *Sph.* 216c, *Plt.* 299b, and *Cra.* 401b. For the
cosmological reading of Plato's "whole," see, for example, Festugière (1948: 62–65), Joly (1961, 1983),
West (1971: 365), Herter (1976), and Mansfeld (1980a).

determines its particular *dunamis*, thereby mirroring the classificatory use of the term *phusis* that appears in *Diseases of Unwed Girls*. In other dialogues, Plato refers to physicians who emphasize that one cannot treat one part of the body without also treating the "whole"; for example, it is impossible to treat the eyes without also treating the head (*Chrm.* 156b–c; cf. *Lg.* 10.902d, 903c). Here, the notion of the "whole" recalls the same concepts of "harmony" (ἁρμονία) and "composition" (σύστασις) that, in the *Phaedrus*, Socrates associates with tragedy and music. Whether one is dividing bodies into classes or considering how one part of the body is connected to the rest, doctors who investigate the "whole" must consider the interconnectedness of causal factors. This meaning of "the whole" (τὸ ὅλον) is similar to the claim in *On Places in the Human Being* that "in my opinion, medicine has been discovered as a whole [ὅλη], medicine of the sort that teaches both the tendencies and the *kairoi* in each case" (46.1, 6.342 L.). In both texts, holistic thinking about a topic involves an ability to appreciate its full complexity, employing a strategy of collection and division to understand how causal factors can interact with one another and thereby identify what is fitting in each case. In this respect, the discussion of the "Hippocratic" method in Plato's *Phaedrus* accords quite well with numerous texts from the Hippocratic Corpus, ranging from *On Ancient Medicine* (cf. *VM* 20, 1.620–624 L.) to *Prognostic* (cf. *Prog.* 6, 2.124 L.) to *Diseases of Women II* (cf. *Mul. II* 29, 8.310–312 L.) and even the cosmological *On Breaths* (cf. *Flat.* 6, 6.96–98 L.). Unlike the more specific testimony from the *Anonymus Londiniensis*, Plato's *Phaedrus* is of limited value for answering the so-called Hippocratic Question. When it comes to organizing all the factors that can influence disease, such an approach to "the whole" was a common feature of medical thinking in the fifth and fourth centuries BCE.

At the same time that we acknowledge that investigations into "the whole" do not have to involve the entire cosmos, we must not discount the extent to which this approach to medicine could engender a cosmological impulse. The arrangement of medical knowledge from the common to the particular, the classification of disease phenomena under a hierarchy of "starting points" (ἀρχαί) and "natures" (φύσεις), and the search for stable principles that transcend individual differences all made cosmological principles an attractive target of medical thinking. While balancing such factors as a patient's age, sex, habits, and physical constitution with the changes in the seasons, the geographical location, and the numerous interventions that Greek doctors had at their disposal, medical writers sought to isolate stable principles that could explain the respective "powers" of each factor to both act and be acted upon. In particular, they sought to explain why certain factors were "in accordance with the nature" (κατὰ φύσιν) of each other, which required appeals to analogical thinking that often bordered on the cosmological.[92] In *On the Nature of the Human Being*, Polybus claims that phlegm, being cold, increases during the winter because this humor is "most in accordance with the nature of winter" (τῷ χειμῶνι κατὰ φύσιν ἐστὶ μάλιστα, 7.1, 6.46 L.; cf. 7.4, 6.48 L., 7.7, 6.48 L., 8, 6.52 L.). With this phrase, Polybus implies that phlegm and winter both have a *phusis* that defines their specific powers, and that there is a commonality between their respective natures (i.e., the cold) that links these two items together. In the *Aphorisms*, certain constitutions are said to "have a *phusis* that is well or ill disposed to summer, while others have a *phusis* that is well or ill disposed to winter" (3.2, 4.486 L.). Similarly, different diseases and times of life are said to have "natures" that are well or ill disposed to different seasons, places, and modes of life (3.3, 4.486 L.). Like Polybus's analogy between phlegm and winter, these passages well illustrate how analogical thinking could enable the formulation of cosmological principles, as medical writers responded to concerns about the interconnectedness of causal factors by seeking out high-level commonalities between different categories of natural phenomena.

In addition to investigating how causal factors relate to one another, medical writers also deployed analogical reasoning to understand what is hidden inside the body. A number of these writers assert that one should begin with what is visible and then progress to what is invisible, drawing connections with outside phenomena to understand the hidden interior.[93] When thinking about fluxes, for example, the author of *On Ancient Medicine* says that the nature of this phenomenon is best understood by first observing fluxes that terminate outside the body. Thus, one should begin with fluxes that run out of the nose, then consider fluxes that terminate in the eyes, and finally presume that fluxes inside the body will behave in the same way (18–19, 1.612–620 L.). When the body itself does not provide a fitting analogue, the author encourages his audience to

---

[92] On the use of analogical thinking in early Greek medicine, see Regenbogen (1931), Diller (1932), Lloyd (1966), Lonie (1981: 77–86), Wenskus (1983), Langholf (1989), Schiefsky (2005: 320–327), and Wee (2017).

[93] For example, *VM* 18.1, 1.612 L., 22.3, 1.626 L., *De arte* 12, 6.22–26 L., *Aff.* 47, 6.256 L., and *Vict.* 11.1, 6.486 L. In *On the Art*, the author notes that "what escapes the eyesight is mastered by the eye of the mind" (11.2, 6.20 L., trans. Jones) – a sentiment shared by the author of *On Breaths* (3.3, 6.94 L.). Compare also Heraclit. DK 22 B54, Anaxag. DK 59 B21a, Democr. DK 68 B11, and Erasistr. fr. 77 Garofalo.

look further afield. In chapter 22, he gives his readers an example of the sort of analogical reasoning that doctors should employ (trans. Schiefsky):

> I hold that one must also know which affections come upon the human being from powers [δυναμίων] and which from structures [σχημάτων]. What do I mean by this? By "power" I mean the acuity and strength of the humors; by "structures" I mean all the parts inside the human being, some hollow and tapering from wide to narrow, others also extended, others solid and round, others broad and suspended, others stretched, others long, others dense, others loose in texture and swollen, others spongy and porous. Now which structures would best be able to attract and draw moisture to themselves from the rest of the body: the hollow and extended, the solid and round, or those that are hollow and tapering from wide to narrow? I think it is these, the ones that taper from wide and hollow to narrow. But one must learn these things from evident things outside the body [καταμανθάνειν δὲ δεῖ ταῦτα ἔξωθεν ἐκ τῶν φανερῶν]. For example, if you hold your mouth wide open you will not be able to draw up any fluid, while if you thrust your lips forward and contract and compress them, you will draw some up; and indeed, if you go on to apply a tube to them, you will easily draw up whatever you like. Again, cupping instruments that are applied to the skin and taper from wide to narrow have been crafted for the purpose of attracting and drawing fluid from the flesh; and there are many other examples of this kind.

In this passage, the author lists multiple examples of hollow and tapering structures that draw moisture to themselves, using these examples to establish a general principle about the nature of these shapes. In doing so, he not only arrives at a natural law that borders on the cosmological but he also follows the same method of reasoning we have already seen deployed by the cosmological doctors. His call to learn about the invisible by contemplating the visible can be directly paralleled in both *On Breaths* and *On Regimen*, as the author of *On Breaths* asserts that the universal power of *pneuma* is "invisible to the sight, but visible to reason" (3.3, 6.94 L.), while the author of *On Regimen* claims that we must "investigate the things that are invisible from the things that are visible" (11.1, 6.486 L.). The concluding assertion in *On Ancient Medicine* that "there are many other examples of this kind" (ἄλλα τε πολλὰ τοιουτότροπα) further recalls the arguments of the cosmological doctors. Like the author of *On Ancient Medicine*, the author of *On Breaths* emphasizes the generalizability of his claims by suggesting that many other examples have been omitted from his account, effectively inviting the audience to confirm his generalization by identifying further examples for themselves (15.2, 6.114 L.).

By drawing such analogies across different classes of phenomena, Greek doctors employed a methodology very similar to what we find in the *Epidemics*. They gathered together multiple accounts, noted the similarities and differences between those accounts, and isolated "one similarity" that unites and governs them all. The main difference, of course, is that instead of finding "one similarity" that applies to particular symptoms, these doctors isolated a general principle that applies to natural phenomena. In *On the Seed-Nature of the Child*, the author makes numerous appeals to analogical reasoning, leading him to formulate general principles that bear a striking resemblance to the theories of the cosmological doctors. Among these generalizations are the observations that "everything that is heated acquires breath" (12.2, 7.486 L.), that "everything which is heated is fed by a proportionate quantity of cold" (12.3, 7.486 L.), that "everything which is compressed upon itself grows warmer than what is loosely packed" (24.2, 7.520 L.), that "all winds come from water" (25.1, 7.522 L.), and that "all fluids produce foam when they are agitated" (1.2, 7.470 L., trans. Lonie). The same author also observes that his principles apply to both humans and other animals,[94] constructs arguments from induction very similar to what we find among the cosmological doctors,[95] compares human physiology to cooking, agriculture, and other nonmedical phenomena,[96] and inserts a long excursus on the growth and nutrition of plants,[97] all under the assumption that such observations will be of use to practicing doctors insofar as they point to principles that apply not merely to the phenomena under discussion but to all things in general. Even though the author does not ground his entire system in an explicit theory about the fundamental "powers" that govern the entire cosmos (beyond, of course, his opening assertion that "law governs all things"), he nevertheless could be grouped with the cosmological doctors. By relating his discussion of the body, health, and disease to highly generalized principles about the universe as a whole, the author of *On the Seed-Nature of the Child* exhibits the same cosmological impulse that seems to motivate the medical writers who ground their entire systems in the first principles of the cosmos.

---

[94] *Genit.-Nat. Puer.* 7.3, 7.480 L., 21.3, 7.512 L., 29.2–3, 7.530 L., 30.7–9, 7.536–538 L., 31.1–3, 7.540 L.

[95] *Genit.-Nat. Puer.* 12.2–5, 7.486–488 L.

[96] *Genit.-Nat. Puer.* 4.2, 7.474–476 L., 6.2, 7.478 L., 9.3, 7.482 L., 10.2, 7.484 L., 12.2–6, 7.486–488 L., 18.3–4, 7.502 L., 19.1, 7.506 L., 21.3, 7.512 L., 26.2, 7.526 L.; compare 24.2, 7.520 L., 25.3–6, 7.522–526 L.

[97] *Genit.-Nat. Puer.* 22–27, 7.514–528 L.

The only significant difference between the cosmological doctors and other medical writers from this period is the level of generalization to which they took their accounts. The best evidence for this continuity can be found not only in the structure of their texts, which all show an interest in dividing things into "classes" and then identifying the shared "nature" (φύσις), "power" (δύναμις), and "starting point" (ἀρχή) of everything that falls within each class, but also in the very principles that these doctors choose as the foundations of their systems. As we see in the cosmological principles formulated by the author of *On the Seed-Nature of the Child*, Greek doctors were interested in the fundamental nature of four topics in particular: heat, cold, moisture, and *pneuma*. Moisture and *pneuma* were associated with the "humors and winds" that were the primary agents of both nutrition and disease, while heat and cold were frequently considered the two factors most responsible for creating changes in these substances. We should not be surprised, therefore, to see Greek doctors treating these factors as the first principles of the universe. All four of these topics are combined in the system of Menecrates, who is reported to have held that humans are composed of four elements, two hot (blood and bile) and two cold (*pneuma* and phlegm) (*Anon. Lond.* XIX.19–XX.1). As I will argue in Chapter 5, a preoccupation with heat, cold, and bodily fluids lies behind the assumption in *On Flesh* that the hot, the cold, and the wet are the three elements from which all living things are composed.[98] *On Breaths* focuses on *pneuma*, while even *On Regimen*'s cosmology of fire and water reflects the association of heat/moisture with both life itself and the pathological properties of fevers and humors, which were already being designated with the terms "fire" (πῦρ) and "water" (ὕδωρ) in other texts from the Hippocratic Corpus.[99] These doctors may have elaborated their own theories with ideas and language borrowed from the inquiry into nature,

---

[98] *On Flesh* also describes the production of *pneuma* at 6.1–2, 8.592–594 L.

[99] Compare especially *Nat. Mul.* 2.1, 7.312 L. (καὶ πῦρ καὶ ὕδωρ αὐτὴν λαμβάνει, "both fire and water seize her") and the opposition between fire and water at *VM* 13.3, 1.600 L., *Nat. Hom.* 5.2, 6.42 L., *Morb. IV* 49.3, 7.580 L., and Arist. [*Pr.*] 1.57, 866b4–6. See also *Morb. II* 2.1, 7.8 L., *Aff.* 22, 6.232 L., and *Cord.* 12.2, 9.92 L., and the "fiery" conditions described at *Acut. App.* 13, 2.420–422 L. and *Morb. III* 7, 7.124–126 L. For similar references to heat, cold, moisture, and *pneuma* as the principal topics for doctors to study, compare Pl. *Plt.* 299d, where high-minded doctors are said to investigate "the truth about winds and things hot and cold," *Aër.* 1.2, 2.12 L., where doctors are instructed to learn the powers of both "winds" and "waters," with winds divided into the "hot" and the "cold," and *Morb. Sacr.* 18.1, 6.394 L., where the sacred disease is said to arise "from the things that enter and leave the body, and from the cold, the sun, and the winds changing and never staying still." Note also *Praec.* 9, 9.266 L., where "the healthy condition of a human being" is defined as "a nature that has naturally attained a movement, not alien but perfectly adapted, having produced it by means of breath, warmth and coction of humours" (πνεύματί τε καὶ θερμασίῃ καὶ χυμῶν κατεργασίῃ, trans. Jones). I will come back to this method for developing first principles in my discussion of *On Flesh*.

but their primary reason for engaging in cosmology was not to imitate the great thinkers of their day but to participate in the search for stable generalizations that defined the very essence of medical inquiry in this period.

4.7   The Limits of Medical Thinking

In light of this analysis, it seems safe to conclude that the cosmological doctors are not the intellectual outliers that many scholars have presumed them to be. Not only do these authors' theories of human pathology accommodate preexisting beliefs about anatomy and physiology, but their search for first principles is also rooted in the belief that medical knowledge advances when doctors gather together multiple accounts and look for commonalities that transcend individual differences. Of course, not all of their contemporaries would have been supportive of their conclusions, or even have endorsed their decisions to take their inquiries as far as they did. As we see most clearly in *On Ancient Medicine*, some Greek doctors were questioning precisely how far their colleagues should take their generalizations. One red line was apparently the contemplation of "the things on high" (τὰ μετέωρα), which became a buzzword in the Classical period for speculating about topics that are irrelevant and ultimately irresolvable.[100] In *Airs Waters Places*, the author preemptively defends his work against the charge of *meteorologia*. He asserts that anyone who makes this complaint should adjust their thinking and realize that "astronomy contributes a not inconsiderable part, but a very great one, to medicine" (2.3, 2.14 L.).[101] Similarly, the author of *On Flesh* assures his audience that he will only consider "the things on high" insofar as they pertain to his investigation of human beings (1.2, 8.584 L.). On the one hand, these authors acknowledge that they are engaging in inquiries that extend beyond the traditional limits of medicine. At the same time, they claim that such "outside" knowledge is directly relevant to the subject at hand. They might not dive as deeply into these topics as those who treat them as their primary area

---

[100] The classic study of how the Greeks talked about "the things on high" is Capelle (1912). For a more recent survey as it relates to *On Ancient Medicine*, see Schiefsky (2005: 137–139).

[101] For the meaning and use of "astronomy" in early Greek medicine, see Hulskamp (2012). A close echo of this passage can be seen in the discussions of medicine and helmsmanship at Pl. *R.* 6.488d–489c and *Plt.* 299b.

of expertise, but that does not mean that such inquiries do not, in some way, overlap with medical thinking.[102]

From these references to *meteorologia*, it becomes apparent that one reason for the pushback against "the things on high" was an increasing awareness of medicine's status as a set discipline. Medicine is delineated from other fields of learning by its subject matter and methods of inquiry, and it should only draw on other subjects insofar as they directly contribute to the treatment of patients. We have already noted that *On Ancient Medicine* seeks to distinguish medicine as a "craft" (τέχνη) from the speculations the author calls "philosophy." In *On the Nature of the Human Being*, Polybus similarly distinguishes his own account of human beings from "those who speak about human *phusis* beyond its application to medicine" (1.1, 6.32 L.). Like the author of *On Ancient Medicine*, Polybus associates nonmedical debates with issues that cannot be verified through perception, but he differs from this author insofar as he places elements labeled the "hot," the "cold," the "dry," and the "wet" squarely within the limits of the perceptible.[103] Polybus and the author of *On Ancient Medicine* come to different conclusions about what sort of speculations are permissible in medicine, but both authors agree that whatever generalizations one makes should be directly relevant to treatment. It is not until Polybus addresses theorists who talk about the humors that he refers to his opponents as "doctors." Similarly, when the author of *On Ancient Medicine* discusses the doctors and "sophists" who assert that medicine must be grounded in "what a human being is from the beginning, how it originally came to be, and from what it was compounded" (20.1, 1.620 L.), he asserts that such accounts "tend toward philosophy" (τείνει ἐς φιλοσοφίην) and adds that "whatever has been said or written about 'nature' by a sophist or doctor pertains less to the art of the doctor than to that of the painter" (20.2, 1.620 L.).[104] If a subject of inquiry does not in some way contribute to the treatment of human beings, then it obviously falls outside the realm

---

[102] For Aristotle's observation that doctors and natural philosophers have overlapping interests, see *Sens.* 436a17–b1 and *Resp.* 480b21–30, with the discussions of van der Eijk (1995) and Lloyd (2003: 177–179). For a notable instance of hesitating over whether an outside topic ought to be covered in a medical work, see *Art.* 8, 4.96 L., where the author is discussing the tendency of cattle to suffer dislocations after the winter. Compare also the rebuttal of the assumption that troubling oneself with incurable cases lies "outside medicine" (ἔξω ἰητρικῆς) at *Art.* 58, 4.252 L.

[103] See pp. 73–74. The author of *On Ancient Medicine* is not the only thinker who would have disagreed with Polybus's position that the hot, the cold, the dry, and the wet are open to perception: see, for example, Arist. *PA* 648a19–25 and Thphr. *CP* 1.21.4.

[104] For my interpretation of this sentence, see note 97 in Chapter 1. On the author's use of the term "philosophy," which probably does not hold the same resonance it has today, see p. 62.

of medicine. If, however, we can show that this information is clinically relevant, then a doctor is permitted to include even cosmological theories under the umbrella of "the physician's art" (ἡ ἰατρικὴ τέχνη).[105]

As we see in *On Ancient Medicine*, another reason for the pushback against "the things on high" was a fear of oversimplification. In the opening of this work, the author balks at the idea that all diseases can be attributed to "one or two" principles, and he repeatedly asserts that medical knowledge should be getting more, not less, complex. The author is concerned about oversimplification because, as we have already noted, Greek doctors were just starting to grapple with the "problem" of individualization, taking this issue so seriously that they were rethinking the very means by which they organized medical knowledge. For a profession that was rejecting older forms of medical writing because they insufficiently accounted for the differences between individual patients, to hear someone claim that all diseases are caused by a limited number of principles does not initially sound like a step in the right direction. As we noted in Chapter 1, the author of *On Fractures* takes aim at "wisdom-mongering" doctors who follow a preconceived notion instead of adjusting their treatments to fit the needs of individual situations. Such references to oversimplifying doctors were in fact a common trope in medical literature, as we also see attacks on such doctors in *Diseases I, On Regimen in Acute Diseases*, and even the cosmological *On Regimen*.[106] These passages suggest that the biggest contention in Classical Greek medicine did not center around whether or not doctors should engage in "philosophy," but rather the extent to which medical writers should engage in *generalization* and what forms these generalizations should take.

---

[105] There is another passage that has traditionally been cited in discussions of how Greek doctors started to separate medicine from "philosophy" (an overly simplistic dichotomy, as I hope this discussion is making clear). In *On Flesh*, the author observes that "there are some who, while compiling a written account of *phusis*, have said that the brain is the part that echoes" (15.4, 8.604 L.). Many scholars have taken the reference to "those who compile a written account of *phusis*" (φύσιν συγγράφοντες) as a synonym for "natural philosophers" (e.g., Willerding 1914: 50–51; Deichgräber 1935: 25; Kahn 1960: 6n2; Jouanna 1992: 96; Schiefsky 2005: 22n65; Laks 2008: 257; Holmes 2010: 3n15). As Jouanna (2002: 223) correctly observes, however, the author is probably not using *phusis* to denote "the nature of all things" but is instead employing this term in the more restricted sense of "(human) nature" – the regular meaning of *phusis* in the Hippocratic Corpus. Thus, the author is not citing "natural philosophers" such as Diogenes of Apollonia but rather the broader category of writers who have discussed the anatomy and physiology of human beings. For the use of *phusis* (without an adjective) to denote *human* nature, see *VM* 20.3, 1.622 L., *Epid. II* 6.15, 5.136 L., and *Epid. VI* 5.1, 5.314 L., and compare *Mul. III* 8.10, 8.442–444 L. It is also worth noting that *On Places in the Human Being* opens its account of human *phusis* with a discussion of hearing (2.1, 6.278 L.) – the same topic that is mentioned in this passage from *On Flesh*.

[106] *Morb. I* 16, 6.170 L., *Acut.* 7, 2.238–240 L., 43–44, 2.314–318 L., and *Vict.* 39, 6.534–536 L.

In all likelihood, there was no single reason why some Greek doctors would have been more ambitious with their generalizations than others. Some may have simply been more optimistic regarding the potential for this new mode of inquiry. Discussing a similar disagreement over the extent to which medicine could make use of exact numbers, Lloyd (1991b: 259) observes that "while some might suppose, and some did suppose, that there was nothing to stop medicine being turned into an exact inquiry, others resisted that ambition and insisted that though not perfectly exact, it was a *techne* nevertheless."[107] Another contributing factor for these high-level generalizations may have been an intellectual culture that rewarded some doctors for grounding their systems in a limited number of principles. Cosmological inquiries were a familiar part of Greek culture in the late fifth century BCE. Investigations into "the things on high" are referenced in popular genres such as comedy and tragedy, and we have already seen that some thinkers could captivate audiences with their presentations about the cosmos. In the *Protagoras*, the doctor Eryximachus is among those asking Hippias questions about "astronomical matters concerning nature and the things on high" (315c), and one can imagine that some Greek doctors who were already interested in these topics would have been more inclined to draw connections between medicine's own search for high-level commonalities and the first principles of the universe as a whole. In doing so, these doctors may have even earned the approbation of contemporary intellectuals who were eager to incorporate the *phusis* of human beings into their discussions of the cosmos and of everything within it.[108] Aristotle, for his part, refers to doctors who take their first principles from the study of nature as "clever and curious" (κομψοὶ καὶ περίεργοι, *Resp.* 480b21–30; cf. Iamb. *Protr.* 10, 54.13–16 Pistelli). He also distinguishes the "master physician"

---

[107] On this point, compare especially the acceptance of medicine's limited *akribeia* at *VM* 9–12, 1.588–598 L. and the attempt to push past this limited *akribeia* at *Vict.* 2.3–4, 6.470–472 L., 67, 6.592–594 L. For further references and discussion, see Lloyd (1987: 253–270).

[108] A few examples: Parmenides, and many after him, explored the nature of human embryology (DK 28 A52–54, B17–18). Empedocles discoursed on anatomy and physiology while narrating the creation of human beings (DK B96–109). Anaxagoras identified bile as the cause of acute diseases (DK 59 A105), and he centered his entire metaphysics around questions of nutrition and growth. Metrodorus of Lampsacus allegorized the *Iliad* in terms of both cosmic and biological principles, identifying Apollo as bile, Demeter as the liver, and Dionysus as the spleen (DK 61 A4). Diogenes of Apollonia mapped the vascular system and explained how doctors traditionally relieve pain by cutting into specific vessels (DK 64 B6). Philolaus attributed all diseases to blood, bile, and phlegm, and he further claimed that the purpose of respiration is to cool the body's innate heat (DK 44 A27, A28). Democritus used atomic structures to account for the effects of different flavors on the body (e.g., the moistening *dunamis* of the sweet) (DK 68 B135), and he also said that "inflammation" (φλεγμονή) is so named because it originates in phlegm (φλέγμα) (DK 68 A159).

from the "ordinary practitioner" (*Pol.* 1282a3–7), while Plato similarly differentiates "master" and "servant" doctors according to their ability to provide high-level explanations to their patients (*Lg.* 4.720a–e, 9.857c–e). By the late fifth century BCE, the concept of a "universal expert" or a "master of all knowledge" was being promulgated by such thinkers as Protagoras, Prodicus, Hippias, and Antiphon. Some of these theorists expressed views about the body, health, and disease alongside broader speculations about an impressive array of topics.[109] Some thinkers from this period even claimed to be universal experts in the "crafts" (τέχναι), thereby popularizing the idea that craft-knowledge can form part of a comprehensive understanding of all things.[110] Antiphon and Archelaus both combined cosmological speculations with discussions about *phusis* and *nomos*, the just and the shameful. In doing so, they showed that cosmology can serve as a foundation for more human-centered fields of inquiry.[111] Likewise, the use of cosmological specula-tions in eschatological contexts, most notably among the Orphics and Pythagoreans, would have provided yet another illustration of how cosmological principles could hold relevance for human lives. If Greek doctors were already immersed in these intellectual currents, it should come as little surprise that some practicing healers, driven by the growing interest in generalization within their own profession, would have thought that they, too, should begin their own inquiries by defining the first principles of all things.

One area where the definition of first principles would have been especially encouraged was the competitive context of public debates. In these exchanges, it was expected that the participants would advance bold theses in opposition to other thinkers. *On Breaths* was either written for such an occasion or at least modeled on the language and arguments of a public *epideixis*, while Eryximachus's speech boldly responds to the "incomplete" account of an argument offered by Pausanias. A familiarity with public debates is also apparent in *On Ancient Medicine, On the Nature of the Human Being, On Flesh,* and *On Regimen,* all of which invoke the need to situate one's own

---

[109] For the medical interests of these theorists, see Prodic. DK 84 B4 and Antiphon DK 87 A6, B2, B33–39, fr. 29A Pendrick. For their cosmological interests, see Protag. DK 80 B1–2, Gorg. DK 82 A10, B1–5, Prodic. DK 84 A5, A10, B3, Hipp. DK 86 A11, B7, Antiphon DK 87 B25–32, and *Dialex.* 8.

[110] For claims of universal expertise, see Protag. DK 80 B8, Gorg. DK 82 A19–20, Hipp. DK 86 A2, A6, A12, and *Dialex.* 8. Compare the *phusis-techne* analogies in *On Regimen* (11–24, 6.486–496 L.) and Eryximachus's presentation of himself as competent to speak not merely about medicine but about all the arts in general.

[111] For Archelaus, see Betegh (2016). For Antiphon's *On Truth*, see Pendrick (2002: 32–38).

"account" (λόγος) either in opposition to or in agreement with the claims of other thinkers.[112] Within this intellectual context, the first principles of health and disease would have been an especially fruitful topic for disagreement. We have already mentioned the beginning of *Diseases I*, where the first entry in a list of debate topics is the same question that was contemplated by the cosmological doctors: "whence all diseases arise in human beings." The author of *On the Art* shows how this format was primed to encourage cosmological thinking, as he defends medicine against the charge of not existing with a sweeping claim about the impossibility for anything that has a name to "not be" (2, 6.2–4 L.). After this surprising foray into Eleatic reasoning, the author assures his audience that "if anyone has not reached a sufficient understanding from what has been said, they can receive clearer instruction in other accounts. But regarding medicine – for this is what my discourse pertains to – concerning this, then, I will make my demonstration" (3.1, 6.4 L.). The author of *On the Art* leverages cosmological principles as part of a familiar rhetorical strategy – the argument *a fortiori*. Another *a fortiori* argument, also appealing to cosmological principles, appears in *On the Sacred Disease*, as the author asserts that the south wind must wield significant influence over the human body since its heat and moisture even dim the sun, moon, and stars (13.3, 6.384–386 L.).

It is important to stress, however, that whatever role such rhetorical considerations may have played in encouraging the formulation of cosmological principles, they were not the sole, or even the primary, inspiration for the daring generalizations of the cosmological doctors. These debates were not closed universes, divorced from all other forms of intellectual discourse, but arenas in which the participants both published and defended beliefs that were then applied in other contexts. The public *epideixis* encouraged the formulation of bold theses, but there is a significant difference between a thesis that is *bold* and a thesis that is *insincere*. In *On Ancient Medicine*, the author makes a number of bold statements, including his assertion that "it is impossible to have any clear knowledge about *phusis* from any other source than medicine" (20.2, 1.620–622 L., trans. Schiefsky, modified). This aggressive stance is presented in the sort of absolutist terms that were encouraged by the competitive context of public debates, but it also seems to have coincided with what this author genuinely believed about the acquisition of

---

[112] For further evidence of these authors' familiarity with public debates, see Lloyd (1979: 92–95).

knowledge about the body. If these debates were insincere, neither Polybus nor the author of *On Ancient Medicine* would have perceived their participants as such a threat to the art of medicine. Indeed, both Polybus and the author of *On Ancient Medicine* present their own arguments in the form of an *epideixis*, revealing just how central this format was for the exchange of ideas. These debates encouraged the advancement of bold theses, but they would not have been the only or even the primary reason why Greek doctors would have formulated such theses in the first place.

A similar response can be made to the suggestion that Greek doctors engaged in cosmological speculations primarily because they wanted to ingratiate themselves with wealthy clients. Social prestige may have been an *added* benefit for such high-level speculations, but to view concerns over one's place in society as the primary impetus for cosmological medicine is to ignore the changing priorities in medical thinking that I have surveyed over the course of this chapter. A "social climbing" explanation also fails to account for the limitations that medical writers often put on their own accounts (avoiding, for example, unnecessary speculations about "the things on high"), and it generally feeds into the tendency, still commonplace in modern scholarship, to prioritize "philosophy" over "medicine," effectively minimizing the ability of practicing doctors to set their own intellectual agendas.

As I have argued, the key factor for the turn to cosmological medicine in the fifth and fourth centuries BCE was the reorientation of medical inquiry around a search for commonalities. Like other medical writers from this period, the cosmological doctors believed that individual variation constituted a serious impediment to the art. They also believed that medical inquiry should proceed by sorting patients, diseases, and treatments into groups, and then comparing those groups with each other in order to isolate stable principles that are inherent to each. These doctors assumed that the most useful generalizations apply to the widest range of cases, and they strongly believed that the identification of these principles would bring the art of medicine to a state of near perfection. As the author of *On Regimen in Acute Diseases* asserts when introducing his own collection of general principles:

> I am confident that this inquiry is wholly profitable, being bound up with most, and the most important, of the things embraced by the art. In fact, it

has great power to bring health in all cases of sickness, preservation of health to those who are well, good condition to athletes in training, and in fact realization of each man's particular desire. (9, 2.244 L., trans. Jones)

For the cosmological doctors, the identification of first principles was a natural endpoint for these inquiries. Other factors may have encouraged them to be bolder with their generalizations than others, but the very drive to generalize originated in medicine itself.

CHAPTER 5

On Flesh

5.1 The Hot, the Cold, and the Wet (but Not the Dry)

Up to this point, our analysis has revealed some important observations about the cosmological doctors. First, we have seen that, contrary to the testimony of *On Ancient Medicine*, these doctors did not replace humors with *hupotheseis*, but they employed the treatment of "opposites with opposites" within a framework that considers both remote and proximate causes. We have also seen that the cosmological doctors frequently wrote about commonality and difference, emphasizing both the many differences between individual cases and the high-level commonalities that transcend these particular differences. Finally, we have offered an explanation for why these doctors were so interested in cosmology in the first place. On the one hand, they used their first principles to understand what is happening in the body, to predict the effects of certain actions, and to construct systems of preventive medicine that can ward off a disease before the patient falls ill. At the same time, these doctors were also motivated by a broader "cosmological impulse." Like other medical writers from this period, they believed that high-level generalizations are inherently desirable, and that the investigation of first principles is the best way to overcome the many variables that can change from one case to the next.

Having arrived at a reasonable explanation for how the cosmological doctors came to be, I would now like to look more closely at the structure of their systems. So far, we have encountered cosmological doctors whose theories about the cosmos were not worked out in any significant detail. Neither Eryximachus nor the author of *On Breaths* identified the physical elements from which all things are composed, as they instead prefer to focus on a single principle that has more "power" (δύναμις) than anything else. Polybus explicitly limits his own discussion of the cosmos to what can be verified through appeals to the senses, and he does not describe how anything other than the humors are composed of his four fundamental principles of the hot, the cold, the dry, and the wet. Our last two texts, *On Flesh* and *On Regimen*, develop more elaborate theories about the cosmos. In this chapter, I will focus on the first of these works, a short text that has long intrigued modern scholars with its curious intermixture of anatomy and anthropogony.[1]

The author of *On Flesh* begins by observing that the universe is divided into the hot, the cold, and the wet. He then describes how each part of the body, with the aid of the "fatty" (τὸ λιπαρόν) and the "glutinous" (τὸ κολλῶδες), arose from these three substances. In all, *On Flesh* describes the construction of over twenty different parts of the body. They include the bones, the sinews, the vessels, the windpipe, the esophagus, the stomach, the intestines, and the bladder (ch. 3); the brain and spinal marrow (ch. 4); the heart (chs. 5–6); the lungs (ch. 7); the liver (ch. 8); the spleen, the kidneys, the flesh, and the skin (ch. 9); the joints and synovial fluid (ch. 10); the nails (ch. 11); the teeth (chs. 12–13); and the hair (ch. 14). Each of these parts is constructed from different combinations of the hot, the cold, the wet, the "fatty," and the "glutinous." These ingredients are not just mixed with one another but acquire new characteristics through "cooking" and "congealing." The following passages provide a good illustration of the types of explanations this author constructs:

> The lung arose beside the heart in the following way: the heart, quickly heating the most glutinous of the wet, dried it out like foam, made it porous, and produced many small vessels in it. It produced small vessels because of this: whatever in the glutinous was cold was melted by the hot and became wet, while that from the glutinous itself became the tunic. (7, 8.594 L.)

---

[1] My translation of the title Περὶ σαρκῶν as *On Flesh* is to be preferred over the non-English *On Fleshes*. In Greek, both the singular and plural of σάρξ can be used to denote "flesh." Even a cursory reading of the Hippocratic Corpus will confirm this point. *Pace* Zwinger (1579: 124), Ermerins (1864: lxvii, lxxxiii), Adams (1886: 97), Kind (1936: 625), and Naddaf (2005: 29), there is no need to emend the title to Περὶ ἀρχῶν (*On First Principles*). Democritus is said to have written a work entitled *On the Nature of the Human Being, or On Flesh* (Περὶ ἀνθρώπου φύσιος ἢ Περὶ σαρκός, DK 68 A33), and in all likelihood the title *On Flesh* was shorthand for either a general account of the human body or, more specifically, an account of the "framework" of the body as distinguished from its moving parts. Compare Plato's reference to diseases befalling the "fleshy body" (σάρκινον σῶμα) at *Lg.* 10.906c. For the dating of *On Flesh* to the late fifth or early fourth century BCE, see Willerding (1914: 73–75), Deichgräber (1935: 27n4), Diller (1936: 377), Joly (1978: 182–183), Jouanna (1999: 391–392), de la Villa Polo (2003: 140–145), and Craik (2015: 47–48).

The liver came together in the following way: when much of the wet was left behind with the hot and without the glutinous or the fatty, the cold overpowered the hot and it congealed. (8.1, 8.594 L.)

The kidneys came together in the following way: a little of the glutinous, very much of the hot, and very much of the cold [were left behind], and the organ was congealed by this [cold] and became very hard and the least red, since much of the hot did not come together. (9.2, 8.594–596 L.)

In between these accounts of how the various parts of the body came to be, the author inserts several digressions on the structure of the vascular system (ch. 5), on the production of *pneuma* under the influence of heat (ch. 6.1–2), on nutrition in the womb (ch. 6.2–4), and on the means by which nutritive juices are distributed through the body (ch. 13). He also explains the workings of hearing, smell, sight, and speech (chs. 15–18) and concludes with the claim that all aspects of human life are governed by the number seven (ch. 19), an argument from induction that we have already mentioned in our discussion of *On Breaths* (see Chapter 3, pp. 85–86).

The author's specific decision to identify the hot, the cold, and the wet as the first principles of all things has never been properly explained. His cosmology is so poorly understood, in fact, that many scholars have not even reported these principles correctly. It is quite common, for example, to encounter the report that *On Flesh* constructs the body from the hot, the cold, the wet, *and the dry*, even though a separate substance labeled "the dry" (τὸ ξηρόν) is never actually mentioned in this text.[2] Many scholars have also reported that the author adopts a four-element theory of fire, air, water, and earth, and that he anticipates Aristotle in assigning pairs of qualities to each of these elements.[3] When we turn to the author's cosmogony, however, it becomes clear that he is not describing the four Empedoclean elements, treating these principles as the material basis of all things. Instead, he is narrating how the universe came to be separated into three major divisions (*aither*, earth, and *aer*), which are themselves large collections of other, more basic substances (2, 8.584 L.):

> I think that what we call "hot" is immortal; that it apprehends, sees, and
> hears all things; and that it knows all things, both what is and what is going

---

[2] Compare Dümmler (1889: 230), Gomperz (1901: 292), Lloyd (1963: 117), Schöner (1964: 53), and Oser-Grote (2004: 28).

[3] Compare Zeller (1862: 334n5), Dümmler (1889: 229), Spät (1897: 24), Heidel (1914: 185, 1941: 19), Willerding (1914: 55), Reinhardt (1916: 227), Deichgräber (1935: 32), Kind (1936: 628), Kahn (1960: 127, 150n1), Jouanna (1961: 453), Schöner (1964: 53), Lloyd (1963: 116–117, 1964: 93, 1966: 19n2, 76, 1979: 150), Ferguson (1969: 11), Hahm (1977: 127n8), Lonie (1981: 100), Thivel (1981: 256, 298), Longrigg (1993: 225), Schiefsky (2005: 22), and van der Eijk (2008: 401). See also Jones (1946: 25).

to be. Now most of this, when all was thrown in disturbance, withdrew to the uppermost circuit, and I think the ancients named this *aither*. The second portion below it is called "earth," cold, dry, and †causing much motion† (πουλὺ κινοῦν MS: *fortasse* πυκινόν Camden),[4] and much of the hot is actually within it. The third portion is that of the *aer* very close to the earth, very wet and very thick.

On reading this passage, one may wonder why so many scholars have claimed that *On Flesh* adopts a four-element theory very similar to that of Empedocles. This error can be traced back to a sixteenth-century interpolation, which adds a fourth "portion" so as to make the passage conform to the doctrines of Aristotle:[5]

> The third portion of the *aer* <took the middle position, being hot and wet. The fourth portion> is closest to the earth, very wet and very thick.

In 1936, Diller showed that this interpolation originated in the Latin translation of Calvus (1525), who is notorious for making insertions (some Christianizing) into his renderings of the Hippocratic Corpus.[6] By an unfortunate series of events, Calvus's expansion made its way

---

[4] The puzzling πουλὺ κινοῦν ("causing much motion") has long drawn suspicion, since (1) "fire, not earth, is the active element" (Heidel 1914: 180), (2) the earth is traditionally viewed as the most stable of cosmic masses (Hes. *Th.* 117, Emp. DK 31 B21.6, Archel. DK 60 A4.3, Diog. Apoll. DK 64 A5), and (3) even if the earth is conceived as being moved *by* something, we would expect κινούμενον, not κινοῦν. Betegh (2020: 58) suggests that the source of this motion is the hot that is present within the earth itself. Thus, the following clause would be an explanation of this unusual detail. Betegh's interpretation is further supported by *Carn.* 6.3, 8.592 L., where the hot is said to "provide the movement" (τὴν κίνησιν παρέχει) for all things. Although I have some sympathy with this reading, I also wonder whether πουλὺ κινοῦν may simply be a corruption of πυκινόν ("dense"). Earth is described as "dense" at Anaximen. DK 13 A5, A7, A8, Heraclit. DK 22 A1, A5, Parm. DK 28 A22 (cf. B8.56–59), Emp. DK 31 B21.6, Anaxag. DK 59 A42, B15 (cf. B16), Democr. DK 68 A95, Diog. Apoll. DK 64 A6 (cf. A1), Pl. *Ti.* 49b–c, Xenocr. fr. 161 Isnardi Parente, Chrysipp. fr. 527, 619 von Arnim, *Genit.-Nat. Puer.* 24.1, 7.518 L., Hp. [*Epist.*] 16, 9.344 L., and Gal. *Elem.* 1.453–454 K. Note also *Carn.* 3.8, 8.588 L. (quoted on p. 181), where the author explicitly associates "the cold" with the power to condense. This entire passage is very similar to Anaxag. DK 59 B15: "the dense, the wet, the cold, and the dark came together where the earth presently is, while the rare, the hot, and the dry withdrew to the farthest part of the *aither*." Paleographically, it is not difficult to see how ΠΥΚΙΝΟΝ could have been erroneously divided (ΠΥ-ΚΙΝΟΝ) and then expanded to Π[ΟΥΛ]Υ ΚΙΝΟ[Υ]Ν. For other attempts to emend, delete, or transpose πουλὺ κινοῦν, see Dümmler (1889: 228–229: [τὸ] πουλὺ κενεὸν *vel* κοῖλον), Heidel (1912: 222: πουλὺ κεινόν, 1914: 180: πολύκενον), Pohlenz *apud* Willerding (1914: 57n1: transpose καὶ πουλὺ κινοῦν to the end of the sentence – καὶ ἐν τούτῳ ἔνι δὴ πουλὺ τοῦ θερμοῦ <καὶ πουλὺ κινοῦν>), Deichgräber (1935: 2: πολὺ κινούμενον), and Kind (1936: 628–629, 635–637: transpose πολὺ κινοῦν to 6.1, 8.592 L. – θερμὸν <πολὺ κινοῦν> ἐστι τὸ πνεῦμα).

[5] I say Aristotle instead of Empedocles because it was Aristotle who assigned pairs of qualities to each element, associating air with the hot and the wet, earth with the cold and the dry, fire with the hot and the dry, and water with the cold and the wet.

[6] For a thorough review of Calvus's fabrications, including this one, see Witt (2018). This particular interpolation has also been discussed by Joly (1978: 205), Spoerri (1983: 61), and Primavesi (2009: 40n9).

into the Greek edition of Cornarius (1538), which was later copied out as *Parisinus graecus* 2255 (= E). For a long time, the pedigree of this manuscript "E" was unknown, and the interpolation thus made its way into the editions of Littré (1853 [1839–61]), Ermerins (1864), and Deichgräber (1935). Diller (1936: 371–372) finally set the matter straight in his review of Deichgräber's commentary, but by that time a good deal of damage had already been done. Deichgräber's commentary quickly became the standard edition, so even though Joly (1978) and Potter (1995) have both published corrected texts, many scholars still refer to a "four-element" theory when discussing this author's views. Given the enduring legacy of Calvus's interpolation, which still lives on in databases like the Thesaurus Linguae Graecae, it cannot be stressed enough that *On Flesh* identifies *three* portions of the cosmos. The author is not describing the four elements of fire, water, earth, and air; he is rather postulating a tripartite universe that comprises *aither*, earth, and *aer*.[7] Furthermore, it should be stressed that these three "portions" (μοῖραι) are not elements in themselves but are simply large collections of other, more basic stuffs.[8] The author's true first principles are the hot, the cold, and the wet, as we see in his subsequent anthropogony.

Of course, if all that survived of *On Flesh* were the opening cosmogony, we would not know for certain that the author's three principles are really the hot, the cold, and the wet. After all, instead of simply stating that "the cold moved to the center, while the wet surrounded it," this passage refers to the earth as both "cold" and "dry," while *aer* is "very wet" and "very thick." On the basis of these statements, it is tempting to place the "dry" and the "thick" on the same level as the hot, the cold, and the wet. It is critical to note, however, that when we turn to the author's anthropogony, the "dry" is never mentioned as an ingredient in human beings. Below, I have appended a full list of the mixtures that the author of *On Flesh* uses to construct the different parts of the human body. In this list, note that, in addition to the supplemental principles of the "fatty" (τὸ

---

[7] Compare Joly (1978: 181): "The author expresses very rapidly a physical vision of the Universe with three tiers: *aither*, air, earth."

[8] In other words, the author does not refer to "earth" as an element but rather "Earth" as a division of the cosmos. See Kahn (1960: 121–126) for this distinction between elements (earth, water, air, fire) and cosmic masses (Earth, Sea, Air, and Sky). Jouanna (1992: 100, 1999: 69–70, 278, 282) confuses these two categories when he calls the hot, earth, and *aer* "three constitutive principles of the whole" and "three elements." On the popularity of dividing the cosmos into earth, *aer*, and *aither*, see Guthrie (1962: 466, 470–471).

λιπαρόν) and the "glutinous" (τὸ κολλῶδες), the only other components are the hot, the cold, and the wet. A substance labeled "the dry" is nowhere to be found:[9]

hot + fatty + very little wet	=	bones (3.2, 8.586 L.)
hot + glutinous + not much cold	=	sinews (3.3, 8.586 L.)
hot + glutinous + much cold	=	vessels, windpipe, esophagus, stomach, intestines, bladder (3.3–5, 8.586–588 L.)
hot + fatty + cold	=	hard bones (3.7, 8.588 L.)
hot + fatty ι glutinous + cold	–	spongy bones (3.7, 8.588 L.)
cold + glutinous	=	brain, spinal marrow (4.1–2, 8.588 L.)
hot + much glutinous + much cold	=	heart (5.1, 8.590 L.)
hot + much glutinous + wet	=	lungs (7.1, 8.594 L.)
hot + much cold	=	liver (8.1, 8.594 L.)
much hot + glutinous + little cold	=	spleen (9.1, 8.594 L.)
much hot + glutinous + much cold	=	kidneys (9.2, 8.594–596 L.)
glutinous + much cold	=	flesh (9.3, 8.596 L.)
hot + glutinous + much wet	=	synovial fluid (10.2, 8.596–598 L.)
hot + glutinous + much wet	=	nails (11, 8.598 L.)
hot + fatty + glutinous	=	teeth (12.1, 8.598 L.)
hot + glutinous	=	hair (14, 8.602 L.)

For the author of *On Flesh*, dryness and density are not substances in themselves but secondary characteristics that arise from the presence of the hot and the cold. In chapter 3, the author writes that "the cold condenses, the hot disperses, and over a long time it also dries." Density, rarity, and dryness, in other words, do not come from the presence of the "dense," the "rare," or the "dry." Instead, they are produced by the actions of the hot and the cold on other substances. If I am correct in suggesting that the author referred to the earth as "cold, dry, and *dense*" (πυκινόν), we should expect that this reference to density would have something to do with the presence of the cold. Similarly, when the author describes *aer* as "very wet and very *thick*" (παχύτατον), we are probably to attribute this thickness to the fact that the *aer* is "very close to the earth" (ἐγγυτάτω πρὸς τῇ γῇ) and is thus colder than the *aither* up above.[10] As for dryness, the author of

---

[9] In this list, the reader should be aware that not all of these ingredients are present in the final product. For some of these recipes, the hot and the cold are what an Aristotelian would call "efficient causes," cooking or condensing the other materials before leaving them behind. This is why so many entries contain the "hot" as an ingredient. As the agent of cooking, the hot is essential for transforming other components.

[10] Note especially the repetition of the same two adjectives πυκνός and παχύς at Anaxag. DK 59 A70: τὸ μὲν μανὸν καὶ λεπτὸν θερμόν, τὸ δὲ πυκνὸν καὶ παχὺ ψυχρόν ("the rare and thin is hot, the dense and thick is cold").

On Flesh never refers to the "dry" as a substance in itself. This, too, is a secondary characteristic, but its relationship with the hot, the cold, and the wet is sufficiently complex to merit a longer discussion.

For the author of *On Flesh*, drying can arise in one of two ways: either the hot can consume the wet and thereby cause it to disappear, or the cold can congeal it to the point that it is completely solidified. The first of these processes is described in chapter 3, where the author claims that the hot, when applied for a long time, has the power to dry (3.8, 8.588 L.).[11] The second process by which drying can occur is mentioned later on in the text. In chapter 17, the author writes about the fluid in the eye: "If it is still hot, it is wet, but after it is cooled, it becomes dry like transparent frankincense" (17.3, 8.606 L.). In this passage, the author explains that the moisture in the eye maintains its fluidity by virtue of the body's innate heat. Once this fluid exits the body, the cold overpowers the hot and causes the fluid to dry out. Similarly, the author notes in chapters 8 and 9 that blood becomes dry when it is cooled after flowing outside the body:

> Whenever someone slaughters a sacrificial animal, the blood is wet as long as it is hot. But when it is cooled, it congeals. (8.2, 8.594 L.)

> If someone is willing to cut whatever part of the human body he wants, blood will flow hot, and it will be wet as long as it is hot. But after it is cooled by the internal and external cold, a skin and membrane arises. (9.5, 8.596 L.)[12]

From these passages, we can see that the author of *On Flesh* views drying as the product of both heating and cooling. The former involves the removal of moisture through evaporation, while the latter involves the removal of fluidity through congealing. A similar approach to drying can be found in *Diseases I*, in which the author writes that "both pleurisy without expectoration and pneumonia without expectoration arise from the same thing, from dryness; and both the hot, when it makes anything too hot, and the cold, when it makes anything too cold, dry" (28, 6.196 L., trans. Potter). Wittern (1974: 98–99) has observed in reference to this passage that the author of *Diseases I* does not require a separate substance labeled the "dry" to

---

[11] See also *Carn.* 3.1, 8.586 L., 3.3, 8.586 L., 7.1, 8.594 L., and 11.1, 8.598 L.

[12] Compare Democritus's explanation of how antlers are formed (DK 68 A153): "The damp material projecting outside the body is dried and hardened by the air and becomes horny, while the stuff which is still shut up inside remains soft; the former is hardened by the cold outside, the latter stays soft because of the heat inside" (trans. Taylor).

account for the production of dryness. The same applies to the author of *On Flesh*, for whom drying exists at both extremes of the very hot and the very cold.[13]

For the author of *On Flesh*, rarefaction is due to the presence of the hot, condensation to that of the cold. *Both* heat and cold, meanwhile, can account for an object becoming dry. As for "wetness," this is substantially different. Instead of existing at the two extremes of the hot and the cold, the "wet" arises from the simultaneous presence of both the hot and the cold. As the author observes in chapter 9, "The hot is in all the body, and the body has very much of the cold as well, much [of this cold being] in the wet. There is as much of the cold as can congeal the wet but has been conquered by the hot, with the result that it has been liquefied." In this passage, the author invokes an important doctrine regarding the relationship between the cold and the wet: the "wet" is not an independent principle, irresolvable into other substances, but it is in fact a melted form of the cold, a physical manifestation of the struggle between the cold and the hot. When the hot is stronger than the cold, it dissolves the cold to produce the wet. When the cold prevails, the wet is congealed and hence becomes "dry" (i.e., solid, non-fluid). The author cites the drying of blood as a "demonstration" (ἀπόδεξις) of this principle: "if someone is willing to cut whatever part of the human body he wants, blood will flow hot, and it will be wet as long as it is hot. But after it is cooled by the internal and external cold [τοῦ ἐνεόντος ψυχροῦ καὶ τοῦ ἐκτός], a skin and membrane arise" (9.5, 8.596 L.). Inside the body, the cold has been "conquered" by the hot and made to liquefy (νενίκηται, ὥστε διακέχυται, ὑπὸ τοῦ θερμοῦ, 9.4, 8.596 L.). Outside the body, the cold within the blood joins forces with the cold in the surrounding air, allowing the cold, in its turn, to conquer the hot. The end result of this "victory" is the cooling, drying, and condensation of the blood, since the cold is now more abundant and hence "stronger" than the hot.

---

[13] Compare Arist. *Mete.* 382b1 ("solidification is a form of drying," τὸ πήγνυσθαι ξηραίνεσθαί πώς ἐστιν). Aristotle also writes that "all things are dried either by being heated or being cooled" (*Mete.* 382b16–17), although the precise mechanisms by which he describes "drying" are not the same as what we find in *On Flesh*. A similar attribution of drying to both the cold and the hot appears at *Vict.* 49.1, 6.550–552 L. On the question of why blood remains fluid inside the body but solidifies outside the body, compare Arist. *PA* 651a4–12. As noted earlier (note 22 on pp. 13–14), the term that we normally translate as "dry" (ξηρός) can denote any situation where there is an absence of fluidity. This can involve either the removal of water (what we now tend to think of as "drying") or the transformation of a liquid into a solid.

The author's initial division of the cosmos into *aither*, earth, and *aer* can therefore be read, at least in part, as a reflection of these physical doctrines. Whatever contains a sufficient amount of the cold is *by default* both dry and dense. Whatever is "very wet," meanwhile, is also "very thick," since it is partially condensed by the cold, though not as much as to make it freeze and stop flowing:

EXTREME COLD	COLD + HOT	EXTREME HOT
(cold, dry, and dense) <====>	(wet and thick) <====>	(hot, dry, and rare)
"earth"	"*aer*"	"*aither*"

For a similar placement of the wet between the two extremes of the cold and the hot, we may compare the following passage from the *Aphorisms* (5.62, 4.554–556 L., trans. Jones):

> Women do not conceive who have the womb dense and cold [πυκνὰς καὶ ψυχρὰς]; those who have the womb watery [καθύγρους] do not conceive, for the seed is drowned; those who have the womb over-dry and very hot [ξηρὰς μᾶλλον καὶ περικαέας] do not conceive, for the seed perishes through lack of nourishment. But those whose temperament is a just blend of the two extremes prove able to conceive.

In his commentary on this passage, Galen complains about the reference to "two" extremes. Assimilating this passage to his own theories about nature, Galen prefers that we talk about *four*: the hot, the cold, the dry, and the wet (17b.864–865 K.). However, the author of this aphorism seems to adopt a view not unlike what we find in *On Flesh*. The cold and the dense lie at one pole, the hot and the dry at another, while the wet occupies a place in the middle, not a healthy point *exactly* in the middle, but another form of excess that would presumably lie closer to the cold and the dense (ψυχρὸν καὶ πυκνόν) than it would to the hot and the dry (θερμὸν καὶ ξηρόν). Since the author of *On Flesh* says that the wet and thick *aer* is "very close to the earth," it appears that he, too, views the universe in terms of two extremes: the hot and the cold.

5.2   The Body and the Cosmos

The obvious question that arises at this point is why the author of *On Flesh* would have wanted to isolate these principles in the first place. What makes him identify the hot, the cold, and the wet as the basic constituents of all things, and why does he not include the "dry" within this cosmic

framework? To understand the origin of this system, I suggest that we start
by recalling Polybus's stipulation that, for generation to occur, all four
elements must be present simultaneously, and that no single element can be
much stronger than the rest. In my discussion of that passage (pp. 70–71),
I noted that Polybus's primary frame of reference for this stipulation is what
happens within the body. When he turns to consider the universe as
a whole, he adopts a theory about the cosmos that mirrors his thinking
about the humors. Along the same lines, I would like to suggest that
a similar tendency to draw analogies between the body and the cosmos
lies behind *On Flesh*'s selection of the hot, the cold, and the wet as the first
principles of all things. The author specifically associates the "wet" with the
humors, while the powers he attributes to the "hot" and the "cold" are
influenced by his own professional use of these principles to manipulate
bodily fluids.

To start, we may note that Greek doctors commonly used the terms
"moisture" or "the wet" (τὸ ὑγρόν) when speaking about the humors.[14] In
On the Seed-Nature of the Child, the author introduces his discussion of
blood, bile, water, and phlegm by describing these humors as "four forms
of the wet" (τέσσαρες ἰδέαι τοῦ ὑγροῦ, 3.1, 7.474 L.; cf. *Morb. IV* 32.1,
7.542 L.), while the author of *On Places in the Human Being* first designates
the humors in the body as "the wet" (τὸ ὑγρόν) before formulating
a highly generalized principle about how "everything that is wet" (πᾶν
τὸ ὑγρόν) becomes thinner when it is heated (9.2, 6.292 L., trans. Potter,
modified):

> Fluxes also arise from excessive heat, when the flesh, on becoming rarefied,
> develops passages, and the wet [τὸ ὑγρόν], being heated, becomes thinner,
> for everything that is wet becomes thinner on being heated, and all flows in
> the direction of least resistance.

Not only did Greek doctors refer to the body's humors as "the wet," but
they also regularly identified heat and cold as the two most important
principles in therapeutics. A good example of this tendency to elevate the
hot and the cold can be found in *On the Application of Liquids*, a text in
which the author writes at length about the external application of these
two powers. Regarding heat, the author observes (1.1–2, 6.118 L.):

---

[14] Compare *VM* 22.6, 1.628–630 L., *Aph.* 5.63, 4.556 L., *Epid. VI* 5.5, 5.316 L., *Flat.* 10.2, 6.104 L., *Morb. I* 20, 6.178 L., *Aff.* 34, 6.246 L., *Loc. Hom.* 1.3, 6.276 L., 4.1, 6.282 L., 9.1, 6.292 L., *Morb. Sacr.* 16.4, 6.392 L., *Morb. II* 7.2, 7.14–16 L., *Int.* 43, 7.272 L., *Genit.-Nat. Puer.* 3.1, 7.474 L., *Mul. I* 57, 8.114 L., 73, 8.154 L., *Gland.* 2, 8.556 L., 5.2, 8.560 L., 7.3, 8.562 L., and *Cord.* 12.2, 9.92 L.

Heating of the body, all or a part, [is good for the following]: softening of hard skin, slackening of what is tense, extraction of fluid from flesh, evacuation of sweat; moistening through stimulation [προκλήσει Camden: προκλήση MSS: προκλύσαι edd.][15] e.g. nostrils, bladder, winds; to promote flesh, to tenderize, to melt, to reduce, to call back color, to dissipate color; it is promoting of sleep [when poured] both over the head and other parts; it is soothing of spasms and convulsions; it dumbs pains of the ear, eyes, all such things; warming what is cold, like pitch; for sores, except the ones that are bleeding or about to bleed, for fractures, for dislocations, for whatever else a physician uses linen bandages, for heaviness in the head.

Just after this passage, the author writes that when deciding on the temperature of an external application, "it is necessary to employ the instances of harm and helping as standards [κανόσι Camden: κἂν ὦσι MSS edd.], [keeping watch] up to the point of the [application] helping or harming" (1.2, 6.118 L.).[16] "Now moistening," the author continues, "is weak, while cooling and warming are strong, as from the sun" (1.3, 6.120 L.). The patient himself judges the right temperature, for "either of these causes harm" (1.3, 6.120 L.), and the harm that comes from heat and cold includes the following (1.4, 6.120 L.):

The hot causes harm in those who use it too much or too often [through creating] a softening of the flesh, powerlessness of the sinews, numbing of the mind, hemorrhages, swoonings – even to the point of death. The cold [causes harm through creating] spasms, convulsions, blackenings, febrile chills.

After describing the general effects of the hot and the cold on the body, the author describes their effects on specific parts. In chapter 2, he claims that some parts of the body are more "hostile" to these qualities than others. In general, this varying hostility depends on the preexisting inclination of the "nature" (φύσις) of each part to the hot or the cold (2.1, 6.122 L.):

The brain and all that [comes] from such [parts] is distressed by cold and takes delight in [the] hot, even though it is colder and more solid by nature, because most of these [things] are far from the [body's] own heat. For this reason the cold is hostile [πολέμιον] to bones, teeth, and sinews, while the hot is friendly [φίλιον], because it is from these parts that spasms, convulsions, and feverish chills arise, things which the cold produces and the hot stops.

---

[15] In favor of this emendation, compare *Liqu.* 2.2, 6.122 L.: "the hot is also [a source of] pleasures and stimulations [προκλήσιες] for the genitals, while from the cold pains and repulsions [arise]."

[16] On the notion of a "standard" that comes from the patients themselves, compare *Fract.* 1, 3.412 L., *Art.* 10, 4.102 L., *Off.* 16, 3.322 L., and *Loc. Hom.* 34.1, 6.326 L.

In another passage, the author writes about the ability of heat to relax the flesh, while the cold causes it to condense, comparing these powers to the effects of the hot and the cold on water (2.7, 6.126 L.):

> [Note] that after a hot [affusion] the body, being more dispersed [διαχυθέν], cools off, and after a cold [affusion], being more contracted [συσταλέν], heats up, just as waters that are to be cooled or heated do, on account of their fineness.

This passage closely recalls the assertion in *On Flesh* that the cold condenses while the hot disperses. This text also recalls *On Flesh* in its statement that dryness can arise from both the hot and cold (6.2, 6.130–132 L.):

> Any lesions that arise from the cold, or that become rough like millet, and then ulcerate, are harmed by cold and benefited by warmth. Things that are benefited by both are swellings in the joints, gout without ulceration, most spasms. Copious cold affusions over them dry up the sweating and numb the pain; moderate numbness resolves pain. Heat too dries and softens.

Taken together, these passages suggest that such fundamental powers as the hot, the cold, and the wet – powers that the author of *On Flesh* would elevate to the rank of first principles – were an integral part of medical thinking even for doctors who had little interest in cosmology.

Further supporting a clinical origin of *On Flesh*'s three principles is the fact that other doctors from this period were already reducing both the origin and treatment of disease to various interactions between heat, cold, and bodily fluids. In *On Places in the Human Being*, the author writes that fluxes from the head occur "when the flesh is excessively cooled or heated, or has an excess or a deficiency of phlegm" (9.1, 6.290–292 L.). In *Diseases II*, the author observes that the brain mortifies "if it is made too hot or too cold, or becomes more bilious or phlegmatic than usual" (5.2, 7.12–14 L.), while the author *On Regimen* notes that hot and cold baths have different effects on the body's moisture: hot baths cause this moisture to expand, while cold baths make the moisture contract (57, 6.570 L.). An even closer parallel to *On Flesh*'s cosmology can be found in the *Anonymus Londiniensis*. In this text, Hippon is said to have observed that the moisture in our body "changes through excess of heat and excess of cold, and so brings on diseases" (XI.35–38, trans. Jones). Hippon is also said to have held that this moisture changes "in the direction of the wetter, or of the drier, or of the thicker, or of the finer" (XI.39–41), echoing the same notions of fluidity (wet and dry) and density (thick and fine) that we find in *On Flesh*. As is the case with *On Flesh*, this testimony for Hippon does not attribute the qualities of dryness and density to separate substances labeled the "dry" and the "dense." Instead, dryness and density are outcomes of the hot and the cold acting upon the moisture in our bodies. In light of these passages, it is not difficult to imagine how a Greek doctor could have elevated the hot, the cold, and the wet to the rank of cosmic elements. When discussing the first principles of health and disease, many Greek doctors were already writing about the interactions between heat, cold, and bodily fluids.[17]

On Flesh's cosmology is so deeply informed by medical thinking that the other properties the author attributes to these principles can also be paralleled in humoral theory. We have already mentioned the author's description of a "struggle" between the hot and the cold (p. 183). This passage recalls a similar struggle between blood and black bile in *Diseases II*, in which blood is identified as naturally hot, while black bile is naturally cold (6a.3, 7.14 L., trans. Potter, modified):

> If this patient gains the upper hand [κρατήσῃ], so that his blood is heated either as the result of what is administered or by itself, the blood is lifted, dispersed [διαχεῖται], and set in motion [κινεῖται], it takes in vapor, foams, and separates itself from the bile, and he recovers. But if he does not gain the upper hand, the blood is cooled even more; when it has been cooled completely and given up its heat, it congeals [πήγνυται] and can no longer move, and the patient dies.[18]

What is most interesting about this passage is the author's use of the verbs διαχεῖν and πηγνύναι when referring to the dispersal and congelation of blood. These are the same verbs that appear in *On Flesh*'s observation that "the cold condenses [πήγνυσι], the hot disperses [διαχεῖ], and over a long time it also dries" (3.8, 8.588 L.).[19] The specific assertion that heat dries "over a long time" (ἐν δὲ τῷ πολλῷ . . . χρόνῳ) may have also originated in the author's own clinical experience. In *On Regimen in Acute Diseases*, the author writes, "If the pain is not dissolved by the hot applications, you

---

[17] Compare *Aër.* 3–4, 2.14–22 L., where the author opens his discussion of environmental factors by describing the effects of hot and cold winds on the waters that people drink. The qualities of the waters, in turn, are directly connected to the humors in our bodies, with some populations producing more phlegm as a result of the waters that they drink, and others producing more bile.

[18] Similar struggles between heat and cold – this time between blood and phlegm – are described at *Morb. Sacr.* 7–9, 6.372–378 L. and *Morb. II* 8.2, 7.16 L. Compare also *Morb. I* 24, 6.188 L., where both phlegm and bile are said to be colder than blood, and *Flat.* 7.2, 6.100 L., 8.2, 6.100–102 L., 8.5, 6.102 L., 14.6, 6.114 L., where a similar battle takes place between hot blood and cold *pneuma*.

[19] For the use of διαχεῖν and πηγνύναι to refer to the dispersal and condensation of the humors, see also *Aër.* 10.7, 2.48 L., *Morb. I* 24, 6.188–190 L., 33, 6.204 L., *Aff.* 16, 6.224 L., 34, 6.244 L., *Morb. Sacr.* 7.11, 6.374 L., 8.1, 6.376 L., *Fist.* 10.2, 6.460 L., *Vict.* 56.6, 6.568 L., 57.1, 6.570 L., 60, 6.572–574 L., 78.1, 6.622 L., *Morb. II* 8.2, 7.16 L., *Genit.-Nat. Puer.* 1.2–3, 7.470 L., *Morb. IV* 42.2, 7.562 L., 45.3, 7.568–570 L., 52.5, 7.592 L., 53.2, 7.594 L., and *Mul. II* 75, 8.366 L.

should not apply heat for a long time [πολλὸν χρόνον], for such a procedure is drying of the lung and productive of internal suppuration" (22.1, 2.272 L.). Similarly, the author of *On Affections* warns against the untimely application of heat to the patient, noting that "this is not useful, as the material only becomes dry" (7, 6.214 L., trans. Potter).

5.3 The Fatty and the Glutinous

So far, we have restricted our attention to the hot, the cold, and the wet. One of the most unusual aspects of this text, however, is the author's combination of these three factors with two auxiliary principles: the "fatty" (τὸ λιπαρόν) and the "glutinous" (τὸ κολλῶδες). Both of these principles are said to have arisen from the putrefaction of the cold under the influence of heat (3, 8.584–586 L.):

> When these things [i.e., the hot, the cold, and the wet] were thrown in disturbance [συνεταράχθη], they moved in a circle and much of the hot was left behind [ἀπελείφθη], here and there, in the earth, some in a great amount, others less so, and still others in a very small amount but many in number. As the earth was dried over time by the hot, these things, left behind [καταλειφθέντα], made putrefactions around themselves like tunics. And whatever from the earth's putrefaction happened to be fatty and to have a very small portion of the wet, as it was heated over time, it very quickly burnt up and became bones. Whatever happened to be more glutinous and to have a share of the cold, meanwhile, could not be burnt up when it was heated, nor could it become dry. For it did not have any of the fatty, so as to be burnt up, nor any of the wet, so as to become dry upon being burnt up. It consequently acquired a form [ἰδέην] rather different from the rest, and became sinews and vessels.

By claiming that putrefaction occurs when pockets of the hot are "left behind" in the earth, the author constructs yet another analogy between the elements and humoral theory. In medical texts, the humors were often said to stagnate, grow hot, and undergo putrefaction whenever they are "left behind" in the body. In *On the Seed-Nature of the Child*, blood that lingers in the uterus for five or six months is said to putrefy and turn to pus (15.6, 7.496 L.). Similarly, the author of *Internal Affections* observes that "when the head is filled with phlegm, it develops a disease and heat is produced, after which the phlegm putrefies in the head because it cannot move and flow away" (10, 7.190 L.). For the use of the verb καταλείπειν ("to leave behind") to describe "residues" of humors, there are many parallels in the Hippocratic Corpus. In both *Epidemics* and *On Joints*, it is noted that material that has been "left behind" after a purge (ἐγκαταλειφθέντα) regularly gives rise to additional complications.[20] In *On Humors*, diseases of the spleen are attributed to bile that has been "left behind" after the summer (ἐγκαταλειφθῇ, 13, 5.494 L.), while the author of *Diseases IV* specifically refers to a "fatty and light substance" (τὸ λιπαρὸν καὶ κοῦφον) that is "left behind" (καταλείπεται) when the body is heated from the outside (49.3, 7.580 L.).[21] This notion that residual fluids undergo putrefaction was so central to his thinking that the author of *On Flesh* returns to this analogy several times in this text. In chapter 3, he writes that the bladder was formed when much cold was "left behind" (ἀπολειφθέν) and the surrounding portion was heated and became a tunic (3.5, 8.586 L.). In chapter 8, he observes that the liver was formed "when much of the wet was left behind [ἀπολειφθέν] with the hot and without the glutinous or the fatty" (8.1, 8.594 L.). In chapter 13, he claims that excrement is produced when the thickest part of nutriment "is left behind [καταλείπεται] as a sediment and undergoes putrefaction" (13.2, 8.600 L.), closely paralleling the process that is said to have given rise to the fatty and the glutinous in chapter 3.

These two auxiliary principles of the fatty and the glutinous add an extra layer of complexity to the author's system. As we see in the above-quoted description of how bones, sinews, and vessels come to be, the fatty and the glutinous account for levels of dryness and density that cannot be explained by the powers of the hot and the cold to disperse and to condense, respectively. The fatty feeds and intensifies the hot, causing quick drying and hardening. The glutinous keeps matter "glued together," shrinking and condensing as it is heated. In chapter 4, the author supports these observations by drawing an analogy with the cooking of meat: "If someone is willing to roast the sinewy and the glutinous parts [i.e., the muscles and tendons], as well as the other parts [i.e., the fat], the other parts are quickly roasted, while the sinewy and glutinous refuse to be roasted, since they have a very small portion of the fatty. The very greasy and very fatty parts are very quickly roasted" (4.3, 8.590 L.).

Like the author's three main principles of the hot, the cold, and the wet, his two supplementary principles of the "fatty" and the "glutinous" seem to have a certain basis in medical thinking. In the Hippocratic Corpus, the adjective κολλώδης is frequently applied to bodily fluids. *On Glands* refers

---

[20] *Epid. II* 1.11, 5.82 L. (= *Epid. VI* 3.21, 5.302 L.), *Epid. VI* 2.6–7, 5.280–282 L., 7.7, 5.340 L., and *Art.* 50, 4.222 L., 63, 4.274 L.

[21] See also *Aff.* 31, 6.244 L., *Loc. Hom.* 10.6, 6.296 L., *Ulc.* 24, 6.428 L., *Vict.* 35.3, 6.514–516 L., *Morb. IV* 49.4, 7.580 L., and *Prorrh. II* 20, 9.48 L.

to a pungent and "glutinous" flux from the head (7.3, 8.562 L.), *Epidemics VII* to a sticky and "glutinous" fluid pressed out from a wound (61, 5.426 L.), *Diseases II* to a thin, scanty pus like barley juice, "glutinous" to the touch (60.2, 7.94 L.), *Diseases of Women I* to thick, sticky, and "glutinous" menses (3, 8.22 L.), *Diseases of Women II* to a "glutinous" flux from the joints (5, 8.246 L.), and the so-called appendix to *On Regimen in Acute Diseases* to a cold and "glutinous" flux from the head (9.1, 2.408–410 L.). As for λιπαρός, this adjective appears over a hundred times in the Hippocratic Corpus. It is applied to bodily evacuations (e.g., stools, urine, menses, and sweat),[22] to medical treatments (e.g., clysters, poultices, ointments, and fomentations),[23] and to various types of food.[24] Particularly noteworthy are the numerous passages in which patients are told to eat foods that are "fatty" while others are instructed to abstain.[25] These passages suggest that Greek doctors were actively attributing specific properties to the fatty, and that there were some physical conditions in which these properties were desirable and others in which they were not.

The fact that Greek doctors were already talking about the glutinous and the fatty in general terms suggests that the author of *On Flesh* did not invent these principles out of the blue. But what made him select these two principles in the first place, and why does he pair these principles with each other? Empedocles, Plato, and Aristotle all refer to "glutinous" (κολλώδης) or "sticky" (γλίσχρος) material that holds the body together,[26] while the Aristotelian *Problemata* include three passages in which the "glutinous" (τὸ κολλῶδες) responds to heat in a manner very similar to what we find in *On*

---

[22] Stools: *Prog.* 11, 2.138 L., *Epid. I* 27.2, 2.686 L., *Epid. III* 1.3, 3.40 L., 8, 3.86 L., 14, 3.98 L., 17.1, 3.104 L., 17.13, 3.140 L., 17.16, 3.148 L., and *Coac.* 621, 5.728 L. Urine: *Prog.* 12, 2.142 L., *Aph.* 7.35, 4.586 L., and *Coac.* 564, 5.712 L., 571, 5.716 L. Menses: *Hum.* 3, 5.478 L., *Mul. I* 26, 8.70 L., and *Mul. II* 6, 8.248 L. Sweat: *Prorrh. II* 4, 9.16 L.

[23] Clysters: *Acut. App.* 51, 2.494 L., *Nat. Hom.* 20.4, 6.78 L., *Mul. I* 109, 8.230–232 L., and *Mul. II* 48, 8.334 L. Poultices: *Aff.* 38, 6.248 L. Ointments: *Acut. App.* 65, 2.520 L., *Liqu.* 6.4, 6.132 L., *Nat. Mul.* 58, 7.398 L., *Mul. I* 35, 8.84 L., and *Mul. II* 24, 8.288 L., 36, 8.322 L., 38, 8.324 L., 40–41, 8.326 L. Fomentations: *Morb. III* 12, 7.132 L.

[24] *Aff.* 47, 6.258 L., 55, 6.266 L., *Vict.* 39.1, 6.534 L., 42.3, 6.540 L., 45.3, 6.544 L., 51, 6.554 L., 55.5, 6.564 L., 56.2–8, 6.566–570 L., and *Int.* 6, 7.180 L. For more passages, see note 25.

[25] Eat τὰ λιπαρά: *Aff.* 23, 6.234 L., 40, 6.250 L., *Loc. Hom.* 18, 6.310 L., 28.1, 6.320 L., *Vict.* 59.2, 6.572 L., 68.5, 6.596 L., 82.4, 6.632 L., *Morb. II* 27.6, 7.44 L., 47a.5, 7.66 L., 47b.2, 7.68 L., 48.4, 7.74 L., 64.5, 7.98 L., 68.2, 7.104 L., *Morb. III* 15, 7.140 L., 17, 7.156 L., *Int.* 1, 7.168 L., 20–21, 7.216–218 L., 29, 7.244 L., 40–42, 7.266–270 L., 51, 7.296 L., *Mul. I* 16, 8.54 L., 45, 8.104 L., 66, 8.138 L., and *Mul. II* 6, 8.250 L. Abstain from τὰ λιπαρά: *Art.* 50, 4.220 L., *Epid. VII* 68, 5.432 L., *Vict.* 81.2, 6.628 L., *Morb. II* 47b.2, 7.68 L., 53.3, 7.82 L., 55.6, 7.86 L., 71.2, 7.108 L., 72.2, 7.110 L., *Morb. III* 16, 7.148 L., *Int.* 2–3, 7.174–176 L., 10, 7.190 L., 30, 7.246 L., *Nat. Mul.* 9–10, 7.324–326 L., 12, 7.330 L., and *Mul. II* 9, 8.254 L., 60, 8.350 L. Note also the many prescriptions to eat or abstain from foods that are "greasy" (πίων) and "oily" (ἐλαιηρός).

[26] Emp. DK 31 B96.4, Pl. *Ti.* 82d–e, and Arist. *GA* 737a35–b7; compare Emp. DK 31 B34.

Flesh.[27] "Fatty" substances are often said to fuel and intensify heat, most notably in reference to the addition of oil to a fire.[28] In the *Cratylus*, λιπαρός and κολλώδης are mentioned side by side, but only within a list of adjectives in which the letter lambda conveys a sense of slipping and gliding (427b). A great deal of energy has been spent on trying to identify the source of these two principles.[29] Building off of the many uses of these adjectives to describe biological fluids, I would like to suggest that *On Flesh*'s two principles of the "fatty" and the "glutinous" reflect the common opposition between bile and phlegm.

In the Hippocratic Corpus, bile is frequently associated with substances that are "fatty,"[30] while phlegm is described as "glutinous" or "sticky."[31] Both bile and the "fatty" can fuel and intensify heat,[32] while phlegm has a tendency to condense and harden when it is heated.[33] In *Diseases IV*, there are two passages that perfectly illustrate both of these associations:

> With the phlegm acting as a glue [κόλλης γινομένης τοῦ φλέγματος], what is melted [sc. by the heat] is expelled by the urine, while the sediment falls together, grows dense, and becomes solid like iron. (55.4, 7.602 L.)

> As the body is heated, it is primarily the watery component, which is most hostile to fire, that is evaporated as a result, while what is left behind [καταλείπεται] is the fatty and light component [τὸ λιπαρὸν καὶ κοῦφον], which is bilious [χολῶδες], and which is the primary nutriment for fire. (49.3, 7.580 L.)

---

[27] Arist. [*Pr.*] 2.22, 868a35–b11, 21.6, 927b6–14, 21.12, 928a11–33.

[28] For example, Arist. [*Col.*] 791b22–24, [*Pr.*] 23.15, 933a19–20, *Metaph.* 1046a24–25, and Thphr. *Ign.* 21.

[29] Compare Willerding (1914: 62), Heidel (1914: 185–186), Deichgräber (1935: 35), Kind (1936: 631–632), Thivel (1981: 251n285, 266n329), Orelli (1998: 135), and Oser-Grote (2004: 29).

[30] For example, *Prog.* 11, 2.138 L., *Epid. III* 8.1, 3.86 L., *Epid. VI* 5.8, 5.318 L., 6.1, 5.322 L., *Aff.* 47, 6.258 L., and *Morb. IV* 49.3, 7.580 L., 51.2–3, 7.584 L. Compare the claim at *Acut.* 53, 2.336–342 L. that melicrat (a beverage mixed with honey) contains "something fatty" (σμηγματῶδές τι) and assists in the evacuation of bile.

[31] For example, *Epid. VII* 84, 5.442 L. ("sticky like phlegm," γλίσχρος ὡς φλέγμα). See also *Acut.* 16.2, 2.258–260 L., 17.2–3, 2.262 L., 53.1, 2.336–338 L., *Art.* 40, 4.174 L., *Nat. Hom.* 7.2, 6.46 L., *Nat. Mul.* 17, 7.336 L., *Morb. IV* 35.2, 7.548 L., 55.4, 7.602 L., *Mul. I* 58, 8.116 L., Arist. *HA* 515b16–18, and especially the "glutinous" and "sticky" fluxes from the head at *Acut. App.* 9.1, 2.408–410 L., *Epid. III* 13.4, 3.94 L., *Epid. IV* 18, 5.156 L., and *Gland.* 7.3, 8.562 L. For the classification of specific humors as "glutinous," see also Praxag. fr. 38, 53 Steckerl.

[32] For the ability of the fatty to fuel and intensify heat, see *Aff.* 38, 6.246–248 L., *Vict.* 45.3, 6.544 L., 51, 6.554 L., 55.5, 6.564 L., 56.1, 6.564 L., *Morb. IV* 49.3, 7.580 L., and *Hebd.* 24. For the attribution of this same property to bile, see *VM* 19.5, 1.618 L., *Aër.* 9.5, 2.40 L., *Nat. Hom.* 15.2, 6.66 L., *Morb. I* 29, 6.198 L., *Morb. IV* 49.3–4, 7.580 L., and *Hebd.* 28.

[33] *Morb. I* 28, 6.196–198 L., *Vict.* 54.2, 6.558 L., *Int.* 14, 7.202 L., and *Morb. IV* 55.4, 7.602 L.

Not only do these two passages specifically identify phlegm as "gluey" and bile as "fatty" but they also describe the responses of bile and phlegm to being heated in terms remarkably similar to what we see in *On Flesh*. As in *On Flesh*, the author claims that phlegm acts as a "glue" (κόλλα), holding matter together and causing it to shrink when it is heated. Bile, meanwhile, is "fatty and light" (λιπαρὸν καὶ κοῦφον; cf. *Morb. IV* 51.2–3, 7.584 L.), and it contributes the same fuel for intense burning that we see in *On Flesh*.

These connections between bile and the "fatty" and between phlegm and the "glutinous" help to explain why the author of *On Flesh* decided to pair these two principles with each other. These associations can also shed light on one of the most obscure passages in *On Flesh*. In chapter 4, the author defines two "mother-cities" within the body, one of which gives rise to "the cold and the glutinous," while the other gives rise to "the fatty":

> The brain is the mother-city [μητρόπολις] of the cold and the glutinous, while the hot is the mother-city of the fatty. For on being heated, the first of all things to arise when being dispersed is the fatty.

So far as I am aware, no one has adequately explained what the author is trying to say in this passage. Ermerins (1864: 505) marks the whole passage as "altogether absurd" and pointedly asks, "Who would oppose the brain with the hot?" Other scholars have been equally perplexed, often complaining about the text's egregious lack of parallelism.[34] In particular, it has been pointed out that the author invokes a specific part of the body (i.e., the brain) to serve as the "mother-city" for two of his fundamental principles (the cold and the glutinous), while two other principles (the hot and the fatty) are not attached to a specific part but are rather arranged *hierarchically* so that one of them (i.e., the hot) is the "mother-city" of the other (i.e., the fatty). In light of this asymmetry, many scholars have concluded that the text must be defective, with Ermerins (1864) inserting "the marrow" (ὁ μυελός), Heidel (1914) "the heart" (ἡ καρδίη), and Kind (1936) "the fat" (ὁ σίαλος) as a more appropriate "mother-city" for the fatty. Heidel and Kind also change the nominative τὸ θερμόν to the genitive τοῦ θερμοῦ, thereby making their preferred reservoirs the "mother-city" of the fatty *and* the hot. If we accept that the author associates the glutinous with phlegm and the fatty with bile, however, then we can not only explain how the brain may be called the

---

[34] For example, Heidel (1914: 183–184), Deichgräber (1935: 37), Kind (1936: 678–680), and Huffman (1993: 195–197).

"mother-city" of the cold and glutinous while the hot is the "mother-city" of the fatty, but we can also understand – and this seems more important – why the author of *On Flesh* would have cared about these mother-cities in the first place.

That "cold and glutinous" phlegm was thought to flow from the head is widely recognized and hardly needs further discussion. The author of Diseases II plainly states that "phlegm descends from the head" (11, 7.18 L.), and we have already cited a passage from the "appendix" to *On Regimen in Acute Diseases* in which the author refers to a "cold and glutinous" flux that originates in the head. From these passages, we can surmise that the brain is the "mother-city" of the cold and glutinous insofar as diseases that are caused by the "cold and glutinous" humor (i.e., phlegm) have their origin in the brain. This is where the humor "separates out," and any treatment that targets a phlegmatic disease must consider both the humor and this source.[35] On analogy with this description of the brain as the "mother-city" of the cold and glutinous, we should assume that by calling the hot the "mother-city" of the fatty, the author of *On Flesh* intends to say three things: (1) that diseases that are caused by the fatty humor (i.e., bile) have their origin in the hot, (2) that this is where the bile "separates out," and (3) that any treatment that aims to eradicate bilious diseases must target both the humor and this source. When we look to other texts from the Hippocratic Corpus, this is precisely what we find.

We are repeatedly told that bilious diseases are set in motion by heat, that this heat engenders diseases by causing the bile to "separate out," and that doctors should combine the purging of bile with the application of cooling treatments to counteract the source of this *apokrisis*. We see as much in the above-quoted passage from *Diseases IV*, in which the author writes that the heating of the humors causes the watery component (τὸ ὑδρωποειδές) to evaporate, while the bilious (τὸ χολῶδες) is left behind (49.3, 7.580 L.). Other works in the Hippocratic Corpus also refer to this process of bile-production, most notably in reference to the heating of moisture in the belly. In Chapter 3, we noted that the heating of stagnant moisture in the belly was commonly thought to produce "breaths" (p. 105). As these breaths make their way to the head, they leave a residue behind, and this residue is concentrated bile.[36] Other texts refer to the production of bile in the lungs, the bladder, the uterus, and other parts, associating its

---

[35] For the treatment of diseases at their "source," see pp. 76–79.

[36] Compare *Acut.* 50, 2.332 L., *Acut. App.* 48–51, 2.486–496 L., *Aff.* 11, 6.218–220 L., 20, 6.228–230 L., 47, 6.258 L., *Morb. II* 69, 7.104–106 L., *Morb. III* 14, 7.134 L., *Nat. Mul.* 89, 7.408 L., *Mul. I* 2, 8.18 L., 8, 8.36 L., 16, 8.54 L., and *Judic.* 5, 9.276 L. See also *VM* 19.5, 1.618 L., *Aër.* 7.2, 2.26 L., *Epid. III*

appearance with the separating out of a watery exhalation from a fatty, bilious residue.[37] Once the watery component is separated out, it can be thickened and transformed into phlegm.[38] The bile, meanwhile, causes fevers to flare up, producing both intermittent paroxysms and the constant burning of "ardent" fevers.[39]

Since the lower cavity was thought to be a major site of bile-production, Greek doctors carefully inspected the vomit, stools, and urine of their patients, checking whether the bile was still mixed with other humors or whether it had become "unmixed" (ἄκρητος) and "concentrated" (κατακορής).[40] In some of these passages, "unmixed" evacuations are described as fatty (λιπαρός),[41] while evacuations that contain a mixture of bile and phlegm are said to be sticky (γλίσχρος).[42] An analogy with the

17.3, 3.116 L., 17.13, 3.138 L., *Aph.* 7.42, 4.588 L., *Epid.* V 18, 5.218 L., *Epid.* VII 1, 5.364–366 L., and *Prorrh. I* 117, 5.548–550 L.

[37] *Morb. I* 18, 6.172 L., 29, 6.200 L., *Mul. II* 12, 8.262 L., *Cord.* 11, 9.88–90 L., and *Oss.* 17, 9.192 L.

[38] Many authors in the Hippocratic Corpus seem to have envisioned the "separating out" of phlegm as a two-stage process involving an alternation of heat and cold: the heat first separates out the watery component, then the cold makes this watery component condense into phlegm. Compare *Aër.* 3.1–2, 2.16 L., 7.2, 2.26 L., *Acut.* 16.2, 2.258–260 L., 17.2–3, 2.262 L., *Epid.* VII 11, 5.382 L., *Nat. Hom.* 7.6, 6.48 L., *Flat.* 10.1–2, 6.104–106 L., *Morb. Sacr.* 10.2, 6.378 L., 13.4, 6.386 L., and *Morb. IV* 52.1–2, 7.590 L. This two-stage process may be reflected in *On Flesh*'s assertion that "on being heated, *the first of all things* [τὸ πρῶτον πάντων] to arise when being dispersed is the fatty" (4.1, 8.588 L.). Note also the description of rainwater at *Aër.* 8, 2.32–36 L., where the production of rain follows the same two-stage process of evaporation and condensation. The author of this text in fact seems to draw an implicit analogy between rainwater and phlegm, as he observes that rainwater contains certain impurities that can give rise to a sore throat, coughing, and hoarseness. For an explicit expression of this rain–phlegm analogy, see *Anon. Lond.* XVIII.36–37 (Philolaus) and Arist. *PA* 652b33–653a8. At *Vict.* 89.2, 6.644–646 L., an *apokrisis* of phlegm is said to produce dream visions of a mist or a cloud.

[39] *Nat. Hom.* 15.2, 6.66 L., *Morb. I* 29, 6.198 L., *Morb. IV* 49.4, 7.580 L., and *Hebd.* 28.

[40] The adjectives "unmixed" (ἄκρητος) and "concentrated" (κατακορής) are only applied to bilious evacuations, never to evacuations that are phlegmatic (the only exception appears to be the highly schematized discussion of purgative drugs at *Nat. Hom.* 6.3, 6.44–46 L.). For references to bilious evacuations as "unmixed," see *Acut.* 53.2, 2.340–342 L., 54.1, 2.342 L., *Epid. I* 2.3, 2.608 L., 27.2, 2.684–686 L., 27.4–5, 2.692–694 L., 27.9, 2.704 L., 27.13, 2.714 L., *Epid. III* 1.1, 3.26 L., 1.5–6, 3.48–52 L., 17.3, 3.116 L., 17.13, 3.140 L., *Fract.* 43, 3.554 L., *Art.* 19, 4.132 L., 31, 4.146 L., *Mochl.* 9, 4.354 L., *Epid. IV* 2, 5.144 L., *Epid. V* 61, 5.242 L., 79, 5.248 L., 88, 5.252 L., 98, 5.256 L., *Epid. VII* 1, 5.364 L., 29, 5.400 L., 33, 5.402 L., 43, 5.410 L., 67a, 5.430 L., 92, 5.448 L., *Coac.* 39, 5.594 L., 389, 5.668–670 L., 437, 5.682 L., 549, 5.708 L., and *Nat. Hom.* 6.46 L., and compare *Prog.* 18, 2.158 L. Contrast the references to "watery bilious" (ὑδατόχολος) evacuations at *Epid. I* 27.10, 2.706 L., *Epid. III* 17.2, 3.110 L., *Prorrh. I* 81, 5.530 L., and *Coac.* 67, 5.598 L., 131, 5.610 L., and the designation of watery stools as "non-bilious" (ἄχολος) at *Epid. II* 3.1, 5.100 L., *Epid. IV* 5, 5.152 L., 45, 5.186 L., and *Prorrh. I* 98, 5.536–538 L.

[41] For example, *Epid. I* 27.2, 2.686 L. (διαχωρήματα ἄκρητα, χολώδεα, λεῖα, λιπαρά, "stools unmixed, bilious, smooth, fatty"). See also *Epid. III* 14.3, 3.98 L., 17.1, 3.104 L., 17.16, 3.148 L.

[42] For example, *Prog.* 11, 2.138 L., *Epid. IV* 18, 5.154 L., 26–27, 5.170–172 L., and *Coac.* 564, 5.712 L., 612, 5.726 L. Note also *Epid. II* 3.11, 5.114 L. ("He passed sticky material on the eleventh day, and the little surrounding fluid was bilious," trans. Smith), and the description of evacuations as "gluey" (γλοιώδεις) at *Epid. VII* 2, 5.368 L.

practice of mixing water with wine probably reinforced this theory about "mixed" and "unmixed" bile. Just as wine is "stronger" and more likely to heat the body when not diluted with water, so bile is "stronger" and more likely to cause problems when separated out from its watery component. Many texts in the Hippocratic Corpus actually prescribe either unmixed wine (οἶνος ἄκρητος) or mixed/watery wine (οἶνος κεκρημένος/ὑδαρής) for problems in the belly, where unmixed wine counteracts a concentration of water, while watery wine counteracts a concentration of bile. These prescriptions can be reversed, however, when the wine is followed by a purge, as Greek doctors often thought that purges draw out humors through the principle of "like to like."[43]

Once the bile becomes fully unmixed (i.e., fully separated from the watery component), many authors suggest that the disease has reached a critical point. Depending on the circumstances, the bile could now be fully evacuated, it could migrate to another location in the body, or it could be further heated and dried to produce black bile. In *Airs Waters Places*, the author describes the production of black bile in the same manner that *Diseases IV* describes the production of bile: "of the bile, the wettest and most watery part is consumed [sc. by heat], while the thickest and most pungent part is left behind" (10.12, 2.50 L.).[44] From these passages, we can see that bile and its derivatives were commonly believed to arise from the heating and drying of fluids within the body. This is in fact why bile came to be associated with dryness,[45] why it was said to arise most abundantly in the summer,[46] and why bilious diseases were often

---

[43] Compare especially *Nat. Hom.* 6.3, 6.44–46 L. and S. fr. 854 Radt.

[44] For the transformation of bile into black bile, see also *Prog.* 14, 2.144–146 L., *Epid. II* 3.15, 5.116 L., *Epid. VI* 6.1, 5.322 L., 6.14, 5.330 L., *Morb. I* 30, 6.200 L., *Anon. Lond.* XIX.33–40 (Menecrates of Syracuse), and Arist. [*Pr.*] 1.12, 860b15–25. Compare also *Nat. Hom.* 7.9, 6.50 L.

[45] Among the tell-tale signs of bilious affections were thirst and a dry, bitter tongue: *Epid. III* 17.3, 3.112–116 L., 17.9, 3.128 L., *Epid. V* 80, 5.250 L., 98, 5.256 L., *Epid. VI* 5.8, 5.318 L., *Epid. VII* 3, 5.368–370 L., 84–85, 5.442–444 L., *Morb. I* 29, 6.198 L., *Aff.* 11, 6.218–220 L., 15, 6.222 L., *Vict.* 82.1, 6.630 L., *Superf.* 34, 8.504–506 L., and *Hebd.* 28. Compare also *Aër.* 10.6, 2.46 L., Arist. [*Pr.*] 1.9, 860a27–28, and Polybus's assertion that both yellow bile and black bile are "dry" (p. 71). Note, however, that the inherent dryness of bile is independent of the question of whether bile is naturally hot or cold. To say that bile is the residue left behind after another humor has evaporated does not necessitate a natural temperature for bile itself. For disagreement over the inherent temperature of bile, see Arist. *PA* 648a31–33.

[46] At *Hum.* 14, 5.496 L., the summer is explicitly said to be χολοποιός ("productive of bile"). Since the summer, being hot and dry, lacks moisture of its own, the only way that it could *make* bile is by heating and drying bodily fluids. The association of black bile with autumn (see pp. 71–72) may also have something to do with the fact that autumn is a "dry" season. Thus, the bile that arises in the summer will be further dried and transformed into black bile in the autumn.

treated with cooling agents.[47] These cooling agents were not directed against the bile itself but against the heat that was separating the bile out. In the same way that a flux of phlegm would be counteracted by attending to the head, an excessive production of bile was counteracted by attending to the heat.[48] And it is precisely with an eye to treatment that the author of *On Flesh* refers to the brain as the "mother-city" of the cold/glutinous and to the hot as the "mother-city" of the fatty. Just as a mother-city can always send out another colony, a disease will continue to ravage the body until the doctor has treated both the affection and its source.[49]

5.4 Anthropogony As a Guide to Treatment

If a theory of pathology lies behind this riddling passage, we should ask to what extent the rest of *On Flesh* is written with an eye to pathogenesis. To start, it is worth noting that the specific parts that the author describes all have special significance within Greek theories of health and disease. Not only does the author describe the vessels and hollows through which both *pneuma* and humors can travel (3.3–6, 8.586–588 L.), but most of the other parts that he emphasizes (e.g., the lungs, the flesh, the liver, the spleen, the joints, and the spinal marrow) are places into which humors were

---

[47] For example, *Epid. V* 42, 5.232 L., *Nat. Hom.* 20.3, 6.78 L., *Aff.* 11, 6.218 L., 14, 6.222 L., *Morb. II* 19.2, 7.32 L., 40.5, 7.56–58 L., 41.3, 7.58 L., 46.4, 7.64 L., 67.3, 7.102 L., 68.2, 7.104 L., 74.2, 7.112 L., *Morb. III* 17, 7.156–160 L., *Int.* 4, 7.178 L., 39, 7.262 L., and *Mul. I* 52, 8.110 L.

[48] Once the bile-production was shut off by cooling down the belly, the bile could then be treated by either removing it completely, such as with vomiting or laxatives, or by breaking it up and re-diluting it with other humors. A popular method for breaking up bile was to administer acidic foods and drinks (e.g., vinegar). According to the author of *On Regimen in Acute Diseases*, acidic humors break up bile and help it mix back into phlegm (ἐκφλεγματοῦται, 61, 2.356–358 L.). Compare Herodicus of Cnidos's opposition between the "acid" (τὸ ὀξύ) and the "bitter" (τὸ πικρόν) at *Anon. Lond.* IV.40–V.34.

[49] For other "mother-city" analogies, see Huffman (1993: 195–197), who concludes that "to say that something is the 'mother-city' of something else is to suggest not only that it is the origin or starting-point of that other thing, but also that it has a continuing relationship with its 'colony' which accounts for the essential characteristics of that 'colony.'" The idea that bile arises from heat would eventually be elaborated by Galen. See especially Gal. *Nat. Fac.* 2.107–125 K. A variation on the process I have described in this section could have bile produced not simply by the separation of an inherent component from a mixture but by the *transformation* of the residual moisture under the influence of heat. Recall how the author of *On Flesh* attributes the production of the fatty and the glutinous to the drying and putrefaction of the earth (3, 8.584–586 L.). Similarly, Thrasymachus of Sardis is said to have believed that bile and phlegm arise from the putrefaction of blood (*Anon. Lond.* XI.43–XII.8). Thus, the author of *On Flesh* may have believed that after the components of a mixture have been separated off from one another, the moisture that stays behind is putrefied and turned into bile, while the moisture that gathers in the head undergoes a parallel form of putrefaction and transforms into phlegm.

commonly thought to flow and get stuck. In *On Places in the Human Being*, the author lists seven fluxes from the head, each of which gives rise to a different class of ailments. The destinations of these fluxes are the eyes, the ears, the nose, the lungs, the flesh, the spine, and the joints, while a similar list of seven fluxes in *On Glands* replaces the flux to the flesh with one to the throat. Other texts describe fluxes that originate in the belly and travel not only to the parts listed above but also to the liver, the spleen, the kidneys, the bladder, the intestines, the skin, and the teeth. All of these parts, together with the hair and the nails, were commonly inspected for signs of disease. They were the parts in which humors and *pneuma* were most likely to become fixed, and hence the most important parts for diagnosis and treatment.

This connection between *On Flesh*'s anthropogony and humoral theory opens up many interesting avenues for our analysis of this text. The author may not simply be accounting for the color, shape, texture, and density of the parts but also, and more importantly, for their role in pathogenesis. Consider, for example, the author's description of flesh, which is said to have arisen when "the cold stopped, congealed, and produced flesh, while the glutinous became caverns" (9.2, 8.596 L.). In this passage, the author is not simply describing the physical appearance of flesh; he is also providing the necessary background for explaining its most common affections. In particular, there are two affections of the flesh that seem to be explained by this passage. The first is the tendency of flesh to melt and flow away, which flesh was commonly thought to do when exposed to excessive heat.[50] The second relates to the author's claim that flesh contains "caverns" (τρῶγλαι). Medical writers often assert that if a flux is directed toward the flesh, the foreign moisture will be retained, and that some patients (e.g., women and the elderly) will retain more moisture while others (e.g., men and the young) will retain less moisture, owing to the fact that the flesh of the first group is more porous, while the flesh of the second group is more dense.[51]

---

[50] On the melting of flesh under the influence of heat, see *Aër.* 7.3, 2.26 L., *Flat.* 12, 6.108–110 L., *Morb. I* 15, 6.168 L., *Aff.* 22, 6.232–234 L., *Loc. Hom.* 7.1, 6.290 L., 9.2, 6.292 L., 24.1, 6.314 L., *Vict.* 54.2, 6.558 L., 60.1, 6.572 L., 65, 6.582 L., 76.1, 6.618 L., *Morb. II* 57.2, 7.88 L., *Int.* 22, 7.220 L., and *Morb. IV* 45.2, 7.568 L. I have already discussed this process as it pertains to dropsy in my analysis of *On Breaths* (p. 115). Since the author of *On Flesh* identifies flesh as a congealed mass of the cold, he would have attributed its melting to a simple overpowering of the cold by the hot.

[51] On the retention of fluids by the flesh, see *De arte* 10.3, 6.16–18 L., *Morb. I* 20, 6.176–178 L., *Aff.* 19, 6.228 L., *Loc. Hom.* 10.3–6, 6.294–296 L., 21, 6.312–314 L., 27.1, 6.318 L., 29, 6.322 L., and *Morb. II* 1.2, 7.8 L. On the distinction between women and men, see *Nat. Hom.* 21.2, 6.82 L., *Mul. I* 1, 8.10–14 L., and *Gland.* 16, 8.570–572 L. On the old versus the young, see *Morb. I* 22, 6.184–186 L.

On Flesh's descriptions of other parts of the body may be similarly tied to their role in pathogenesis. Quick heating of the glutinous creates bones that are "spongy" (3.7, 8.588 L.), a class of bones that *On Head Wounds* singles out for their tendency to suppurate after injury (18.1, 3.250 L.). The same combination of the glutinous and extreme heat gives rise to the lungs, which are also described as "spongy" (7.1, 8.594 L.), and which were similarly notorious for their ability to attract and retain morbid humors.[52] In *On Flesh*, the spleen and the joints are both said to contain glutinous material in the form of fibers and synovial fluid, respectively (9.1, 8.594 L., 10, 8.596–598 L.). This glutinous material would explain the well-known ability of the spleen and the joints to swell and harden to an excessive degree, as any foreign moisture that enters these parts would become stuck and unable to flow away, while the glutinous material would dry and harden when exposed to excessive heat.[53] In the Aristotelian *Problemata*, the presence of glutinous matter in the joints is said to be responsible for precisely these conditions: "Our strength is in our joints, and they are relaxed by south winds (as is shown by the fact that things which have been glued together [τῶν κεκολλημένων] creak); for the viscous matter [γλίσχρον] in the joints, if it hardens, prevents us from moving, whereas, if it is too moist, it prevents us from exerting ourselves" (1.24, 862a30–33, trans. Forster *apud* Barnes).[54] As for the spleen, Greek medical writers often refer to its ability to attract fluids to itself. The author of *Diseases IV* makes the spleen one of the body's four "reservoirs," noting that any water in the body is both collected in the spleen and distributed therefrom (33.2, 7.544 L., 37, 7.552–554 L.). In *Airs Waters Places*, the flesh is said to melt and flow into the spleen (7.3, 2.26 L.). In *Internal*

---

[52] For example, *VM* 22.6, 1.628–630 L., *Morb. I* 22, 6.186 L., and *Oss.* 13.2, 9.184–186 L. In *Diseases IV*, the author says that the spongy nature of the lungs is what makes them especially prone to ulceration (56.4, 7.606 L.). Plato suggests that drinks are drawn into the lungs because of their spongy nature, with the ultimate purpose of the lungs' porosity being to surround the heart with cooling moisture (*Ti.* 70c–d).

[53] Swelling and hardening of the spleen: *VM* 22.6, 1.628–630 L., *Aër.* 7.3, 2.26 L., 24.4, 2.88 L., *Acut.* 50.1, 2.332 L., 62.3, 2.360 L., *Acut. App.* 4.1, 2.400 L., *Epid. II* 2.7, 5.86 L., 2.22, 5.94 L., 2.23d, 5.94 L., *Epid. IV* 7, 5.146 L., 13, 5.150–152 L., 25, 5.166 L., *Epid. VI* 6.4, 5.324 L., *Prorrh. I* 125, 5.554 L., *Coac.* 321, 5.652–654 L., *Aff.* 20, 6.228–230 L., *Loc. Hom.* 24, 6.314–316 L., *Int.* 25, 7.230–232 L., 30–34, 7.244–252 L., *Mul. I* 61, 8.122–126 L., and *Prorrh. II* 35–37, 9.66–68 L. Swelling and hardening of the joints: *Prog.* 24.2, 2.180 L., *Aph.* 5.25, 4.540 L., *Epid. VI* 1.12, 5.272 L., 1.15, 5.274 L., *Liqu.* 6.2–3, 6.132 L., *Int.* 41, 7.266–268 L., *Mul. III* 18.7, 8.442 L., and *Prorrh. II* 15, 9.40 L. At *Epid. II* 3.8, 5.110 L. (= *Epid. VI* 2.7, 5.282 L.), material left after a crisis is said to produce "swelling in the spleen, unless it terminates in the joints."

[54] For a similar explanation of swelling and hardening, see *Gland.* 7.2–3, 8.560–562 L. In this passage, the author claims that an influx of pungent and "glutinous" (κολλῶδες) material will make the tonsils fill up with fluid (φλεγμαίνει), swell (συνοιδίσκεται), and become tense (συντείνει).

Affections, the spleen "draws bile to itself" (30, 7.244 L.). *On Ancient Medicine*, *Diseases IV*, and *Diseases of Women I* all attribute the spleen's attractive powers to its porosity (*VM* 22.6, 1.628–630 L., *Morb. IV* 33.2, 7.544 L., 40, 7.560–562 L., and *Mul. I* 61, 8.122 L.). The author of *On Flesh* invokes the same belief when he observes that the spleen is "soft" (μαλακός, 9.1, 8.594 L.), a term usually applied to porous, moisture-filled flesh.[55] The author of *On Flesh* further notes that both the spleen and the liver contain large quantities of the hot, which might explain their common association with the two "hot" humors, blood and bile.[56] In chapter 6, the author observes that "the hot is located mostly in the vessels and the heart," apparently associating blood with "the hot."[57] Two major vessels, the *hepatitis* and the *splenitis*, were commonly thought to run to the liver and the spleen, explaining why diseases in the spleen tend to coincide with bloody noses, and why other symptoms involving these organs seem to travel along predetermined paths.[58] The liver in particular was often said to be full of blood. Empedocles describes the liver as "rich in blood" (DK 31 B150), while *On Anatomy* observes that the liver contains more blood than any other part of the body (3, 8.538 L.).[59] According to the author of *On Ancient Medicine*, it is the soft, bloody nature of the liver that makes it especially prone to sharp pains (22.8, 1.632 L.). The author of *Diseases IV*, meanwhile, states that the heart does not feel pain, "the reason being that the heart is a hard and dense object" (38.1, 7.554 L.). Similarly, the author of

[55] For the tendency of "soft" flesh to attract and retain fluids, see *Aër.* 20.1, 2.72–74 L. and *Gland.* 16.2, 8.572 L. At *Carn.* 16.1, 8.604 L., the brain is said to absorb odors through the nostrils by way of "a soft cartilage, like a sponge" (χονδρίον μαλακὸν ὅπωσπερ σπόγγος). At *Cord.* 9, 9.86 L., we find this principle formulated in general terms: "the soft is more attractive" (τὸ γὰρ μαλακὸν ἑλκτικώτερον). Note also the tendency of some doctors to prescribe "soft" foods for moistening regimens (e.g., *Nat. Hom.* 16.1–2, 6.72–74 L., 17.3, 6.74 L. and *Vict.* 68.10–11, 6.600–602 L., 73.2, 6.614 L., 89.6, 6.648 L., 90.5, 6.656 L.).

[56] On the innate heat of these humors, see *Nat. Hom.* 7.4–5, 6.46–48 L., but see my comments in note 45 on p. 196.

[57] Blood is said to be hot at *Carn.* 9.5, 8.596 L. Compare also *Carn.* 5.2, 8.590 L., 6.2, 8.592 L., 7.1, 8.594 L., and especially 8, 8.594 L., where the process by which the liver is formed ("when much of the wet was left behind with the hot and without the glutinous or the fatty, the cold overpowered [ἐκράτησε] the hot and it congealed") is compared to the process by which blood congeals outside the body.

[58] On these vessels, see *Epid. II* 4.1, 5.120 L., *Epid VI* 7.2, 5.338 L., *Nat. Hom.* 11, 6.48–60 L., *Morb. I* 26, 6.194 L., *Aff.* 20, 6.230 L., *Morb. Sacr.* 6, 6.370–372 L., *Oss.* 10, 9.178 L., and Diog. Apoll. DK 64 B6. At *Epid. II* 2.22, 5.94 L., an enlarged spleen is accompanied by a pulsing of the *splenitis*. For the association of bloody noses with diseases in the spleen, see *Prog.* 7, 2.124–130 L., *Epid. II* 2.6, 5.86 L., 2.23d, 5.94 L., *Aff.* 20, 6.230 L., 3.8, 5.110 L., *Epid. IV* 7, 5.146 L., 13, 5.150–152 L., 23, 5.162 L., 37, 5.180 L., *Epid. V* 2.5, 5.278 L., *Prorrh. I* 125, 5.554 L., *Coac.* 321, 5.652–654 L., and *Prorrh. II* 35–36, 9.66–68 L.

[59] In this context, note also *Epid. VI* 2.25, 5.290 L., where the right side of the body (the location of the liver) is said to be "more bilious and more blooded, to the extent that that is the warmer area in animals" (trans. Smith).

On Flesh asserts that the heart arose when much of the glutinous and the cold were heated by the hot and became "hard and sticky flesh" (5.1, 8.590 L.). In *On Flesh*, the heart does not contain any of the hot within its flesh. The hot is used to harden the two main ingredients of the heart (the cold and the glutinous), but the hot only remains in the heart insofar as it constitutes the blood that fills the heart's hollows. The hot is also absent from the nails and the hair (11, 8.598 L., 14, 8.602 L.), while it remains in abundance in the liver and the spleen (8, 8.594 L., 9.1, 8.594 L.). Perhaps the author of *On Flesh* intended for the presence of the hot (i.e., blood) to explain why some parts of the body (e.g., the liver and the spleen) are more susceptible to pain, while others (e.g., the heart, the nails, and the hair) are less susceptible or even wholly insensate.[60] The large quantity of the hot in both the vessels and the liver may also explain why bile tends to be generated in these places. As we have already noted, the author specifically observes that the hot is the "mother-city" of the fatty.[61]

An interest in pathology may also explain why *On Flesh* follows its anthropogony with discussions of hearing, smell, sight, and speech (15–18, 8.602–608 L.), as the disruption of these functions was commonly associated with fluxes to the ears, the nose, the eyes, and the throat.[62] In the Classical period, medical writers often comment on the normal functioning of these parts when discussing their impairment. The author of *On Places in the Human Being*, for example, opens his general account of human *phusis* with discussions of hearing, smell, and sight (2, 6.278–280 L.), a passage that anticipates his later description of three fluxes to the nose, the ears, and the eyes (11–13, 6.296–302 L.). Similarly, the author of *Diseases II* describes both sight and hearing when discussing diseases of the eyes and the ears (1.1, 7.8 L., 4.2, 7.10–12 L.), while the author of *Diseases IV* briefly explains how humans emit and articulate sound before noting that "I have given a better explanation of this matter in my discussion of

---

[60] For the author's association of the hot with perception, see *Carn.* 2.1, 8.584 L. (quoted on pp. 178–179).

[61] For the generation of bile in the vessels and the liver, compare Galen's critique of Erasistratus at *Nat. Fac.* 2.114–116 K.: "[Erasistratus] ought surely to have added something about [bile's] genesis in the liver and veins, seeing that the old physicians and philosophers declare that it along with the blood is generated in these organs" (trans. Brock, modified).

[62] Compare *Acut. App.* 6.1, 2.402–404 L. (speech), *Epid. VII* 9, 5.380 L. (speech), *Morb. I* 3, 6.144 L. (sight and hearing), *Loc. Hom.* 10.3, 6.294 L. (sight), *Morb. Sacr.* 14, 6.386–388 L. (sight and hearing), *Morb. III* 2, 7.120 L. (hearing), 4, 7.122 L. (hearing and speech), 10, 7.128–130 L. (sight and hearing), *Int.* 12, 7.194 L. (speech), 18, 7.212 L. (sight and hearing), 40, 7.264 L. (speech), 48, 7.284–286 L. (sight), and *Prorrh. II* 27, 9.60 L. (sight and hearing). Wenskus (1995) draws a similar conclusion about the purpose of this section.

pneumonia" (56.1, 7.604–606 L.).[63] There is even a passage in *On Flesh* in which the author seems to explicitly connect his discussion of hearing, smell, sight, and speech with the pathological conditions that impair these functions. "Whenever the nostrils are made wet," he writes, "they cannot smell, since the brain does not draw the air to itself. Along the same lines, when the brain melts and sends very much fluid from itself to the palate, the windpipe, the lung, and the rest of the cavity, people recognize this and say there is a downward flux from the head" (16.3, 8.604 L.).[64]

Such, I think, is the spirit of *On Flesh*. The author's goal is not simply to speculate for the sake of speculation, but to give the doctor insight into the origin and treatment of disease.[65] This is why the author never explains how the parts of a human being ultimately come together to form a single whole. His interest is not to construct a complete anthropogony in the manner of Empedocles or Archelaus. Instead, his goal is to understand the inherent properties of each part, since a knowledge of these properties will be directly relevant for the art of healing.[66] This interpretation should come as little surprise to anyone who has read the opening of this text. In his introductory remarks, the author explicitly notes that his discussion of "the things on high" will only extend to what is relevant for medicine (1, 8.584 L.):

> Regarding the things leading up to this account [τὰ μέχρι τοῦ λόγου τούτου], I make use of common opinions held by others before me as well as myself. For it is necessary to set down a common starting point for my opinions when intending to compile this account on the physician's art. Concerning the things on high I also need not speak, except insofar as I will make an exposition on humans and the other animals, how they grew and came to be, on what soul is, on what being healthy is, on what being sick is, on what is bad and good for humans, and from what they die; but now I publish opinions that are my own.

---

[63] On the ability of pneumonia to change a patient's voice, note the reference to a "pneumonic voice" at *Epid. VII* 85, 5.444 L.

[64] On this author's selection of hearing, smell, sight, and speech as the four processes impaired by fluxes from the head, compare *Anon. Lond.* VIII.35–IX.4, where Abas (or Aias?) is said to have claimed that "the brain is purged by way of nostrils, ears, eyes, and mouth."

[65] Contrast Lo Presti (2016: 165), who writes that *On Flesh* is "a cosmological-anthropological project with no necessary link with medical practice." Similar statements have been made by Oser-Grote (1997: 334, 2004: 27), who claims that *On Flesh* "is not pathologically or therapeutically oriented," and Dümmler (1889: 225), who asserts that *On Flesh* "certainly did not grow on medical ground." Recall also the assessment of Peck (1936: 62), quoted on p. 4.

[66] That said, we should not discount the importance of thinkers such as Empedocles for modeling the sorts of explanations that we find in *On Flesh*. Empedocles's elemental recipes for bones and blood, for example (DK 31 B96, B98), provide a clear parallel for *On Flesh*'s construction of different parts of the body from the hot, the cold, and the wet.

In this passage, the author refers to two *logoi* ("discourses" or "accounts") that lie outside the limits of his own account. The first leads up to his account both chronologically and intellectually, as it comprises the common opinions that the author shares with his predecessors and which provide the "starting point" (ἀρχή) for his own contribution to the art.[67] The second *logos* lies outside the author's account inasmuch as it is *irrelevant* to medicine. "Concerning the things on high," he writes, "I also need not speak [οὐδὲ δέομαι λέγειν], except insofar as I will make an exposition on humans and the other animals, how they grew and came to be, on what soul is, on what being healthy is, on what being sick is, on what is bad and good for humans, and from what they die; but now I publish opinions that are my own."[68] Interestingly, the author only fulfills the first of his announced topics ("humans and the other animals, how they grew and came to be"). The soul is never mentioned,[69] nor do we get explicit definitions of health and sickness[70] or of what is "bad" and "good" for human beings,[71] or an explanation of how our bodies transition from life to death.[72] Together with the author's statement in chapter

---

[67] For the sentiment, compare *VM* 2.1, 1.572 L., *De arte* 4, 6.6 L., *Vict.* 1, 6.466–468 L., Diog. Apoll. DK 64 B1, and X. *Eq.* 1.1.

[68] Incidentally, this reading of the author's proem as the identification of two *logoi* that lie outside his own *logos* – one because it is *implicit* and the other because it is *irrelevant* – speaks in favor of the manuscript's οὐδὲ δέομαι λέγειν, which many scholars have attempted to emend, changing the adverbial οὐδέ either to οὐδέν or to οὐ. In chapter 19, the author repeatedly follows δέ with an adverbial καί ("and ... also"), while δὲ ... οὐδέ ("and ... also not") is simply a negation of this phrase.

[69] The description of the "hot" at 2.1, 8.584 L. suggests that the author may have drawn some connection between this principle and the soul, associating the soul within our bodies with the cosmic heat that governs the entire universe. The evidence of 6.1–2, 8.592–594 L. suggests four additional details about the soul: (1) it is centered in the heart, (2) it is the hottest part of a human being, (3) it is constantly in motion, and (4) it is closely associated with both blood and *pneuma*. As we will see in the next chapter, these beliefs about the soul can all be paralleled in *On Regimen*.

[70] Considering the author's anthropogony, one presumes that his system would have focused on interactions between heat, cold, and bodily fluids, with the two most important humors for pathogenesis being the "fatty" (i.e., bile) and the "glutinous" (i.e., phlegm). As for the other humors, the author mentions the "sweet" and the "bitter" at 13.3, 8.600 L. and blood at 8.2, 8.594 L., 9.5, 8.596 L. Note also the reference to women who are "phlegmy" (βλεννώδης) at 19.1, 8.610 L., and to a downward flux from the head at 16.3, 8.604 L. As I argued earlier, the specific details in this author's anthropogony seem to have been designed to explain common narratives of pathogenesis. Taken together with the reference to critical days at 19.4, 8.612–614 L., these observations suggest that the author of *On Flesh* likely held the same beliefs about the humors that we find in other texts from this period, giving special emphasis to the notions of *apokrisis*, flux, coction, and crisis.

[71] Levin (2014: 60) cites many parallels for this language in the Hippocratic Corpus, concluding that the author means "what holds the promise of benefit or the specter of harm respecting symptoms and medical treatment."

[72] Compare *Morb. IV* 16, 7.574–576 L., *Hebd.* 52, and the explanations of how patients die from pleurisy, pneumonia, ardent fever, and phrenitis at *Morb. I* 32–34, 6.202–204 L. In *On Ancient Medicine*, the author claims that his opponents established a limited number of principles as the

19 that he will discuss some matters on another occasion (ἐγὼ φράσω ἐν ἄλλοισιν, 19.7, 8.614 L.), these omissions suggest that *On Flesh* originally formed part of a series of texts, not unlike the works of Aristotle or the medical treatises *Diseases IV, On the Seed-Nature of the Child*, and *Diseases of Women I–III*, all of which contain multiple cross-references to other works within their series.[73]

Although the author of *On Flesh* claims to omit irrelevant speculations about "the things on high," what he defines as medically relevant goes well beyond what a modern reader might expect. For example, there does not appear to have been any practical need for the author to claim that the hot, the cold, and the wet are the first principles of everything in the universe, let alone for him to postulate the existence of three cosmic strata that divide the universe into *aither*, earth, and *aer*. There is also no clear therapeutic reason for the author to have claimed that the fatty and the glutinous arose from the putrefaction of the earth, or for him to have argued at length that the number seven plays a *universal* role in regulating the lives of human beings. Such details suggest that the author of *On Flesh*, like the author of *On Breaths*, is at least partly driven by a separate "cosmological impulse," a belief that high-level generalizations – the absolute highest one can find – are inherently desirable and directly relevant to the medical art.

As we turn to our final work by a cosmological doctor, we will see this cosmological impulse taken to its extreme. *On the Nature of the Human Being, On Breaths*, and *On Flesh* all equate the first principles of medicine with the first principles of the universe, but none of these authors attempts to create a truly comprehensive account of the sort that we traditionally associate with the inquiry into nature. This is not the case with *On Regimen*, whose author constructs the most detailed,

---

cause "of both diseases and death" (1.1, 1.570 L.). Given the importance of the hot in *On Flesh*, which the author may have identified with the soul itself, one possibility is that he associated death with a final "victory" of the cold over the hot, which could conceivably arise in several ways: (1) from the cold "overpowering" the hot (9.4, 8.596 L., with which cf. *Nat. Hom.* 12.6, 6.64 L., *Epid. I* 12.3, 6.638 L., and *Morb. II* 6a.3, 7.14 L.), (2) from the hot burning up all its nutriment (6.2, 8.592 L., with which cf. *Vict.* 29.2, 6.504 L. and *Morb. IV* 16, 7.574–576 L.), or (3) from the hot being gradually breathed out through respiration (5.2, 8.590 L., 6.1–2, 8.592 L., with which cf. *Vict.* 25, 6.496–498 L., 29.2, 6.504 L., 44, 6.542 L. and *Hebd.* 52). As we will see, all of these explanations also appear in the treatment of death in *On Regimen*, a text that has many affinities with *On Flesh*.

[73] Other texts that have sometimes been attached to this series include *Diseases of Unwed Girls, Superfetation*, and *On Glands*. *On Flesh* contains numerous affinities with these texts, including a passage in *On Flesh* (19.1, 8.610 L.) that repeats the same claim to have seen an aborted fetus that appears in *On the Seed-Nature of the Child* (13, 7.488–492 L.).

non-fragmentary description of the cosmos that survives from the pre-Platonic period. My investigation of this text will necessarily range farther than the analyses I have offered for other works by cosmological doctors, but, as we will see, such scope is required just to skim the surface of this complex and extremely important work.

CHAPTER 6

On Regimen

6.1 The Self-Sufficiency of Fire and Water

On Regimen is the longest and by far the most complicated text by a cosmological doctor to have survived from the Classical period. It originally circulated in three "books" (i.e., three papyrus scrolls), although there is a modern tendency – here discarded – to divide the third book into two, thereby bringing the total to four.[1] Already in antiquity, some readers of *On Regimen* were attempting to identify its author. Other than Hippocrates, the most commonly cited candidates were Ariston (the "student" of Petron) and Philistion of Locri,[2] although Galen says that others attributed it to Euryphon, Phaon, Philetas, or Pherecydes, the last of whom may be identical with the sixth-century cosmologist from Syros.[3] Modern attempts to attribute *On Regimen* to Herodicus of Selymbria, the supposed "inventor" of regimen, have found few endorsements,[4] and even less has been made of Pfleiderer's (1896: 551–553) suggestion that the author was Eryximachus. Some have postulated that the author is not a practicing doctor but rather a "health expert," although this contention depends

[1] On the inappropriateness of this division, see Jouanna (1989), who concludes that "we should no longer speak of Book IV of *On Regimen*, which has been an invention of modern editors since Littré."
[2] Ariston and Philistion are included in all of Galen's lists of potential authors of *On Regimen*. As I noted in Chapter 1, Philistion was widely recognized as an authority on dietetics, and he may have also emphasized the same two principles of fire and water as the author of *On Regimen* (see p. 31). As for Ariston, his identification as the "student" of Petron suggests at least a tangential connection with cosmological medicine.
[3] On Pherecydes, see Schibli (1990). On Euryphon, see Manetti (2008a). Phaon and Philetas are otherwise unknown and could well be ancient corruptions of "Philistion."
[4] For the attribution of *On Regimen* to Herodicus or to one of his "students," see Spät (1897: 22–23), Jones (1947: 49), Bourgey (1953: 129n2), Kahn (1960: 189n2), Ducatillon (1977: 118), López Morales (2001: 24–28), and Lebedev (2014: 29–31), with the rebuttals of Jüthner (1909: 14–16) and Joly (1960: 203–205, 1967: xiii–xiv, 1984: 34–36). Manetti (2005) discusses the various testimonies about doctors named Herodicus, who are in fact very difficult to tease apart. On the problems with identifying Herodicus as the "inventor" of regimen, see Bartoš (2015: 29–35), who also notes that the tendency of modern scholars to attribute *On Regimen* to Herodicus depends largely on Diels's (1893a) speculative reconstruction of *Anon. Lond.* IX.20–36. Without Diels's reconstruction, the case is very weak.

largely on arguments from silence and ignores the restricted focus of the author's subject matter ("human regimen in its relation to health," 1.1, 6.466 L.).[5] At the opposite end, Smith (1979: 44–60, 1999) has argued that the author was none other than Hippocrates. Smith's thesis has failed to gain much traction in modern scholarship, primarily because he does not adequately show how the testimony from the *Anonymus Londiniensis* could have been feasibly extracted from *On Regimen*.[6]

As for the date of *On Regimen*, a potential *terminus ante quem* is provided by Aristotle. In *Divination in Sleep*, Aristotle describes an approach to dream interpretation that is remarkably similar to what we find in *On Regimen*, down to what appears to be a reference to prodiagnosis – that is, the method of identifying "the diseases and other affections about to occur in our bodies" (463a18–20) – that the author of *On Regimen* proudly claims to have invented.[7] Peck (1928), Olerud (1951: 64–66), Jouanna (1966), Sisko (2006), and Bartoš (2015: 231–241) have all claimed that Plato makes use of *On Regimen* in the *Timaeus*. If this is correct, then the *terminus ante quem* would be pushed back to around 360 BCE, the conventional date for Plato's dialogue. Joly (1984: 44–49) suggests a date of around 400 BCE, while Jaeger (1938: 171, 1944: 33–40) argues that the work was written by a contemporary of Plato, well into the fourth century. In the end, we do not need to worry too much about assigning *On Regimen* to this or that decade in the fifth or fourth century BCE. So long as this text can be placed in the Classical period, what really matters is not when it was written but rather what it presupposes.

The author of *On Regimen* claims that all animals, including humans, are composed of fire and water. In chapter 3, he writes that "fire has the power to move everything in every circumstance [πάντα διὰ παντὸς

---

[5] For the designation of the author as a "health expert," see Jones (1931: xlvi, n5), followed by Bartoš (2015: 47–48). Compare Farrington (1953: 138), who suggests that the author was a "director of a gymnasium," and van der Eijk (2008: 401), who calls *On Regimen* "a work apparently written by a trainer or supervisor of athletes." Lloyd (1968: 90n57) also takes it for granted that the author is not a practicing doctor. As we will see, the author of *On Regimen* identifies the same disease categories that were maintained by other authors in the Hippocratic Corpus, and like the other doctors who turned their attention to cosmology, he was deeply concerned with the inability to generalize prognoses and treatments in the face of many variables. It is important to remember that this author is focusing on (1) high-level commonalities and (2) the prevention of disease. Thus, he has little reason to discuss either the fine details of human anatomy or the treatment of specific patients.

[6] For explicit rejections of Smith's thesis, see Mansfeld (1980a) and Lloyd (1991a: 195–196). Smith identifies *Vict.* 74, 6.614–616 L. as the source of the Peripatetic report on Hippocrates, but it is difficult to see how this passage could have inspired the specific details we find in this doxography.

[7] Note, however, the attribution of a similar use of dream interpretation to the Pythagoreans at D.L. 8.32. For a more detailed discussion of Aristotle's potential knowledge of *On Regimen*, see van der Eijk (1995: 454–455) and Bartoš (2015: 241–289).

κινῆσαι], while water has the power to nourish everything in every circumstance [πάντα διὰ παντὸς θρέψαι]." In establishing these principles, the author draws on traditional associations between heat and movement and between moisture and nourishment that were frequently invoked in early Greek thought.[8] Some scholars have tried to identify a single source for *On Regimen*'s two principles of fire and water. Gomperz (1901: 287) suggests an origin in Parmenides's distinction between "light" and "night," while Burnet (1930: 150n2) points to Heraclitus's oscillations between fire and sea. Others have tried to establish the author's dependence on either Archelaus or Hippon, both of whom are said to have discussed an opposition between fire and water in their cosmological systems (Archel. DK 60 A7, Hippon DK 38 A3, A5).[9] López Morales (2001: 20) plainly states that, whatever source we ultimately identify, "we can rule out that [the theory of fire and water] is an original doctrine of our author." On the one hand, this statement is correct insofar as an opposition between fire and water was very common in early Greek thought. Theognis writes that "fire and water will never mix together" (1245). *Diseases IV* observes that the watery component in human beings is "most hostile to fire" (49.3, 7.580 L.), while Polybus similarly states that substances with opposite properties must clearly be different things "if in fact fire and water are not one" (5.2, 6.42 L.). At the same time that we recognize these various parallels, however, it must be stressed that no modern attempt to identify a single "source" for *On Regimen* has found a system that perfectly matches what we see in this text. Instead, this author seems to draw on a more general tendency in both medicine and cosmology to isolate two opposing principles, of which the one, being hot, plays the role of an active, architectonic force, while the other, being cold, plays the role of a passive, malleable material. An especially clear example of this division appears in *On Flesh*, where the author's two principles of the hot and the cold closely parallel *On Regimen*'s two principles of fire and water. In *On Flesh*, the cold principle is said to be "nourishment for the hot" (6.2, 8.592 L.), while the hot principle "provides movement to the rest of the body and to all other things" (6.3, 8.592 L.). These statements closely recall the third chapter of *On Regimen*,

---

[8] On the wide acceptance of these associations, see Kahn (1960: 109n2). Betegh (2020) surveys early Greek theories about the relationship between heat and movement. For the idea that water nourishes fire, compare Diog. Apoll. DK 64 A18, A33, Arist. *Mete.* 355a5, *de An.* 416a26–27, [*Pr.*] 1.20, 861b38–862a3, *Metaph.* 983b22–24, and the opposition to this view at *Morb. IV* 51.4, 7.586 L. and *Cord.* 3, 9.82 L. For the nutritive power of water, see also Arist. *GA* 767a32–33.

[9] For the claim that *On Regimen* draws on Archelaus, see Zeller (1892: 697), Weygoldt (1882: 171–174), Fredrich (1899: 129, 135, 138–141), Joly (1960: 19, 89, 1984: 32), and Betegh (2020: 53). For Hippon, see Joly (1960: 20, 31, 1984: 32–33) and López Morales (2001: 21–22).

where we are told that fire, being hot, is the source of all movement, while water, being cold, is the source of all nourishment. A fire–water duality lurks behind Petron's two elements of the hot and the cold (where the hot is conjoined with the dry and the cold with the wet), as well as Polybus's four-humor system in which hot, dry bile (encouraged during summer) is contrasted with cold, wet phlegm (encouraged during winter). It therefore seems likely that the author of *On Regimen* at least partly based his own selection of fire and water not simply on previous models of the cosmos but also, and perhaps more directly, on previous discussions of health and disease. In Chapter 5, we observed that the cosmological doctors tended to center their search for first principles around four topics in particular: heat, cold, moisture, and *pneuma*. Some medical writers were already speaking in general terms about the presence of "fire" or "water" within the body (see p. 167), and we should therefore not be surprised to find these two principles highlighted by the author of *On Regimen*.[10]

In chapter 4, the author observes that fire contains the hot and the dry, and water the cold and the wet. He then adds that these two elements also share certain properties with each other, as "fire has the wet from water, for there is moisture in fire, and water has the dry from fire, for there is dryness in water, too." We have already encountered this tendency to pair the hot with the dry and the cold with the wet in our discussions of both Petron of Aegina and *On the Nature of the Human Being*, where we noted that the hot and the dry tend to be associated with summer, fire, bile, youth, and the male, while the cold and the wet tend to be associated with winter, water, phlegm, old age, and the female. The author of *On Regimen* invokes all of these associations over the course of his text. What is new in this system is the author's assertion that water also contains a certain amount of the "dry," while fire contains a certain amount of the "wet." To understand what the author means by this statement, we should first remember that the Greek words normally translated as "wet" and "dry" do not simply refer to the presence or absence of water. Instead, these adjectives commonly distinguish substances that are "solid" (= ξηρός) from those that are not (= ὑγρός). In chapter 10, the author calls the belly a "storeroom for dry and wet water" (ὕδατι ξηρῷ καὶ ὑγρῷ ταμιεῖον, 10.1, 6.484 L.). By "dry and wet water," the author means solid and liquid nutriment, both of which are presumed to be forms of water because they both provide nourishment to

---

[10]   In light of these parallels, there is no reason to follow van der Eijk (2004: 191) and Craik (2015: xxxi) in supposing a direct connection between *On Regimen*'s fire/water cosmology and the Ayurvedic concepts of *agni* and *soma*. The parallel is worth exploring from a comparatist point of view, but it should not be considered explanatory for the system of *On Regimen*.

the body.[11] In his section on embryology, the author uses the notion of "wet fire" to explain how the fiery soul can take the form of a fluid and circulate through the vessels (9.3, 6.484 L.), while "dry water" becomes compacted when it is heated, thereby giving rise to bones and sinews (9.2, 6.484 L.).[12] As we see in these examples, one of the author's primary reasons for assigning dryness to water and wetness to fire is to account for phenomena that cannot be reduced to a simple choice between cold/wet water and hot/dry fire. When the author notes that wine is "hot and dry" and that certain wines "dry with their heat, consuming the moisture from the body" (52.1, 6.554 L.), he seems to rely on the notion of a "wet fire" that heats, dries, and consumes water as its fuel.[13] On the other hand, when the author says that barley becomes cold and dry when it is "exposed to fire" (πυρωθῶσι) because "the fire makes the wet and purgative component depart, while the remaining component is cold and dry" (40.1, 6.536 L.), he seems to rely on the notion of "dry water," drawing on the same process that he had previously used to describe the creation of bones and sinews in chapter 9.

Further references to "wet fire" and "dry water" appear in two other passages: the author's discussion of healthy and unhealthy constitutions in chapter 32 and his description of soul-mixtures in chapter 35. In these passages, we learn that fire is generally light and quick while water is generally heavy and slow, and that either of these elements can be thick, thin, dense, or strong – adjectives that imply the author is incorporating some aspects of humoral thinking into his discussion of the elements. When the author talks about the "mixing" of these elements, he draws on the notion of humoral "blending," while their "separating out" is described with the same verb (ἀποκρίνεσθαι) that is also applied to an *apokrisis* of harmful humors.[14] In

---

[11] On the designation of nutriment as "dry" (i.e., solid) or "wet" (i.e., liquid), see also *Flat.* 7.1, 6.98 L., *Alim.* 1, 9.98 L., 30, 9.108 L., 49, 9.118 L., E. *Ba.* 274–283, Arist. *Sens.* 444a16–17, *Resp.* 476a30, *HA* 492b20, *PA* 658b35–659a1, *GA* 725b1–2, 737b34, [*Pr.*] 10.56, 897b19–21, 21.13, 928a33, *EN* 1118b10, and Thphr. *CP* 3.6.8.

[12] This property of "dry water" has much in common with the "glutinous" in *On Flesh*. Later on, a similar desire to explain why some fluids thicken when heated would lead Aristotle to claim that fluids only thicken if they contain a certain amount of the "dry" (i.e., earth). Compare Arist. *Mete.* 380a33–34 ("Nothing moist ripens by itself without the admixture of some dry matter") and 383a11–12 ("Thickening occurs when the moisture goes off and the dry matter comes together," trans. Webster *apud* Barnes). Aristotle directly applies this concept of "dry water" to both the hardening of phlegm (*GA* 735b35–37) and the coagulation of blood (*PA* 651a4–12), suggesting that his theory of "dry water" may in fact be inspired by medical texts like *On Regimen*.

[13] For the idea that both wine and vinegar are primarily composed of fire, see p. 223. Note also the reference to the "hot and burning" juice of onions at 54.1, 6.556–558 L.

[14] "Blending": 6.1, 6.478 L., 7.1, 6.480 L., 25.1, 6.496 L., 26.2, 6.498 L., 28.4, 6.502 L., 32.2, 6.508 L., 32.6, 6.510 L., 33.1, 6.510 L., 35.1–2, 6.512–514 L., 35.8, 6.518 L., and 36.1, 6.522 L. "Separating out": 4.1, 6.474 L., 6.3, 6.480 L., and 10.2, 6.486 L. Compare note 77 on p. 46.

fact, the author's notions of "wet fire" and "dry water" may at least partly be intended to account for certain properties of the humors, such as the notion that some humors (e.g., blood) behave like liquid fire, while others (e.g., phlegm) resemble dry water.[15] One final point to consider is the author's assertion in chapter 35 that the "wettest fire" and "driest water" create a soul with the most intelligence. To justify this point, the author states that this combination of elements is the most "self-sufficient" (αὐτάρκης), since each element contains an abundant portion of the opposite on which it depends. This detail suggests that yet another reason for postulating "wet fire" and "dry water" is to illustrate the inseparability of these two elements. Just as fire depends on water, so too does water depend on fire, and it is accordingly impossible to completely isolate one of these elements from the other.

In Book 1, the author uses his principles of fire and water to describe both the shared nature of all human beings (chs. 3–24) and the particular constitutions of different classes of human beings (chs. 25–36). In Book 2, he then applies these same principles to the "powers" of the external factors that can influence a patient's health, including geographical locations (ch. 37), winds (ch. 38), food and drink (chs. 39–56), and different forms of physical activity (chs. 57–66). In Book 3, the author presents his great discovery of "prodiagnosis," a combination of prognosis and diagnosis that identifies an incipient disease before it has a chance to fully manifest (ch. 67). After describing the adjustments that every person must make as one season gives way to the next (ch. 68), the author records the signs, both on the body and in dreams, that will identify an imbalance in either eating or exercise before it gives rise to a full-blown disease (chs. 69–93).

The author of *On Regimen* presents his ideas in an impressively systematic manner. He also makes use of implicit analogies, refers only indirectly to the structure of the universe, and shows an unusual predilection for concise, telegraphic phrases, all of which requires a great deal of unpacking on the part of the reader. For a good introduction to the complexity of this work, we may turn to the following passage, in which the author first introduces his two main principles of fire and water (3.1, 6.472 L.):

> Both the human being and all other animals are composed of two things, different in their power [δύναμις] but complementary in their application [χρῆσις], fire and water. Together, these things are sufficient in themselves

---

[15] Compare *Vict.* 9.3, 6.484 L., where the author directly associates blood with "wet fire," and 89.2, 6.644–646 L., 89.7, 6.648 L., where "fiery" dreams indicate an excess of bile while "watery" dreams indicate an excess of phlegm.

[αὐτάρκεα] both for each other and for all other things; when separated, however, they are not sufficient either for themselves or for anything else.

What is most notable about this passage is the author's reference to "self-sufficiency" (αὐτάρκεια). By calling this combination of elements "self-sufficient," the author implies that they are self-supporting, independent, and not in need of anything else.[16] In chapter 35, he observes that the blend of fire and water that is "most sufficient in itself" (αὐταρκέστατον) is the one in which the wettest fire and the driest water are mixed with one another, since the fire in this circumstance is not "in need of nourishment" (τῆς τροφῆς ἐνδεέστερον) from any other source than the moisture with which it is mixed, while the water is not "in need of movement" (κινήσιος . . . δεόμενον) from any other source than the fire that is its neighbor (35.1, 6.512–514 L.). A similar opposition between self-sufficiency and "being in need" can be found in *On Regimen in Acute Diseases*. In this text, the author complains about doctors who indiscriminately apply the same treatment in every case, chiding them for not applying supplementary treatments to fit the needs of particular situations: "If one does not provide the additional treatments that this mode of treatment . . . needs [δέεται] to be sufficient in itself [αὐτάρκης], manifold harm will result" (16.1, 2.256 L.). The additional treatments that this author has in mind are the emptying of the bowels for those in whom they are obstructed, and the relieving of pains in the side for those afflicted with this condition. If these additional treatments are not applied, the administration of barley gruel will only exacerbate the disease. In another passage, the same author attacks *Cnidian Signs* for allegedly prescribing the same treatment in every case. In response, the author remarks that "if these remedies were good and suited [ἁρμόζοντα] to the diseases for which they are recommended, they would be much more worthy of praise because, while few, they would be sufficient in themselves [αὐτάρκεα]. But as it is, this is not the case" (3.1, 2.226 L.). Again, the author asserts that treatments must be adapted to the individual situation. It is only when they fulfill this requirement of "fitness to the situation" (ἁρμονία) that they can rightly be called "self-sufficient." In other texts, treatments are freely described as "sufficient in themselves."

---

[16] Compare Arist. *Pol.* 1326b27–30: "everyone would agree in praising the territory which is most self-sufficient; and that must be the territory which can produce everything necessary, for to have all things and to want nothing is self-sufficiency" (trans. Jowett *apud* Barnes). For similar definitions of "self-sufficiency," see Pl. *R.* 2.369b, 3.387d–e. Especially close to *On Regimen*'s use of this term is the description of first principles as "self-sufficient" at Pl. *Ti.* 33d, 68e and Arist. *Metaph.* 1091b16–19.

In these cases, the treatments enjoy "self-sufficiency" because they are simple and yet retain their effectiveness even when all other variables change. In *On Joints*, the author writes that "perforating cautery is exceedingly sufficient in itself [αὐταρκέστατον] for all cases of aggravated wounds" (40, 4.176 L.), while *On the Application of Liquids* claims that "sweet wine, applied continuously, is sufficient in itself [αὔταρκες] for all cases of chronic wounds" (5.1, 6.128 L.). In both passages, the authors claim that doctors do not need to apply other treatments when making these prescriptions. These treatments are "sufficient in themselves" inasmuch as they are simple and yet apply *universally* to all members of the specified class.

In light of these parallels, it is worth considering whether the author of *On Regimen* is drawing an implicit analogy between the elements and medical treatments. We might observe that when the author refers to fire and water as different in their "power" (δύναμις) but complementary in their "application" (χρῆσις), he employs two terms that could just as easily be applied to "powers" and "applications" of treatments. The term "power" is frequently associated with treatments in *On Regimen*, as the author observes that different foods, drinks, and exercises all have a different "power" to change what is happening in the body.[17] The word χρῆσις is even more interesting, as both the noun χρῆσις and the verb χρῆσθαι are standard terms in the Hippocratic Corpus for the "use" or "application" of treatments,[18] while the association of this term with *elements* is unusual to say the least.

What really confirms the analogy between the elements and treatments is the second chapter of *On Regimen*, in which the author defines what "anyone who intends to write correctly about human regimen" must consider before treating a patient.[19] First, the doctor should "recognize and

---

[17] On the medical use of the term *dunamis*, which literally denotes a "capacity" (< δύνασθαι) to act or be acted upon, see Plamböck (1964), von Staden (1998), and my discussion on pp. 152–153.

[18] On the verb χρῆσθαι, we may simply note the passage from *On the Application of Liquids* quoted earlier ("sweet wine, applied continuously [συνεχέως χρωμένῳ], is sufficient in itself [αὔταρκες] from all cases of chronic wounds," 5.1, 6.128 L.). The noun χρῆσις is applied to treatment at *VM* 4.1, 1.578 L., *Off.* 4, 3.286 L., *Ulc.* 2.3, 6.404 L., *Mul. II* 4, 8.244 L., *Medic.* 3, 9.208 L., 12, 9.218 L., *Praec.* 7, 9.260 L., and in the title of *On the Application of Liquids* (Περὶ ὑγρῶν χρήσιος).

[19] For the structure of this passage, compare *Prorrh. II* 11, 9.28–32 L.: "Whoever wants to discern about wounds, how each will end, must first know clearly the different constitutions of human beings, those better off with regard to wounds, and those worse off. Then he must know in which ages each of the wounds are difficult to cure, he must observe how the parts of the body differ [διαφέρει] from one another, and he must know which other evil and good things follow upon each. For if a person knows all these things, he will also know how each case will turn out, whereas if he does not, he will not know how the wounds will end" (trans. Potter). Such assertions of "what the doctor should know" are very common in the Hippocratic Corpus. Other examples include *VM* 20.1, 1.620 L., *Aër.*

discern" (γνῶναι καὶ διαγνῶναι) the nature of a person as a whole: he must recognize the "original constitution" (ἡ ἐξ ἀρχῆς σύστασις) and discern the component that has "gained the upper hand" (τὸ ἐπικρατέον, 2.1, 6.468 L.). What the author means in this sentence has been interpreted in different ways. On the one hand, it has been suggested that the author is claiming that one must learn both the common nature of all human beings (= chs. 3–10) and the particular natures of different classes of human beings (= chs. 32–36), not unlike the approach to human *phusis* that is attributed to Hippocrates in Plato's *Phaedrus*.[20] It is also possible, however, that the author is already writing with an eye toward treatment, in which case both "recognizing" and "differentiating" would be activities that the doctor must perform afresh for each patient. On this reading, the "original constitution" would not simply be the common nature of all human beings, but more specifically the aspects of one's *phusis* that remain the same from birth to death, namely one's sex and innate disposition toward a certain blend of fire and water (= chs. 32, 34–36), while "what has gained the upper hand" would denote the aspects of one's *phusis* that change over the course of a person's life; that is, the differences between children, youths, adults, and the elderly, which the author attributes to a cyclical "gaining the upper hand" of fire and water within the body (ch. 33). This second reading would better accord with the other lists of "what the doctor should know" that we find in the Hippocratic Corpus,[21] and it would also correspond with the author's own following of the constitutions of human beings with different age groups at 2.2, 6.470 L. and 67.1–2, 6.592 L.[22]

1, 2.12 L., *Prog.* 25, 2.188–190 L., *Epid. III* 16.2, 3.102 L., *Lex* 2, 4.638–640 L., *Morb. I* 1, 6.140–142 L., and *Oct.* 9.4, 7.448 L.

[20] For this reading, see, for example, Heidel (1941: 12n9). *On Regimen's* reference to the component that has "gained the upper hand" cannot refer to a concentrated humor or an otherwise noxious imbalance, as this would be a part of the patient's *diathesis* rather than their *phusis* (see note 94 on p. 62).

[21] For example, *Prorrhetic II's* list of "what the doctor should know" (quoted in note 19), which similarly follows the "constitutions of human beings" with different age groups (a sequence also found at *Acut. App.* 6.2, 2.404 L., *Fract.* 7, 3.440 L., *Aph.* 2.34, 4.480 L., 7.82, 4.606 L., *Morb. I* 16, 6.168–170 L., *Nat. Mul.* 1, 7.312 L., *Mul. I* 11, 8.42 L., *Mul. II* 2, 8.238–240 L., and *Hebd.* 28). At *Hum.* 1, 5.476 L., a person's "inborn constitution" (ξυγγενὲς εἶδος) is juxtaposed with their "age" (ἡλικίη) as well as other factors such as country, habit, season, and the constitution of the disease, recalling the lists of what the doctor should bear in mind in *On the Nature of the Human Being* (quoted on pp. 80–81). When Polybus writes that "the constituents of a human being are, according to both convention and nature, always alike the same, whether the patient be young or old, or whether the season be cold or hot" (2.5, 6.36 L.), he similarly draws a contrast between the permanent, inborn features of human *phusis* and those aspects of human *phusis* that change over the course of a person's life.

[22] At the end of chapter 32, the author closes his discussion of different blendings of fire and water by noting that "regarding the discerning of the nature of the original constitution [περὶ μὲν οὖν φύσιος

After determining the patient's *phusis*, both what is present "from the beginning" and what is due to the person's age, the author asserts that one must further learn the "powers" of the various foods and drinks that a patient might consume, both the powers that these substances have "by nature" (κατὰ φύσιν) and those they acquire "through compulsion and human art" (δι' ἀνάγκην καὶ τέχνην ἀνθρωπίνην, 2.1, 6.468 L.). "But even when all this is known," the author writes, "the patient's treatment is not yet sufficient in itself [οὔπω αὐτάρκης ἡ θεραπείη τοῦ ἀνθρώπου], since the patient cannot maintain health through eating without also taking exercise" (2.2, 6.468 L.). This claim that neither eating nor exercise is "sufficient in itself" recalls the author's assertion that when fire and water are taken separately, they are not "sufficient in themselves," either in relation to each other or to anything else (3.1, 6.472 L.), and the parallel grows even stronger when the author notes that "foods and exercises have opposite powers [δυνάμιας], but they are complementary [συμφέρονται] in their contribution to health" (2.2, 6.468–470 L.), mirroring his assertion that fire and water are "different in their power [δύναμις] but complementary [συμφόροιν] in their application" at 3.1, 6.472 L. The author continues his account of "what the doctor should know" by claiming that physicians should adjust their prescriptions to fit the needs of individual situations (2.2, 6.470 L.):

> One should discern . . . the due proportions [συμμετρίας] of exercises to the amount of foods, to the nature of the patient, to the ages of individuals, to the seasons of the year, to the changes of the winds, to the situations of the regions where people live, and to the constitution of the year. It is also necessary to recognize the risings and settings of the stars in order to know

διαγνώσιος . . . τῆς ἐξ ἀρχῆς συστάσιος], this is how one must discern [οὕτω χρὴ διαγινώσκειν]" (32.6, 6.510 L.), again suggesting that the "original constitution" is not the common *phusis* of all human beings but rather the original *phusis* we acquire at birth – a *phusis* that is not necessarily the same from one person to the next, but that can involve individualized mixtures of fire and water. In this passage, the repetition of the verb "discern" might suggest that these individual constitutions answer the second portion of the author's instructions, in which he says that one must "discern" (διαγνῶναι) the nature of a human being by identifying the element that has "gained the upper hand." Already in chapter 2, however, the author is inconsistent with his use of the verbs γιγνώσκειν and διαγιγνώσκειν, indicating that he will not necessarily maintain a sharp distinction between these two verbs later on in the text. Indeed, the author uses διαγιγνώσκειν at 32.3, 6.508 L. and γιγνώσκειν at 32.4, 6.510 L., both in reference to the same activity. Moreover, the verb "to gain the upper hand" (ἐπικρατεῖν) never appears in chapter 32, where the author is not speaking of a cyclical "dominating" and "being dominated" of fire and water but rather a "mixture" (σύγκρασις) that stays the same over the course of a person's life (hence the repetition of the phrase "original constitution," ἡ ἐξ ἀρχῆς σύστασις, at 32.6, 6.510 L.). Where we do find the verb ἐπικρατεῖν is chapter 33, where the author is discussing the differences between children, youths, adults, and the elderly. In this section, the verb (ἐπι)κρατεῖν appears three different times.

how to guard against changes and excesses in foods, drinks, winds, and the whole cosmos – the very things from which diseases arise in human beings.

Like other authors in the Hippocratic Corpus, the author of *On Regimen* asserts that treatments must be adapted to fit the needs of particular situations. The doctor must carefully consider all the factors that can influence human health, and then aim for the "due proportion" (συμμετρία) like an archer trying to hit a moving target.[23] Whereas other Greek doctors might have stopped at this point, the author of *On Regimen* pushes the matter even further, claiming that "even when all these things are discerned, the discovery is not yet sufficient in itself" (2.3, 6.470 L.). This repetition of the adjective αὐτάρκης clearly shows that the author is deeply concerned with the concept of self-sufficiency. Medicine is not yet sufficient in itself, he claims, because it is impossible to discover "a measure and proportionate number [μέτρον καὶ ... ἀριθμὸς σύμμετρος] of foods and exercises in accordance with the nature of each patient, without any imbalance toward either excess or deficiency" (2.3, 6.470 L.). Because the doctor cannot accompany a patient at all times, "it is impossible to set down [ὑποθέσθαι] foods and exercises with precision [ἐς ἀκριβείην]," since "if there arises even a slight deficiency of one thing or another, it is inevitable that, over time, the body will be overcome [κρατηθῆναι] by the excess and fall sick" (2.3, 6.470–472 L.).[24] The author uses these observations about the impossibility of precision and about the inevitability of disease to justify his great discovery of prodiagnosis. We will discuss this system in more detail later on, but for the time being, suffice it to say that both the system of prodiagnosis and the author's cosmology of fire and water appear to have been motivated by a similar set of concerns. On both fronts, the author seeks to overcome the many differences that exist between individual cases, uncovering a limited number of principles that are "sufficient in themselves" and not in need of anything else. The cosmology of fire and water is "sufficient in itself"

---

[23] The specific term for this target is the *kairos*, a word that the author employs at 2.1, 6.468 L. and 7.2, 6.480 L. For this concept, see p. 125.

[24] Note the parallel with *On Ancient Medicine*. In both texts, the authors claim that medicine lacks a precise "measure" (μέτρον) and "number" (ἀριθμός) that is the same in every case (cf. *VM* 9.3, 1.588–590 L.), and they also both claim that it is impossible to "set down" (ὑποθέσθαι) treatments without adapting them to particular situations. As we will see later in this discussion, the author of *On Regimen* expresses many of the same concerns about oversimplification and individual variation that we see in *On Ancient Medicine*. Where these authors differ is that the author of *On Ancient Medicine* rejects all *hupotheseis*, equating causal reductionism with therapeutic reductionism, while the author of *On Regimen* "sets down" his first principles as a means of overcoming the doctor's inability to "set down" treatments.

insofar as everything in the universe can be reduced to these two principles, while prodiagnosis is "sufficient in itself" insofar as it provides a reliable guide for preventing all forms of disease.

6.2 The Cyclical Universe

The author continues on this theme of "self-sufficiency" when he describes the powers of fire and water to move and to nourish, respectively (3, 6.472–474 L.):

> Now each of them has the following power [δύναμις]: fire has the power to move everything in every circumstance [πάντα διὰ παντὸς κινῆσαι], while water has the power to nourish everything in every circumstance [πάντα διὰ παντὸς θρέψαι]. Each one dominates and is dominated in turn [κρατεῖ καὶ κρατεῖται], to the maximum and minimum of what is possible. For neither is able to dominate completely for the following reason. The fire, as it advances to the limit of water, lacks nourishment and so turns away [ἀποτρέπεται] to the source from where it will be nourished. The water, as it advances to the limit of fire, lacks motion and so stops at that point, and when it stops, it no longer maintains the upper hand, but it is at once consumed as nourishment for the assailing fire. And it is for these reasons that neither is able to dominate completely. If either of them had been vanquished in the past, none of the things that now exist would be as they are now; but since they *are* as they are now, fire and water will always be the same, and neither of them will fail, either separately or together. So fire and water, as I said, are sufficient in themselves [αὐτάρκεα] for everything in every circumstance [πᾶσι διὰ παντός], to the maximum and minimum alike.

In this passage, the author stresses not only that fire and water can sustain "all things in all circumstances" (πάντα διὰ παντός) but also that they are locked in a continuous cycle of advancement and retreat. The author describes this cycle as one of "dominating" (κρατεῖν) and "being dominated" (κρατεῖσθαι), of one power advancing to its limit before turning around and allowing the other power to dominate in its turn. In the above-quoted passage, the author writes that fire first dominates water, "attacks" it, and grows in strength until it reaches a point where it no longer has sufficient nourishment, at which point the fire loses its dominance and starts to retreat, while the newly dominant water advances to the point where it, too, needs the assistance of its adversary. As we noted earlier (pp. 72–73), a similar principle of opposite interdependence can also be found in *On the Nature of the Human Being*. Both authors support this principle by pointing to the continuing existence of everything in the universe, and they both seem to have applied it, first and foremost, to the regular cycles that exist within the cosmos. In chapter 68, the author notes that the solstices, which the Greeks called "turning points" (τροπαί, the same term for the "routing" of an enemy), are the points in the year when winter and summer have reached their extremes, after which they become "more gentle" (μαλακωτέρη, 68.8, 6.598 L.) and start to give way, reaching a perfect balance at the spring and fall equinoxes before advancing to the opposite extreme. As we see in this example, the pendular cycle between fire and water "dominating" and "being dominated" is governed by two laws that are by no means intuitive, but are nevertheless central to the author's system. The first requires that the element that has "gained the upper hand" must retain its dominance until it has reached its extreme, with no switching of directions midcourse. The second requires that, after this extreme has been reached, the prevailing element must give way to its opposite, even if it still appears to be stronger than its adversary (as would be the case on the first day after a solstice).²⁵ The author sees this cycle of "dominating" and "being dominated" repeated throughout the cosmos. It governs the alternation of day and night, the lengthening and shortening of the days, the waxing and waning of the moon, and what is conventionally known as "life" and "death."

The cycle of life and death is especially interesting as it forms part of a more general cycle of creation and destruction. Fire and water are in constant motion. They move to this or that extreme as each element dominates and is dominated in turn, and at any given moment this ever-changing mixture can experience an *apokrisis*, separating off invisible "seeds" (σπέρματα) and "animals" (ζῷα) that will eventually give rise to visible objects (4.1, 6.474 L.). The constant change in the mixture of fire and water guarantees that the various secretions that separate off from this mixture will have "many different forms" (πολλὰς καὶ παντοδαπὰς ἰδέας) and that the resulting objects will be "by necessity dissimilar" (ἀνόμοια ἐξ ἀνάγκης, 4.1, 6.474 L.). The author also stresses that these secretions are "in no way similar to one another either in appearance or in power" (4.1, 6.474 L.), since different mixtures of fire and water will

---

²⁵ In this respect, the author would be susceptible to the same criticism that Aristotle directs against the alternating supremacies of love and strife in the system of Empedocles (*Metaph.* 1000b12–17).

by necessity give rise to different properties. Just after this statement, the author observes that when human beings talk about "life" and "death," we are not really using the proper terms (4.2, 6.474–476 L.):

> Of all things, nothing perishes, nor does anything come to be that did not exist before, but things change by mixing and separating. Humans, however, hold the belief that what increases, by moving from Hades to the light, comes to be, and what decreases, by departing from the light to Hades, perishes. For they put more faith in the eyes than in reason [γνώμη], though the eyes are incapable of judging even the things that they see. For my part, I will use reason for the following exposition. For there are living things both there [sc. in the realm of the invisible] and here [sc. in the realm of the visible]. And if there is a living thing, death is impossible, unless everything dies along with it. For whither would they go to die? Nor is it possible for what is not [τὸ μὴ ἐόν] to come to be. For whence will it have existence? But all things increase and decrease to the maximum and minimum of what is possible.

As the author stresses in this passage, the process of "coming to be" is simply an increasing in size of some preexisting seed. The seed grows by adding material to its frame, eventually acquiring a size that can be seen with the human eye. "Perishing," meanwhile, is simply a decreasing in size, a passing from the realm of the visible to that of the invisible. The real movement "from the light to Hades" is not a passing from life to death but a passing from the visible to the invisible. Hades, in this instance, is not the irredeemable destruction that we normally call "death," but simply a shrinking in size, a movement from what can be seen by the eyes to what can only be seen by the mind. Behind this statement, there is an obvious play on the name "Hades" (Ἅιδης), which in Greek recalls the adjective ἀϊδής ("invisible").[26] Death is not really "death" but rather one of two extremes in an ever-repeating cycle of growth and diminution, a "separating off" that will later be counterbalanced by a subsequent act of mixture.

This author's emphasis on the cycle of life and death, wherein "death" never really exists, has traditionally been read as an unimportant feature of *On Regimen*. The author, it is said, is simply stressing the bromide that "nothing comes from nothing," while any reference to "life" and "death" can simply be attributed to his unusual decision to mimic the stylings of

---

[26] On the association of Hades with invisibility, compare *Il.* 5.845, Pl. *Phd.* 80d, 81c, *Cra.* 403a, 404b, and *Grg.* 493b.

Heraclitus. Kirk (1954: 21) is especially cold in his assessment, noting that "there are places in these chapters where I would say that the author (unlike Heraclitus) simply did not know what he meant."[27] Joly (1984: 26) usually rushes to this author's defense, but even he thinks the passage is insignificant, writing that "these passages do not play a fundamental role in the overall thought of Book I: it is rather a sort of generalizing parenthesis which departs very temporarily from the specific purpose of the author, which is man, the nature of man." As we will see, however, this passage is in fact extremely significant and indeed *fundamental* to our understanding of this text. It points to an entire eschatological system that lies at the heart of *On Regimen*, a system that must be understood before we can appreciate the full significance of this work.

These references to the permanence of "life" and to the nonexistence of "death" are central to the author's thinking. They are not a stylistic ploy to give the text "philosophical" authority, but a reflection of the author's deeply held beliefs about the soul, the gods, and the overlapping "geographies" of the body and the cosmos. In what follows, I would like to reconstruct what the author believes about each of these topics. I will start with the geography of the cosmos and the general characteristics of animals and plants, after which I will move to the "geography" of the human body, a microcosmic structure that the author explicitly calls a "resemblance of the whole" (ἀπομίμησιν τοῦ ὅλου, 10.1, 6.484 L.). While describing the structure of the body and the nature of health and disease, I will have a good deal to say about the role of the doctor in restoring and maintaining a person's health. I will also, inevitably, focus on the soul, a fiery entity that dominates every aspect of this author's thinking. This discussion of the soul will eventually lead us to consider what this author has to say about the nature of "intelligence" (γνώμη) and about the proper method for both discovering and communicating insights about the "whole" (τὸ ὅλον). It will also bring us to one of the most important aspects of this text: the relationship between humans and the gods and what it means to be divine in a world of constant change.

By providing this general survey, I hope to clarify a number of topics that have not yet been fully explored in modern scholarship. I also hope to give the general reader, who may be encountering this text for the first time, a helpful starting point for approaching this complex and often difficult work, highlighting in particular how the author's cosmological

---

[27] A similar stance is taken by Barnes (1983: 100), who calls these chapters a "breathless and muddled farrago."

theories provide the basis for his "self-sufficient" system of medicine. The author of *On Regimen* adopts a narrow focus for his treatise ("human regimen in its relation to health," 1.1, 6.466 L.), but his thinking about this topic is rooted in a comprehensive understanding of the body and the cosmos, an elaborate and highly unified system whose details he frequently invokes only in passing. The author's fire–water cosmology is difficult to miss, but his system contains many other theories that are largely implicit and that can only be uncovered through a close reading of the text. Some significant work has already been done on this author's theory of the soul, his discussion of dreams, his analogies between "nature" and the crafts, and his general cosmology of fire and water, all of which have so far pointed to an impressive level of consistency and unity,[28] but there is still a great deal that has yet to be unpacked, especially regarding this author's views on the following four topics: (1) the overlapping structures of the body and the cosmos, (2) the origin, treatment, and prevention of disease, (3) the correct process for gaining and communicating insights, and (4) the true nature of divinity. The investigation of these topics has been discouraged, in part, by the sheer length and complexity of *On Regimen*. It has also been hampered by a long tradition of viewing this text as the work of an "eclectic" who cannot be held responsible for all the details in his system. For some scholars (e.g., Fredrich 1899), *On Regimen* was simply a cut-and-paste job by a mindless compiler. Others have resisted such an extreme characterization,[29] but it is still generally supposed that one of the most productive ways to understand this text is to catalog its various "debts." With one passage supposedly attributable to Heraclitus, another to Empedocles, and another to Anaxagoras, there is still some reluctance to approach this work as an interconnected whole. In his study of *On Regimen*, Bartoš (2015) correctly pushes against this view, emphasizing that *On Regimen* is "a text with remarkably strong unity in its structural composition, with precision in its details, and with a coherent theoretical stance pervading all four books," but even he concedes that "there are certainly passages that resist such a reading" and that "an ambition to make 'all the details harmonize exactly' would be rather a futile one" (p. 5). In what follows, I will treat *On Regimen* as the work of an author in full control of his system. By adopting this approach, I hope to clarify

---

[28] Among recent studies, see especially Bartoš (2015), Hulskamp (2016), and Schluderer (2018).

[29] For example, Diller (1959). Note, however, the persistence of the "compiler" designation in Langholf (1986: 26).

many obscurities in this text, opening up new perspectives on the author's system and clearing away any residual hesitance to read this text on its own terms.

Another reason for going into such detail about *On Regimen* is that it is an invaluable resource for the student of Greek cosmology. In a field where so many systems are preserved only in fragments and secondhand summaries, where even the selection of verbatim quotations is determined by the agendas of the ancient authors who cite them, what we need is a fully preserved text that illustrates the sort of cosmological system that could be constructed in this era. I am therefore providing this extended investigation not only to advance our understanding of *On Regimen* and the broader phenomenon of cosmological medicine but also to offer a helpful starting point for readers who might want to compare this text with other thinkers from this period. My discussion will necessarily be far-ranging, but I have throughout endeavored to proceed with clarity and as much concision as a text of this complexity will allow. As we will see, *On Regimen* is not just concerned with a simple back-and-forth between fire and water. Even more fundamentally, its author is guided by the assumption that the immortality of the soul cannot be separated from the discussion of health and disease, and that everything in the universe is guided by a cosmic intelligence that is concentrated in the sun, is composed of the strongest fire, and is the ultimate source from which all other divinities branch off. In this way, *On Regimen* shares many affinities with other thinkers from this era, and it thus provides a critical example of what it means to investigate the cosmos in the fifth and fourth centuries BCE.

6.3 Mapping the Cosmos

The author of *On Regimen* divides the cosmos into two parts. At the center lies the earth, which is primarily composed of water, while at the periphery there are the heavens, which are primarily composed of fire. The author believes that the earth contains two frozen poles and a hot and dry band across its diameter.[30] This central band is hot and dry because it is closest to the sun (i.e., because the sun moves along this line), while the two poles are frozen because they lie farthest from the sun and therefore manifest the extreme ascendancy of water. Between the north pole and the central band, the author places an inhabited zone, the *oikoumene*, which includes the Mediterranean and its encircling lands. There is

---

[30] *Vict.* 37.1, 6.528 L., 38.2–3, 6.530–532 L.

another inhabited zone in the south, although its geography and the nature of its inhabitants are left unspecified. All winds originate from the frozen poles. They start out cold and wet, and then become hotter, colder, drier, wetter, sicklier, or healthier depending on the regions through which they blow (38, 6.530–534 L.). The winds that originate from the south have the effect of cooling and moistening the southern *oikoumene*, while they become hot and dry as they pass the central desert and then change again when they cross the Mediterranean, thereby explaining why south winds are hot and dry in Libya but hot and wet in Greece. The winds that originate from the north pole cool and moisten the northern *oikoumene*. While passing the equator, they lose much of their water to the thirsty desert, and thus arrive in the south with the powers of heating and drying.

Between the frozen poles and the parched central band, the author believes that each *oikoumene* is primarily shaped by a cycle of evaporation and precipitation. As the sun sends its rays down to earth, it draws up moisture from anything that is wet – not only the sea but also animals and plants (37.1, 6.528 L.). For the author of *On Regimen*, the humors that are contained within plants are the same humors that can nourish the bodies of animals. Just as animals "cook" humors in their bellies, so plants "cook" their humors by the heat of the sun. This cooking ripens the juices in fruits, transforming them from acid to sweet, while further coction transforms the sweet juice of grapes into wine, and it ultimately completes the cycle back to acid (ὀξύς) by transforming wine into vinegar (ὄξος). As these juices ripen, the fire within them steadily increases to the point where they no longer contain any nutriment. Acidic fruits cool and moisten, sweet fruits warm and moisten, wine warms and dries, and vinegar cools and dries because its fire consumes all the loose moisture in the body.[31]

In addition to plants, the earth is also home to animals, a category to which we humans belong. Different animals thrive in different environments, while their varying diets, activities, and habitats change the qualities of their humors and flesh.[32] The flesh of animals is constructed primarily

---

[31] Acidic foods cool and moisten: 52.3, 6.556 L., 55.3, 6.562 L. Sweet foods warm and moisten: 55.3–4, 6.562–564 L. Wine warms and dries: 52.1–3, 6.554–556 L. Vinegar cools and dries: 52.4, 6.556 L., 56.1, 6.564 L., 56.8, 6.570 L., 79.2, 6.624 L., 81.2, 6.628 L.; compare 42.1, 6.540 L. For the cooling that comes when the flesh is emptied of moisture, thereby allowing cold *pneuma* to fill the empty space, see 57.1, 6.570 L., 60.1, 6.572 L., 60.4, 6.574 L., 66.7, 6.586 L., 83.1, 6.634 L., and compare Arist. [*Pr.*] 1.29, 862b35–863a5.

[32] *Vict.* 28.4, 6.502 L., 41.2, 6.538 L., 46, 6.544–546 L., 56.4, 6.566–568 L.

On Regimen

out of water, while their growth, movements, sensations, and thoughts are directed by a fiery soul. In chapter 28, the author makes the critical observation that

> soul is the same for everything that is ensouled, while the body of each is different. So soul is always similar both in the larger and the smaller, for it is not altered either naturally or through compulsion, while the body of anything is never the same either naturally or through compulsion, for it dissolves into everything and is mixed with everything. (28.1, 6.500–502 L.)

Since all living things share a single, unalterable soul, what makes one animal differ from another is the specific arrangement of the watery body around this fiery soul.[33] Human reproduction begins with a soul that already possesses all the parts of a human being.[34] When this "portion" (μοῖρα) first separates off from a larger mixture, the watery body dominates the fiery soul and prevents the animal from growing. These invisible seeds of animals float around in the air, and they do not begin to grow until they are breathed into the body of another animal. Once these seeds have been inhaled, they are then nourished by the soul of the larger animal, which feeds the seed a diet of dry water and hot fire.[35] The author specifically says that these seeds are breathed in by animals that are "large" (6.3, 6.480 L.) and in whom respiration occurs (25.1, 6.496 L.), a detail that has puzzled many readers of *On Regimen*. As Bartoš (2015: 210) observes, "it is not exactly clear what the author has in mind when restricting his account only to 'large' animals." Elsewhere, the author observes that the invisible seeds of animals (i.e., animals that are "small") are secreted during the alternating ascendancies of fire and water (4.1, 6.474 L.), and he also remarks that respiration is acquired only after these seeds begin to grow in size (9.1, 6.482 L.). For this author, size is inextricably linked to his cycle of growth and diminution, in which "death" is simply a return to the realm of the invisibly small. Thus, by referring to animals that are "large" and in whom respiration occurs, the author may simply intend to distinguish the invisible, free-floating "seeds" of animals from those that have grown large enough to initiate respiration. Another possibility is that the author is drawing a distinction between different species of fully grown animals. For this point, we may compare Aristotle's claim that insects and fish do not engage in respiration (*Sens.* 444b7–10, *GA* 742a1–5) and the widely attested belief that

---

[33] *Vict.* 6.3, 6.478–480 L.
[34] *Vict.* 6.1, 6.478 L., 6.3, 6.478 L., 7.1, 6.480 L., 25.1, 6.496 L., 26, 6.498 L.
[35] *Vict.* 7.2, 6.480 L., 25, 6.496–498 L.

some small animals are not born through sexual reproduction but are instead generated spontaneously (e.g., Arist. [*Pr.*] 1.16, 861a10–19). To explain why insects and fish are still able to smell and move even without respiration, Aristotle claims that their bodies contain a certain innate *pneuma*, which "is present from the beginning in all of them by nature and not introduced from outside" (*PA* 659b18–19). Thus, the author of *On Regimen* might be thinking about small lungless animals such as insects, which do not participate in reproduction via respiration but are instead spontaneously generated around a free-floating soul.

Regardless of what the author thinks about other animals, he restricts his narrative to human beings in the opening of chapter 7. In human beings, the union of seeds takes place in the womb. After an inhaled soul has grown for a period of time, it makes its way to the womb, and, if everything attains the proper "attunement" (ἁρμονία), it has the potential to be combined with another soul when its host engages in sexual intercourse. Both the male and the female secrete a seed that contains a mixture of fire and water. On its own, the fire in each seed is over-powered by its watery body, but when it falls upon and mixes with the fire in the other seed, they have enough strength to "dominate" the water in turn.[36] This mixture then initiates an ascendancy of fire that lasts from the formation of the embryo to the midpoint of the animal's life, at which point the growing soul will run out of nutriment and yield to the oncoming water.[37] From middle age to "death," the ascendancy of

---

[36] *Vict.* 27.2, 6.500 L., 30.1, 6.504 L. At 9.1, 6.482 L. and 29.2, 6.504 L., the author uses the verb ζωπυρεῖσθαι ("to be imbued with the fire of life"), a term that nicely encapsulates his idea that what we call "life" begins when fire "gains the upper hand" over water. At 27.2–3, 6.500 L., the author also observes that this mixture of two seeds can only occur when the womb is sufficiently dry, and that this dryness only occurs one day each month. The author interestingly states that this "attunement" within the womb is musical in nature, involving the three concordances of the fourth, the fifth, and the octave (see Pelosi 2016). For limits of space, I will save my own thoughts on this analogy for a later publication, as it has far-ranging implications not only for *On Regimen* but also for other thinkers who see musical "attunement" in the arrangement of the cosmos (e.g., Parmenides, Heraclitus, Philolaus, and Plato).

[37] *Vict.* 25, 6.496–498 L., 33, 6.510–512 L. For the consumption of the available nutriment as the cause of this "retreat," see 29.2, 6.504 L. In *Epidemics I*, older people are similarly described as "those in whom the hot is now being dominated [sc. by the cold]" (ὅσοις ἤδη τὸ θερμὸν κρατεῖται, 12.3, 2.638 L.). This passage suggests that *On Regimen*'s conception of aging, wherein heat first "dominates" and then "is dominated" by the cold, draws on a belief that was already circulating among Greek doctors by the late fifth century BCE. Compare *Morb. Sacr.* 9, 6.376–378 L., where the young are said to have blood that is hot and thus able to "dominate" (κρατεῖν) the coldness of phlegm, while the old have blood that is cold and "watery" (ὑδαρές) and thus "dominated" (κρατηθέν) by phlegm. *On the Sacred Disease*'s opposition of hot blood with cold phlegm is strikingly similar to *On Regimen*'s opposition of fire and water, again suggesting that this author's cosmology has deep roots in medical thinking.

water gradually forces the soul out of our bodies. "Death" occurs when the last remnant of the soul separates off into the realm of the invisible (29.2, 6.504 L.). After the soul separates off, it can be inhaled by another animal, thereby starting the whole cycle again.

At a certain point, the soul might be liberated from this cycle, shedding its watery body and rejoining some larger collection of soul-like fire within the *aither*.[38] As the soul travels through the *aither*, it will encounter three "circuits" (περίοδοι) that are located progressively farther from the earth. The circuit that is closest to the earth belongs to the moon, the uppermost circuit belongs to the stars, while the middle circuit belongs to the sun.[39] At the limit of the uppermost circuit, there is a hard shell, the *periechon*, beyond which nothing can pass,[40] while the lowermost circuit is bounded by the *aer*, a layer of moist air that is home to all meteorological phenomena.[41] This strip of moist *aer* is distinct from the dry *aither* that is home to the heavenly bodies, which the author specifically labels as "divine" (5.1, 6.476 L.).[42] Like the winds that change their quality depending on the regions through which they blow, the material that comes down from the *aither* can be either pure or impure, healthy or diseased, presumably acquiring its impurities as it travels through the *aer* (89.12, 6.650–652 L.).[43]

The author of *On Regimen* seems to have believed that the sun is the most important entity in the cosmos. When he prescribes prayers to the gods, it is Helios who comes first (89.14, 6.652 L.), while he equates the "hottest and strongest" fire in our bodies with the circuit of the sun, observing that the central fire in our bodies "steers all things in all circumstances, both these things here and those things there, never staying still" (10.3, 6.486 L.). He also claims that our bodies' hottest and strongest fire contains "soul, mind, thought,

---

[38] The idea that our souls return to the *aither* after death was commonplace in the Classical period. Compare the epitaph for those who died at Potidaea in 432 BCE ("The *aither* received their souls and the earth their bodies"). As we will see, the author of *On Regimen*'s understanding of divinity and the soul strongly suggests that he shared this common belief.

[39] *Vict.* 10.2, 6.486 L., 89.2, 6.644–646 L.   [40] *Vict.* 10.2, 6.486 L.

[41] *Vict.* 10.1–2, 6.484–486 L., 89.2, 6.644 L., 89.13, 6.652 L.

[42] On the dryness of *aither*, note the association of "clear sky" (αἰθρία) with dryness at 89.6, 6.646 L. For a similar distinction between *aither* and *aer*, see *Carn.* 2, 8.584 L. (quoted on pp. 178–179).

[43] On the essential healthiness of the *aither*, note the reference to *aer* corrupting the heavenly bodies at 89.2, 6.644–646 L., and compare *Epid. VI* 4.17, 5.310 L.: "Of natural waters, what is separated off [ἀποκριθέν] from the *aither* with thunder is good, while what comes out of a storm is bad." Compare also DK 64 A19, where Diogenes of Apollonia is said to have contrasted land animals who consume "wetter nutriment" and breathe "air from the earth" with the various birds who breathe the "clean" air in the sky.

movement, growth, diminution, change, sleep, and waking" (10.3, 6.486 L.), and that "from the division of one soul there arise other souls, more and less numerous, greater and smaller in size" (16.2, 6.490 L.). In light of these passages, I would like to suggest that the author views the sun as the equivalent of the soul within our bodies. Its fire is the "one soul" from which all other souls branch off, the director of the universe as a whole. Anything else that possesses either intelligence or movement is merely an emanation of this fire, and it represents a unitary god from which all other divinities branch off. I will elaborate on each of these points over the course of my discussion. Before doing so, however, let me offer some further observations about the cycle of "life" and "death" and the relationship between our bodies and the cosmos as a whole.

We have already mentioned the "ascendancy" and "retreat" of the soul within our bodies. Its ascendancy begins when the male and female seeds are mixed together, and it ends when the animal reaches middle age. At this point, the fire loses its dominance to water, and our fiery soul is gradually forced out of the body from middle age until the moment that we "die." To explain how two souls can initially mix together, the author compares two sets of coals that are burning at different temperatures and then placed next to each other. Even though one set of coals is stronger and the other is weaker, the coals will eventually become indistinguishable from one another, burning at precisely the same intensity (29.2, 6.504 L.). The author then adds that, at a certain point, the fire within these coals will have consumed all the available nutriment. At this point, the fire will "separate off" into the realm of the invisible (διακρίνονται ἐς τὸ ἄδηλον) in the same way that the human soul will separate off after water acquires dominance over fire (29.2, 6.504 L.). Another analogy with the separating off of the soul from the body can be found in chapter 44. In this passage, the author notes that freshly cooked foods are drier than foods that are "old" (παλαιά), since freshly cooked foods are "closer to the fire," while "as they grow old they breathe out the hot component and bring the cold into themselves" (τὸ μὲν θερμὸν ἐκπνεῖ, τὸ δὲ ψυχρὸν ἐπάγεται). The author does not explicitly refer to the soul in this passage, but he is almost certainly drawing an implicit analogy between the aging of food and the lives of human beings. Just as foods become cold and wet as they age, so too do humans grow cold and wet as they approach the ends of their lives. We "breathe out" our fiery soul and replace it with cold water in the same way that foods gradually "breathe out" their heat and replace it with an "inhalation" of watery *pneuma*.

In chapter 25, the author adds a further detail to this process, observing that just as we exhale portions of our soul when water dominates fire, so too can we *inhale* souls and temporarily house them when our bodies are in the prime of life:

> The soul of the human being, possessing a mixture of fire and water and parts of a human being, enters into every animal that breathes and in particular into every human being, both the younger and the older. However, it does not grow in all of them in the same way. In young bodies, because the revolution [of the fiery soul] is rapid and the body is growing, [the incoming soul] is engulfed in fire, thinned out, and consumed for the growth of the body. In older bodies, because the movement [of the fiery soul] is slow and the body is cold, [the incoming soul] is consumed for the diminution of the human being. Bodies that are at their peak and in the fertile period of life are able to provide [these souls with] nourishment and growth. A human potentate is strong when he is able to provide nourishment for many human beings, but he is weaker when they abandon him. A similar circumstance applies to all bodies. They are very strong when they are able to provide nourishment for many souls, but they are weaker when these [souls] depart.

This passage describes the body's inability to nourish souls during two distinct stages in a person's life. The first stage is when the body is young and fire dominates water, while the second stage is when the body is older and water dominates fire. Both younger and older bodies (and, for that matter, both humans and other animals) inhale the free-floating souls of human beings. By "souls," the author technically means the "seeds" of a human being, consisting of a fiery soul and its watery body, relegated to the realm of the invisible. When we are young, the fire in our souls dominates the water in our bodies, thereby causing the soul to move very rapidly. When our souls encounter the inhaled seeds of human beings, they engulf them in fire and cause them to be "thinned out." By saying that these seeds are "thinned out" (λεπτύνεσθαι), the author implies that a lighter component in this mixture is separated off from a heavier component. The lighter component increases the intensity of the fiery soul and contributes to the growth of the body, while the heavier component is expelled from the body, presumably by way of breath. Parallels with other texts suggest that the author locates this entire process in the heart, which receives *pneuma* from the windpipe and is connected to the rest of the body by way of the vascular system. In *On Flesh*, the author writes that "the child in the belly, puckering its lips, suckles and draws both the nourishment and the *pneuma* from the mother's womb into the heart – for this is the hottest part of the child – whenever the mother inhales" (6.3, 8.592 L.). *On the Heart* similarly observes that "whereas a person must of necessity expel the air, after it has fulfilled its office, back through the same passage by which he drew it in, the moisture he partly spits out into the sheath of the heart, and partly allows to go back with the air to the outside" (3.1, 9.82 L., trans. Potter).

According to the author of *On Regimen*, the circulation of our souls slows down when we grow older and our bodies become colder. The water in our bodies acquires dominance over fire, and it initiates the inevitable march toward the dissolution we know as "death." At this stage in a person's life, the human seeds that we inhale contribute to the diminution of the soul. It is not the fire but rather the water that is dominant at this stage, with the result that the watery part of the inhaled *pneuma* gradually pushes out our fiery soul. All the fire that we had previously inhaled is now abandoning the cooling body, eventually reaching a point where the last remnant of our fiery soul is expelled with our final breath. This is what the author means when he refers to the departure of souls that had previously been "nourished" in our bodies. The *pneuma* that we inhale is a mixture of fiery souls surrounded by their watery bodies. Depending on whether fire or water is dominant at a particular stage in a person's life, this ensouled *pneuma* will either increase or decrease our fiery souls whenever we engage in respiration. The analogy with coals is especially enlightening when applied to this process. As with human beings, the coal begins its "life" with an abundance of moisture and a fire that has just established its dominance. The fire continues to grow in strength until all the available nourishment is used up, at which point the fire is slowly "breathed out" until all that is left is cold ash. When the fire is dominant in the first half of the coal's life, a blast of air will make the fire grow stronger and burn hotter. When the fire is receding in the second half of the coal's life, a blast of air will simply hasten the rate at which the fire is peeled off.[44]

Even when reduced to the realm of the invisibly small, our souls are still enveloped in a watery body that contains all the parts of a human being. In chapter 7, the author explains why this has to be: "it is necessary for the things that enter [i.e., the seeds of animals that we inhale] to have all the parts, since whatever does not have a portion of itself from the beginning cannot grow, whether the incoming nutriment is great or small, because the nutriment has nothing to grow onto." Growth proceeds by the

---

[44] See *Vict.* 13, 6.488 L., where the author compares respiration to the stoking of fire in a furnace, and 65, 6.582 L., where ash and dust are specifically labeled as cold.

principle of "like to like," so if a part does not already exist, it cannot increase in size. As the soul moves around the body, it takes substances from one place and deposits them in another, but it never endows the body with a completely new part. One exception to this rule comes in chapter 9, when the author describes a moment in embryogenesis where the fiery soul becomes trapped within the embryo. This happens when the soul's increasing heat causes the body's exterior to harden, producing an impenetrable shell of skin that recalls – but is not quite as impervious as – the *periechon* that surrounds the entire universe. With no other avenue for bringing in nutriment, the fire must consume the moisture in the body. Any water that is "wet," "soft," and dominated by the fire will be completely consumed, giving rise to hollow parts such as the belly and the vessels. The "wettest" part of the fire remains in the vessels and becomes the conveyor of both blood and *pneuma*, while any water that is "dry" cannot be consumed by the fire but it is rather condensed to make sinews, bones, and the membranes around the hollows. In between everything else, there is flesh (σάρκες). The author uses this term interchangeably with "the body" (τὸ σῶμα), and he implies that the flesh is simply a mass of concentrated water that has condensed by virtue of being cold.

6.4   A Resemblance of the Whole

In chapter 10, the author makes his critical observation that "the fire set everything in the body in proper order by itself as a resemblance of the whole [ἀπομίμησιν τοῦ ὅλου], small in relation to large and large in relation to small." The anatomy of the human being, in other words, reflects the "anatomy" of the cosmos, as the soul constructs our bodies in such a way that the geography of the cosmos can be "mapped" onto the body. The author does not explain why this analogy exists, but it may be related to the fact that our soul is merely a secretion of the central fire that governs the universe as a whole. This central fire is ultimately responsible for putting the entire cosmos in order, and we should therefore not be surprised if a portion of this fire, when trapped within a body, shapes the body in such a way as to make the "small" resemble the "large," turning the body into a "resemblance of the whole." There is only one intelligence in the universe, only one "soul," and so it will perform the same actions wherever it is found. This interpretation is supported by the author's claim that the soul of all animals is the same, regardless of the individual species (28.1, 6.500–502 L.). It is also supported by his assertion that there is *pneuma* (i.e., the source of these souls) both in animals and in all other

things (38.1, 6.530 L.), as well as his claim that the hottest and strongest fire
within our bodies "steers all things in all circumstances, both these things
here and those things there, never staying still" (10.3, 6.486 L.). By
mentioning "these things here and those things there," the author refers,
on the one hand, to the parallels between an invisible "seed" of a human
being and a fully grown individual. At the same time, he also seems to
associate our bodies with the universe as a whole, holding that the central
fire in our bodies reflects the heavenly fire that governs the entire cosmos.
In his extended analogy between the body and the cosmos, the author
specifically connects our "central intelligence" with the sun, which likewise
inhabits a central circuit and sends its rays down to earth. Just as the
"hottest and strongest" fire in our bodies is the source of all movement,
growth, and intelligence, so the "hottest and strongest" fire in the heavens
performs all of these same functions on a much larger, cosmic scale. This
implicit analogy appears to be activated already in chapter 6, where the
author claims that the soul, no matter the scale, "revolves around"
(περιφοιτᾷ, 6.3, 6.478 L.) its parts, adding material to some while taking
it away from others, just as the sun shapes the earth through a cycle of
evaporation and precipitation.[45] This soul "does everything [i.e., all the
same things] wherever it goes" (6.3, 6.478 L.), a statement that seems to
encapsulate the idea that wherever fire is located, it will perform the same
actions.

In chapter 10, the author observes that the body, like the cosmos,
contains a bipartite division between "earth" and "sky," in which the
earth is further subdivided into "land" and "sea." He also notes that the
"sky" within our bodies is subdivided into three fiery "circuits" (περίοδοι),
in which the middle circuit contains the hottest and strongest fire and is
associated with the sun, the innermost circuit contains a weaker form of
fire, is engaged in a constant struggle with water, and is associated with the
moon, and the outermost circuit contains fire that is also weaker than the
fire in the middle circuit, is scattered in many directions, and is associated
with the stars. The sky and its three circuits map onto the vascular system,
while the earth maps onto the rest of the body. The body proper (i.e., the

---

[45] For the association of the verb περιφοιτᾶν with the revolution of the heavenly bodies, see Parm. DK
28 B10.4 and compare the references to the "revolutions" (περιφοραί) of both the soul and the
heavenly bodies at *Vict.* 10.2, 6.486 L., 22, 6.494 L., 25.1, 6.498 L., and especially 89.2–3, 6.644–646
L. and 89.10, 6.650 L. In chapter 6, the author also notes that free-floating souls "wander"
(πλανᾶσθαι, 6.3, 6.480 L.), using the same verb that Greek astronomers applied to the "wandering"
planets. At 89.9, 6.648 L., the author observes that dreams about a "wandering" sun, moon, or star
signify a disturbance of the soul.

flesh) correlates with the land, while the belly correlates with the sea. As in the universe as a whole, the "sky" (i.e., the vascular system) contains the highest concentration of fire, while the "earth" and "sea" (i.e., the flesh and the belly) contain the highest concentration of water. The flesh is simply a concretion of cold water, as is the case with the earth. The belly, meanwhile, is a "storeroom for dry and wet water" (10.1, 6.484 L.), and it resembles the sea insofar as it experiences evaporation into a microcosmic *aer*, giving off "thin water and *aer*-like fire" (10.2, 6.484–486 L.) when exposed to external heat. Incidentally, this reference to fire as "*aer*-like" (ἠέριος) suggests a close connection between fire and air. The author tends to associate *pneuma* with fire, as his reference to how "winds" (πνεύματα) are ejected from the frozen poles closely recalls his description of how fiery "breath" (πνεῦμα) is ejected when water dominates fire in both aging bodies and cooling foods.

The most important aspect of this analogy between the body and the cosmos is the author's discussion of the vascular system. As Hüffmeier (1961) has demonstrated in a meticulous analysis of this text, the author places a mixture of blood and *pneuma* in the vessels, associating them both with the soul. Part of this mixture is a distillation of the "thinnest" water and the "wettest" fire that is separated from food and drink,[46] and it is combined with the "thinnest" portion of *pneuma* that is breathed into the heart and is likewise separated off from a heavier component. This soul-mixture is manifested in the form of pulsating blood, and it runs through the body's vessels to provide movement, growth, and sensory perception to all the parts.[47] The soul's speed, perceptiveness, attentiveness, and memory are all determined by the amount of water with which it is mixed, with the ideal mixture having a slight imbalance in the direction of fire, thereby allowing the soul to move at a brisk pace.[48] If the soul is too wet, it will move too slowly and lack perceptiveness, while if the soul is too dry, it will move too quickly and overinterpret all sensory data. Regimen can change the amount of moisture in the vessels but it cannot change the structure of the vessels themselves. It is therefore possible to use regimen to make a person more perceptive or intelligent, but regimen cannot be used to change someone who is "quick-tempered, easy-tempered, deceitful, straightforward, unfriendly, or friendly" (36.2, 6.522 L.), since all of these traits depend on the structure of the vessels through which the soul-mixture flows.

---

[46] *Vict.* 7.2, 6.480 L., 10.2, 6.484–486 L.   [47] *Vict.* 10.2–3, 6.486 L.
[48] *Vict.* 35, 6.512–522 L. On this whole chapter, see Hankinson (1991: 200–206) and Enache (2015).

As we have already noted, the author's analogy between the body and the cosmos divides the vascular system into three "circuits" that mirror the revolutions of the sun, moon, and stars. The innermost circuit extends to the belly and concocts all food and drink. Like the moon, the fire in this circuit is engaged in a constant struggle with water, and it transmits an exhalation from the belly (= the "sea") of "thin water and *aer*-like fire" (10.2, 6.484–486 L.) that seems to reflect the process of evaporation. As for the outermost circuit, this extends to the flesh, branching off in many directions just as the stars are scattered in the sky. The soul in this outermost circuit plays three important roles in the author's physiological system. First, it brings moisture into the flesh and consumes moisture out of the flesh, a cycle that, as we will see, is critical for the maintenance of health. Second, it creates movement in the limbs by sending portions of itself out to the various parts,[49] and third, it picks up sensory data in the form of "hot and cold *pneuma*" (10.1, 6.484 L., 23.2, 6.496 L.) from the eyes, the ears, the nostrils, the tongue, and the skin, after which it transports this information back to the middle circuit for analysis by the body's intelligence (γνώμη). All of these activities are governed by the hottest and strongest fire that is an analogue to the sun and is located in the middle circuit. This circuit seems to comprise the heart and two vessels that run up and down the torso, forming the central trunk from which all other vessels branch off.[50] The other two circuits of the vascular system carry weaker secretions of this central fire to the rest of the body, illustrating the author's principle that "from the division of one soul there arise other souls, more and less numerous, greater and smaller in size" (16.2, 6.490 L.). In this context, the author writes that the body's hottest and strongest fire contains "soul, mind, thought, movement, growth, diminution, change, sleep, and waking" (10.3, 6.486 L.) and that this fire "steers all things in all circumstances, both these things here and those things there, never staying still" (10.3, 6.486 L.).[51] The middle circuit runs both "inward and outward"

---

[49] *Vict.* 10.3, 6.486 L., 16.2, 6.490 L., 86.1, 6.640 L.

[50] On this point, see Joly (1960: 41–43), Hulskamp (2012: 165), and Shcherbakova (2018). The author of *On the Heart* also compares the heart to the sun, describing how the heart first drinks up a distillation of nutriment and then sends out its "rays" (ἀκτῖνες) through the body (11.1, 9.88–90 L.). For the belief that the hottest blood is located in the region around the heart, see also Arist. *PA* 653a29–30.

[51] For this distinction between a "central intelligence," located in the heart, and the rest of the soul, compare *Cord.* 10.3, 9.88 L.: "For the intelligence [γνώμη] of the human being is located in the left ventricle and commands the rest of the soul." See also *Epid.* II 6.19, 5.136 L., *Oss.* 19, 9.196 L., Pl. *Phd.* 96b, and especially the reference to mortals being "steered" by the vessels, "some extending up and some down" (i.e., from the heart), at Antiph. fr. 42 K–A.

(ἔσω καὶ ἔξω, 10.2, 6.486 L.),[52] and the entire vascular system forms something of an interconnected circle.[53] The author also observes that our body's central fire is "untouched by both sight and touch" (10.3, 6.486 L.), representing pure thought (διάνοια), mind (νοῦς), and intelligence (γνώμη) that, under the right conditions, can stand apart from the world of the senses.

As we noted earlier, there are two main divisions of the body in *On Regimen*: the belly and the flesh. These two reservoirs of moisture are connected to each other by way of the vascular system, and problems in either part can threaten the body as a whole. When everything in the body is working according to plan, the innermost circuit concocts food and drink within the belly. It separates out the lightest component of whatever we ingest, and it then transfers this "secretion" (ἀπόκρισις)[54] to the middle circuit before expelling the heavier component through the intestines. The middle circuit then takes up this secretion from the innermost circuit, separates off an even lighter component to nourish its own fire,[55] and then sends out the rest of the nutriment to be distributed to the flesh.[56] As the soul in the outermost circuit moves around the flesh, it consumes any stagnant moisture it encounters and replaces it with a delivery of fresh humors that it has just received from the middle circuit. Each component of the flesh then attracts "like to like" what it needs from this humoral mixture, while the rest is simply left to stagnate. This stagnant moisture then waits until the soul comes back around through the outermost circuit, at which point the soul drinks up the stagnant moisture and starts the whole process again.[57]

---

[52] On vessels that pass "inward" to the belly and "outward" to the rest of the body, compare *Nat. Hom.* 11.5, 6.60 L.

[53] *Vict.* 19, 6.492–494 L.; compare *Loc. Hom.* 1.1–2, 6.276 L., *Oss.* 11, 9.182 L., and Herophilus fr. 115 von Staden.

[54] For this use of the term *apokrisis*, see 10.2, 6.486 L. and 90.1, 6.654 L.

[55] *Vict.* 35.10, 6.520 L., 56.6, 6.568 L., 62.2–3, 6.576–578 L.; compare *Cord.* 11, 9.88–90 L. For the nourishment of the heavenly bodies by evaporated moisture, see Aristotle's arguments against this view at *Mete.* 354b33–355a32.

[56] Inasmuch as the belly is a "storeroom" of nutritive moisture (ταμιεῖον, 10.1, 6.484 L.), this would make the soul the body's "steward" (ταμίας). Compare *Carn.* 5.2, 8.590 L., where the heart, because it contains much of the hot, is said to "distribute" (ταμιεύει) *pneuma* throughout the body. At *Ti.* 84d, Plato likewise calls the lungs the "steward" of the breath, while *Genit.-Nat. Puer.* 26.2, 7.526 L. refers to a "dispensing" (ταμιείη) of cold and heat from a tree's roots. Note also Democr. DK 68 B149, where the belly is said to be a "storeroom and treasury of evils," and the comic reference to the belly as a "storeroom" at Phoenicid. fr. 3 K–A.

[57] Scattered references to this process appear throughout *On Regimen*, although the clearest discussions can be found in the chapters on exercise (61–66, 6.574–588 L.). This cycle of moistening and drying seems to be the primary reason why the author defines human regimen as an act of "moistening the dry" and "drying the moist" at 17, 6.492 L. and 22.2, 6.494 L.

When this system is completely efficient, the body enjoys a state of *summetria* ("due proportion") that the author defines as health. Moisture is distilled from the belly and delivered to the flesh at the same rate that the soul in the outermost circuit empties the flesh of excess moisture. If there is a slight imbalance in one direction or another, the flesh will become too wet or too dry. Pain is produced when a part of the body is emptied to a degree that is contrary to what is accustomed, and it also arises when moisture that is "hostile" to the flesh (πολέμιος) spends too much time in its vicinity.[58] As the hostile moisture stagnates in the flesh, it can disrupt the normal distribution of nutriment to the flesh, and it can even grow hot and attract more moisture to itself.[59] Once these humors have reached a certain volume, they can either stay where they are or move throughout the body, initiating a "flux."[60] Individual diseases such as pneumonia and strangury acquire their particular characteristics from differences in the quality of the humor and the part that it overpowers,[61] although all diseases ultimately come from the same source: a lack of "due proportion."

6.5 Treating and Preventing Disease

Like other doctors from the Classical period, the author of *On Regimen* presents illness as a battle between what is "healthy" and what is "diseased," in which both the healthy parts and the disease struggle to "gain the upper hand."[62] To assist the healing process, the author advises that doctors strengthen the healthy parts while avoiding any treatments that will strengthen the disease – the same procedure that is recommended in the speech of Eryximachus.[63] He also stresses the importance of identifying the cause of a disease, and he explicitly rejects the *post hoc, propter hoc* reasoning of patients who attribute their ailments to whatever they happened to be doing before they fell sick.[64] The specific diseases that the author cites are the same affections that are identified in other texts from the Hippocratic Corpus: fevers, chills, pneumonia, strangury, diarrhea, dysentery, lientery,

---

[58] *Vict.* 66, 6.582–588 L., 76.1, 6.618 L., 78.1, 6.622 L.
[59] On the tendency of humors to stagnate, grow hot, and attract moisture to themselves, see p. 41.
[60] *Vict.* 71.2, 6.610 L., 73.1, 6.612 L., 77, 6.620 L., 78.1, 6.620–622 L.
[61] *Vict.* 70.1, 6.606 L., 71.3, 6.610 L., 72.1, 6.610 L., 73.1, 6.612 L. Compare the explanation of how diseases differ from one another in *On Breaths* (pp. 116–119).
[62] *Vict.* 2.4, 6.472 L., 66.3, 6.584 L. See pp. 42–43.
[63] *Vict.* 2.4, 6.472 L., 66.6, 6.586 L., 72.1, 6.610–612 L., 93.1, 6.660 L.
[64] *Vict.* 72.1, 6.610–612 L., 74.1, 6.614–616 L.; compare *VM* 21.2–3, 1.624–626 L.

cholera, dropsy, tumors, fatigue pains, and mania.[65] The author also resembles other doctors insofar as he holds that stagnant humors can putrefy, acquiring a "pungent" character that ulcerates the flesh,[66] that humors can gather in the head and produce catarrhs,[67] that dropsy arises from a melting of the flesh,[68] that fevers occur when the blood transmits heat from a concentrated humor to the rest of the body,[69] and that diseases are resolved when the patient undergoes a "crisis."[70] The body sometimes removes diseased humors on its own through the action of the soul,[71] and doctors can also intervene to move the offending humor in one direction or another. One of the author's favorite modes of treatment is to purge some part of the body so that the peccant humors will flow into the empty space, a process he calls "drawing back" (ἀντίσπασις). He then follows this "drawing back" with a second purge in order to remove the gathered humors from the body.[72] Bile is attracted "like to like" by a variety of substances, most of them bitter or fatty.[73] It is also counterbalanced by substances that are watery, white, thin, and soft,[74] while phlegm is melted and consumed by substances that are heating, drying, burning, salty, pungent, harsh – in short, anything that resembles fire.[75] If a concentrated humor is allowed to grow strong, it can become very difficult to remove. Sometimes, these

---

[65] *Vict.* 40.3, 6.538 L. (diarrhea), 54.2, 6.558 L. (strangury), 66, 6.582–588 L. (fatigue pains), 70.1, 6.606 L. (catarrhs, fever, chills), 72.1, 6.612 L. (fever, pneumonia), 72.3, 6.612 L. (fever), 74.1–2, 6.616 L. (diarrhea, dysentery), 76.1, 6.618 L. (dropsy), 79.1, 6.624 L. (lientery), 83.1, 6.632 L. (chills, fever), 84.1, 6.634 L. (chills, fever), 89.11, 6.650 L. (fluxes, tumors), 90.7, 6.658 L. (fever), 93.1, 6.660 L. (cholera), and 93.5, 6.662 L. (mania). The dry, bitter tongue at 82.1, 6.630 L. suggests that the author is describing an *apokrisis* of bile (see note 45 on p. 196). Van der Eijk (2004: 202) wrongly characterizes the author's nosology as "primitive" and apparently overlooks his reference to pneumonia in chapter 72. The reason why we do not find so many disease names in *On Regimen* is not because they were not recognized by the author but simply because his entire work is devoted to disease *prevention*, removing diseases at their source before they have a chance to differentiate (71.3, 6.610 L.; cf. Hulskamp 2013: 36n9). When the author refers to fluxes from the head, for example, we must assume that the resulting diseases will be the same ailments we find in other texts; that is, pleuritis, consumption, and all the other conditions that were recognized by his contemporaries.

[66] *Vict.* 74.2, 6.616 L.

[67] *Vict.* 32.4, 6.510 L., 70, 6.606–608 L., 73, 6.612–614 L., 89.11, 6.650 L., 90.2, 6.654 L.; compare 62.3–4, 6.576–578 L., 83, 6.632–634 L., pp. 105–106.

[68] *Vict.* 76.1, 6.618 L.; compare p. 115.

[69] *Vict.* 66.3, 6.584 L.; compare *Flat.* 8.5, 6.102 L., discussed on p. 112.

[70] *Vict.* 70.2, 6.608 L., 72.3, 6.612 L.; compare 90.5, 6.656 L., p. 52.

[71] *Vict.* 15.2, 6.486 L., 66.3, 6.584 L., 70.2, 6.608 L.

[72] For the term ἀντίσπασις, see *Vict.* 56.5, 6.568 L., 63.3, 6.578 L., 66.8, 6.588 L., 73.1–2, 6.612–614 L., 79.3, 6.624–626 L., 89.4–5, 6.646 L., 90.2, 6.654 L. The procedure is also employed at 59.2, 6.572 L., 68.5, 6.596 L., 74.3, 6.616 L., 76.2, 6.620 L., 78.4, 6.622–624 L., 81.4, 6.630 L., 82.4, 6.632 L., 89.8, 6.648 L., 89.11, 6.650 L.

[73] *Vict.* 53, 6.556 L., 54.5–6, 6.560 L., 82.4, 6.632 L., 89.8, 6.648 L.   [74] *Vict.* 89.8, 6.648 L.

[75] *Vict.* 89.4, 6.646 L.; compare 89.8, 6.648 L., 93.1, 6.660 L.

humors have to be purged with special drugs, which are fast acting but also dangerous.[76]

There are three general classes of treatments in *On Regimen*: (1) treatments that manipulate the belly, (2) treatments that manipulate the flesh, and (3) treatments that manipulate the soul's movement through the vessels. The author's food catalog is an especially good source for understanding his treatments of the belly. Contrary to the testimony of *On Ancient Medicine*, the author of *On Regimen* does not simply identify one food as "hot," another as "cold," another as "dry," and another as "wet." Instead, the author focuses on how different foods influence the process of digestion, and especially on how they interact with the three circuits of the vascular system. Foods that are roasted, for example, are said to be constipating because "when they fall into the belly, they attract to themselves the moisture from the belly, closing the mouths of the vessels with their drying and heating, with the result that they block up the passages for the moisture" (56.3, 6.566 L.). Substances that are thin (λεπτός) are quickly evaporated, some being taken up by the soul to be distributed through the body,[77] some being expelled through exhalation,[78] and some being expelled with the urine,[79] while foods that are heavy (βαρύς) are not easily broken down and distributed through the body, as they merely sit in the belly and are especially prone to growing hot and creating a "disturbance" (ταραχή).[80] Foods are strong (ἰσχυρός) when they contain raw and concentrated humors, which are difficult to concoct but can be a source of great nutriment if the soul can overpower them.[81] Foods are nourishing (τρόφιμος) if a large portion of their moisture is received into the innermost circuit, which happens if the food is "pure" (καθαρός),[82] if it contains a large quantity of moisture (including flesh),[83] or if it does not flood the vessels with more nutriment than they can handle.[84] Foods that pass quickly by stool are less nourishing than those that do not, since they provide the vessels with less time to absorb the available nutriment.[85] A food can be light (κοῦφος) if

---

[76] *Vict.* 66.8, 6.588 L., 67.3, 6.592–594 L., 73.2–3, 6.614 L., 76.2, 6.620 L., 89.8, 6.648 L. On the dangers arising from drugs that are too powerful, compare *Epid.* V 15, 5.214 L., 18, 5.216–218 L., Pl. *Ti.* 89a–d.

[77] *Vict.* 25.1, 6.498 L., 56.6, 6.568 L.   [78] *Vict.* 40.2, 6.536 L.

[79] *Vict.* 52.2, 6.554 L., 55.2, 6.562 L.

[80] *Vict.* 46.1, 6.544–546 L., 46.3, 6.546 L., 56.4, 6.566 L., 74.1, 6.616 L.

[81] *Vict.* 45.2, 6.542 L., 45.4, 6.544 L., 54.1, 6.556 L., 56.4, 6.566–568 L., 93.2, 6.660 L.; compare 68.5, 6.596 L. What makes these foods nourishing is presumably the fact that much of the "raw" moisture has not already been consumed by fire.

[82] *Vict.* 42.1, 6.540 L., 55.5, 6.564 L.

[83] *Vict.* 42.2, 6.540 L., 45.1, 6.542 L., 45.3, 6.544 L., 55.5, 6.564 L., 56.1, 6.564 L.

[84] *Vict.* 40.4, 6.538 L., 56.4, 6.566 L.

[85] *Vict.* 40.2, 6.536 L., 42.1, 6.540 L.; compare 40.3, 6.538 L.

much of its nourishment has already been consumed before entering the belly, if it nourishes the soul without nourishing the flesh, or if its moisture is not absorbed by the innermost circuit but rather expelled through other avenues, including the production of breaths.[86] "Breaths" (φῦσαι) are typically manifested in the form of belching and flatulence, and they usually arise from the flooding of the belly with more moisture than it can handle. This moisture is not quickly drawn off either by the vessels or by the intestines, with the result that it stagnates and starts to "steam" within the belly.[87] Foods that happen to be fragrant (εὐώδης) tend to be warmer and lighter than those with "heavy odors" (ὀδμαὶ βαρεῖαι), and they also tend to pass more often by urine than by stool, presumably because they are more easily mastered by the belly's heat.[88]

The author emphasizes that doctors can manipulate the powers of foods by changing their properties within the kitchen. Some ingredients can be added, some removed, and others can be "concocted" or made more or less concentrated "in accordance with what happens to be the *kairos* for the particular situation" (2.1, 6.468 L.). The author specifically says that doctors should make these adjustments "with the knowledge that all things, both animals and plants, are composed of fire and water, that they grow in size by means of these things, and that they undergo separation [διακρίνεται] into these things" (56.2, 6.566 L.). With these two statements, the author illustrates two important points about his physiological system. The first is that, despite his emphasis on the first principles of all things, the author is still deeply concerned with the differences between individual patients. The second is that the author views his cosmology of fire and water as a means of *overcoming* these differences – these principles provide a stable guide for determining what the doctor should do in every case.

In addition to targeting the belly, the author also cultivates treatments that work by manipulating the flesh. These include the manual kneading of the flesh to open up its vessels, the application of substances such as oil (to warm, moisten, and soften) or dust (to cool, dry, and contract), the exposure of the body to heat and cold, the prescription of sleeping on a hard or a soft bed, the bathing of the body in hot or cold water, and the leaving of the skin either covered

---

[86] *Vict.* 40.2, 6.536 L., 42.1, 6.540 L., 42.3, 6.540 L., 46.1, 6.546 L., 56.4, 6.566–568 L., 88.3, 6.644 L., 89.12, 6.652 L., 92.2, 6.658 L.

[87] *Vict.* 40.2, 6.536 L., 40.4, 6.538 L., 42.3, 6.540 L., 45.1, 6.542 L., 52.4, 6.556 L., 54.1, 6.556 L., 55.3, 6.564 L., 55.5, 6.564 L., 56.8, 6.570 L., 74.1, 6.614 L.; compare pp. 105–106.

[88] *Vict.* 54.7, 6.560 L., 55.2, 6.562 L., 78.3, 6.622 L.; compare Arist. [*Pr.*] 1.48, 865a19–24.

or exposed. Exercise, for its part, encourages the movement of the soul through the vessels. It increases the rate at which moisture is consumed from the flesh, and it also quickens the transfer of moisture from the belly to the outermost circuit.[89] The flesh grows harder and stronger by assimilating more humors to itself, but it also runs the risk of melting if it is constantly bombarded by the fiery soul. The author divides all exercises into two groups: the "natural" (κατά φύσιν) and the "violent" (διὰ βίης).[90] Aristotle similarly draws a distinction between "natural" and "violent" movement, associating "natural" movement with what originates inside a body and "violent" movement with what originates from outside.[91] In other contexts, we see the terms "natural" and "violent" used to categorize forms of death (Pl. *Ti.* 81e, Arist. *Resp.* 472a16–18, 478b24–25, 479a32–b4, and Thphr. *CP* 5.11.1–2), disease (Thphr. *CP* 5.8.1), destruction and change (Arist. *Ph.* 230a18–b10 and *Mete.* 379a5–8), governments (Pl. *Lg.* 3.690c), and acquired versus hereditary traits (*Aër.* 14.3–4, 2.58–60 L.), where again the emphasis seems to be on internal versus external causes. For the author of *On Regimen*, "natural" exercises include speaking, thinking, and the use of the senses, all of which gently warm and dry the flesh by making the soul move through the vessels.[92] Walking is partly natural and partly violent, while running is fully violent. What makes running "violent" is presumably the fact that it leverages the *pneuma* outside the body (an external force) via heavy respiration, while what makes speaking, thinking, and sensation "natural" is that these activities leverage the *pneuma* inside the body (an internal force) by making the soul simply circulate through the vessels. Walking, for its part, is partly natural and partly violent, presumably because it both encourages the natural circulation of the soul (sc. to produce movement) and because it gently increases the intake of external *pneuma*. Walking differs from running, however, insofar as it does

---

[89] *Vict.* 61–64, 6.574–580 L. A similar idea may lie behind the curious statement in *Epidemics VI* that "exercise is food for the joints and flesh, sleep for the organs" (5.5, 5.316 L.). For the use of exercise to distribute food and drink throughout the body, compare Hippon. fr. 118 West and Pl. *Phd.* 117a–b. For the use of exercise to counterbalance food and drink, compare *Flat.* 7.1, 6.98 L. and Arist. [*Pr.*] 1.46, 864b36–847a2.

[90] *Vict.* 2.2, 6.470 L., 61.1, 6.574 L.

[91] Arist. *APo.* 94b37–95a3, *Ph.* 215a1–6, *Cael.* 269a7–8, 274b30–31, 276a22–30, 295a7–25, 300a20–301b31, 305a26–28, *GC* 333b26–30, and [*Pr.*] 24.9, 936b23–39.

[92] *Vict.* 61, 6.574–576 L. Compare *Epid. VI* 5.5, 5.316 L., 6.2, 5.322–324 L., 8.23, 5.352 L., and the inclusion of sight and hearing as disease agents in *Diseases I* and *On Affections* (pp. 32–34). At *Sens.* 31, Theophrastus notes that sensation is always "natural" (κατὰ φύσιν) and never involves "violence" (βία).

not leave a person completely out of breath.[93] Running is especially useful when humors invade the vascular system, as it quickens respiration and thus causes the foreign moisture to be pushed out with the breath.[94]

Because eating generally adds moisture to the body while exercise generally consumes moisture from the flesh, the author speaks in broad terms about a "due proportion" between eating and exercise. As we have seen, this simply boils down to the idea that the soul's conveyance of new moisture from the belly and the soul's removal of old moisture from the flesh need to proceed in such a way that the flesh is neither too wet nor too dry. If the flesh becomes too wet, then eating has essentially "gained the upper hand" over exercise, while if the flesh becomes too dry (or if the fiery soul causes the flesh to melt), then exercise has now "gained the upper hand" over eating.

6.6 The Quest for Precision

In a perfect world, the doctor will accompany his patients at all times in order to preserve a healthy balance between eating and exercise. In most cases, however, such constant vigilance is impossible, with the result that "it is impossible to set down [ὑποθέσθαι] foods and exercises with precision," since "if there arises even a slight deficiency of one thing or another, it is inevitable that, over time, the body will be overcome by the excess and fall sick" (2.3, 6.470–472 L.). In this passage, the author is speaking from the perspective of a doctor in the field, one who already knows the individual constitution of the patient, the powers of the available treatments, and the environmental factors that are prevailing in that particular time and place. When the author comes back to this topic in chapter 67 (quoted on p. 124), he writes from a different perspective. He is no longer talking about a doctor in the field but rather a doctor writing a book.[95] We have already noted the similarity between this passage and the deep concern for individual differences that appears in other texts. What is

---

[93] The author apparently believes that the movements involved in running require more *pneuma* than the body contains, meaning that running is "violent" (i.e., externally caused) insofar as the limbs are being moved with the help of the *pneuma* that we inhale.

[94] *Vict.* 62, 6.576–578 L. For the use of exercise to expel foreign moisture, compare Arist. [*Pr.*] 1.47, 865a17–18.

[95] Strictly speaking, the author also takes this perspective of a doctor writing a book at 2.1, 6.468 L. (cf. τὸν μέλλοντα ὀρθῶς συγγράφειν, "whoever intends to write correctly"), but his perspective quickly shifts to a particular doctor with a particular patient, as we see at 2.3, 6.470–472 L. (εἰ μὲν οὖν παρείη τις καὶ ὁρῴη κτλ, "if someone should be present and see . . .").

special about this passage is not simply the repetition of the common refrain that doctors must adapt to changing circumstances, but the author's specific claim that these differences influence the very information that can be reliably committed to writing. In a perfect world, a particular doctor keeping watch over a particular patient could theoretically achieve "due proportion." As soon as we move to the realm of writing, however, that theoretical possibility is unavailable. Writing about medicine involves a transition from the particular to the general. We can divide patients into groups and talk about the shared characteristics of each group, but at the end of the day we are still dealing with *generalized* observations that elide many of the variables that can change from one case to the next. In this passage, the author is especially adamant that even if we were to follow the method of inquiry that is advocated in *On Ancient Medicine*, dividing and subdividing patients into groups and then considering the effects of different foods on each group, there is still too much variation *within* these groups to create a system of medicine that is absolutely "precise." In *On Ancient Medicine*, the author recognizes that a perfect system of medicine has not yet been discovered, but he simply claims that we should continue on the road that has already been established, making finer and finer distinctions between different classes of patients until we have accounted for all the variables that can influence a patient's health. In *On Regimen*, the author accepts this method up to a point. He also claims, however, that such a system will never be fully sufficient in itself. There are simply too many differences between individual cases, too many variables to account for every conceivable permutation. If we want to achieve true precision in medicine, we need a system that rises above all the variables that can change from one case to the next.

In the immediate context, the author uses this passage to justify his system of prodiagnosis. At the same time, however, it could just as easily be applied to his cosmology of fire and water. It seems quite likely, in fact, that this is the sort of thinking that motivated our author to base the art of medicine on the first principles of all things. Like the author of *On Ancient Medicine*, the author of *On Regimen* is deeply concerned with the many differences that exist between individual cases. The author also recalls *On Ancient Medicine* insofar as he stresses the impossibility of "setting down" (ὑποθέσθαι) generalized treatments without taking account of individual differences. Where these authors part ways is the extent to which they are willing to isolate high-level commonalities that transcend these particular differences. In *On Regimen*, the author tends to start with what is general (κατὰ παντός) before moving to what is particular (καθ᾽ ἕκαστα). He sometimes even comments on the extent to which generalization is possible, as we see in the preface to his food catalog (39, 6.534–536 L.):

> Those who try to speak generally [κατὰ παντός] about the powers of substances that are sweet, fatty, salty, or anything else of such a sort do not possess correct recognition. For the same power is not shared by the sweet, the fatty, or anything else like this. Of sweet substances, many pass easily by stool, while others are constipating. Some are drying, while others are moistening. It is the same with everything else. Of the substances that are astringent, some pass by stool, others pass by urine, and still others do neither of these things. It is the same with the substances that are warming and everything else: one has one power, another has another. Concerning the whole category [περὶ μὲν οὖν ἁπάντων], it is impossible for their properties to be made clear. I will accordingly give instruction about the powers that each substance has individually [καθ' ἕκαστα].

At the same time that the author warns against overgeneralization, especially as it applies to the "powers" of foods and drinks, he explicitly states that the "powers" of fire and water are the same for "all things in all circumstances" (πάντα διὰ παντός, 3.1, 6.472 L.). In other words, the properties of these elements remain the same even when all other variables change. They provide a stable guide for everything in the cosmos, and they can be referenced in any particular situation, regardless of the other factors that distinguish one case from the next.

In Book 3, the author presents his system of prodiagnosis as another way to overcome the many variables that can change from one case to the next. Whereas medical writers can set down general principles that *explain* particular situations, there is no way for them to write down generalized, step-by-step instructions that will maintain *summetria* in all cases. The author provides his best approximation of such instructions in chapter 68. This passage has a great deal in common with the final section of *On the Nature of the Human Being*, inasmuch as the author describes the adjustments one should make as one season gives way to the next. At the winter solstice, we should employ a regimen that is heating and drying, while at the summer solstice we should employ a regimen that is cooling and moistening. The rest of the year should be devoted to slowly building up to one extreme or the other, thereby avoiding the sudden changes that can potentially give rise to disease. In other passages, the author describes the adjustments one should make for different physical constitutions, dividing patients into groups and considering the specific needs of each group. In chapter 32, he lists six different constitutions and provides general instructions on how to maintain the health of each. In the end, however, these are only rough approximations. No two seasons are exactly the same, and no two constitutions are exactly the same, even though we may give them the same name.

Because there are so many differences between individual cases, it is inevitable that an imbalance will occur. This is where the author brings in his system of prodiagnosis, presenting it as a way to overcome the many variables that can change from one case to the next (69, 6.606 L.). In this system, the author reduces all diseases to a limited number of starting points (ἀρχαί), each of which determines a different "class" of imbalance. His use of the term "class" (εἶδος) recalls *On Breaths'* assertion that all categories of disease can be traced back to a single cause and, as a result, ultimately belong to one "class" (2, 6.92 L.). The author of *On Regimen* claims to have uncovered the signs (τεκμήρια) that will tell a doctor which type of asymmetry he is dealing with. These signs are the same for every patient who falls within the specified class, and they can be opposed with simple treatments that are more or less the same in every case.[96] In the first part of Book 3, the author describes fifteen classes of imbalance, each of which gives rise to a different set of affections. These include a common origin for both catarrhs and fevers (ch. 70), the invasion of the middle circuit by foreign moisture (ch. 71), the beginnings of pneumonia (ch. 72), the attraction of moisture to the head (ch. 73), the stagnation of heavy food within the belly (ch. 74), the indigestion caused by an overcooling of the belly (ch. 75), two forms of acid-belching (chs. 76–77), an *apokrisis* from the flesh (ch. 78), a cold and wet belly (ch. 79), a cold and dry belly (ch. 80), a hot and wet belly (ch. 81), a hot and dry belly (ch. 82), and two forms of dry flesh (chs. 83–84). On several occasions, the author specifically observes that the ultimate form that a disease will take depends on the supervention of additional factors, but he stresses that the doctor should not let the matter get to that point, correcting the imbalance while the disease is still undifferentiated.[97] A similar attitude carries over into the second half of Book 3, where the author specifically talks about the signs that can be drawn from a patient's dreams. What enables the author to construct this system is his observation that "diseases do not supervene in human beings right away, but they gather together a little at a time before manifesting

---

[96] We have already encountered this idea that diseases are easier to treat when the doctor intervenes as close to the "starting point" (ἀρχή) as possible (p. 149).

[97] *Vict.* 70.1–2, 6.606–608 L., 71.3, 6.610 L.; compare 83.1, 6.634 L., 84.1, 6.634 L. For the stability that arises from treating diseases at this point, see especially 85.1, 6.636 L.: "In some cases not all the symptoms are experienced, but only some of them. But with all these symptoms exercises overpower food, and the treatment is the same" (trans. Jones).

themselves in a mass" (2.4, 6.472 L.). In our discussion of *On Breaths* (pp. 113–114), we saw a similar reference to humors that "gather together" over time in the author's explanation of catarrhs. We compared that passage with a similar one in *Prognostic*, where the lag between an *apokrisis* and flux is said to last for up to twenty days. These parallels are significant insofar as they suggest that the author of *On Regimen* did not invent his system of prodiagnosis out of the blue. In fact, Greek doctors cultivated elaborate systems of prognosis, which they used to determine whether a patient would recover or die, when a crisis would occur, and even the patient's expected reaction to a particular treatment. Such systems of prognosis involved the cataloging of signs (τεκμήρια) that are the same across a wide range of cases, and they similarly encouraged doctors to act quickly before the patient developed a more difficult disease. What distinguishes the author of *On Regimen* from his peers is not that he looks for the signs of an impending disease but that he organizes these signs into a comprehensive system. He claims to have found the starting points for *all* diseases, and he assumes that anyone who has mastered every detail in his system will never run the risk of falling ill.

6.7 The Nature of Intelligence

Now that we have clarified this author's theories about disease, we can return to his discussion of the soul and its relationship with the cosmic fire that is the source of all intelligence. As we have mentioned, the author believes that sensation occurs when effluences of "hot and cold *pneuma*" enter the body's pores and "fall upon" the soul as it moves through the outermost circuit.[98] When these effluences hit the soul, they make an impression that is then carried back to the middle circuit for analysis by the body's "intelligence" (γνώμη). The fiery soul in the middle circuit is "untouched" by the senses (10.3, 6.486 L.), and it can thus submit them to objective analysis. Sight and hearing can be improved by purging moisture from the head,[99] but they can also be harmed by too much purging,[100] just as perception in general is corrupted whenever the soul is either too wet or too dry (p. 232). If a concentrated humor enters the middle circuit, then the patient will suffer from mental illness. Bile, for example, provides excessive fuel for the fiery soul, making it burn hotter and give rise to nightmares.[101]

---

[98] For discussions of this theory, see Hüffmeier (1961), Jouanna (1966, 2003b, 2007), Brisson (2013), and Lo Presti (2016).

[99] *Vict.* 61.3–4, 6.576 L., 62.3–4, 6.576–578 L.; compare 90.1–2, 6.652–654 L.

[100] *Vict.* 83.1, 6.634 L.   [101] *Vict.* 89.7, 6.648 L., 93.1, 6.660 L.

When the body is awake, the soul is the body's servant, dividing its attention and literally giving a "part" of itself to "hearing, seeing, touching, walking, the activities of the body as a whole" (86.1, 6.640 L.). When the body is asleep, the soul is still moving and awake, although the body is still and its sensory receptors are closed off. Without any distractions from the outside world, the soul "tends its own household" (διοικεῖ τὸν ἑωυτῆς οἶκον, 86.2, 6.640 L.). It interacts with the body and perceives what falls upon it in the same way that, when the body is awake, the soul interacts with and perceives the external world. During sleep, the soul sees, hears, and feels what is happening in the body; it walks, runs, and experiences emotions such as grief, fear, anxiety, and desire.[102] What we see in dreams directly corresponds to the first-person experiences of the soul. Sometimes, dreamers see visions as if they themselves are the soul and the body is their home,[103] while at other times the three "circuits" of the soul are represented by the three divisions of the heavens.[104] If the soul does not meet any impediments in its journey, it will retain all the same impressions that it acquired during the day.[105] When it travels around the flesh, it will see images that correspond to the land, while it will see images that correspond to the sea when it travels around the belly.[106] It is healthy to have visions that are "clean" (καθαρός), "bright" (εὐαγής), "shining" (λαμπρός), "translucent" (διαφανής), and "white" (λευκός), while it is unhealthy to have visions that are "black" (μέλας), "obscure" (ἀμυδρός), and "unclean" (οὐ καθαρός),[107] presumably because darkness is associated with unhealthy humors, while light is associated with moisture that is "pure."[108] The relative intensity of an image reflects the strength of whatever the soul has encountered,[109] while movement reflects the transfer of material from one place to the next.[110]

According to this author, the innermost and outermost circuits of the soul originate in a middle circuit that is analogous to the circuit of the sun. In dreams, "outbound" souls (i.e., souls that are moving *away* from the

---

[102] *Vict.* 86.2, 6.640 L., 89.9, 6.648–650 L., 89.12, 6.650–652 L., 90.1–2, 6.652–654 L., 93.1–3, 6.660 L., 93.5, 6.662 L.; compare *Epid. VI* 8.10, 5.348 L.: "Even the mind's consciousness, itself by itself, distinct from the organs and events, feels misery and joy, is fearful and optimistic, feels hope and despair" (trans. Smith).

[103] *Vict.* 86.2, 6.640 L., 90.5, 6.656 L., 92.2, 6.658 L.   [104] *Vict.* 89.1–2, 6.644–646 L.

[105] *Vict.* 88.1, 6.642 L.   [106] *Vict.* 89.10–11, 6.650 L., 90.1–6, 6.652–656 L.

[107] *Vict.* 88.1, 6.642 L., 89.1, 6.644 L., 89.10, 6.650 L., 89.12–13, 6.650–652 L., 90.1, 6.654 L., 90.3–4, 6.654 L., 90.6, 6.656 L., 91, 6.658 L., 92.1, 6.658 L., 93.3, 6.660 L.

[108] Two exceptions to this explanation are 90.6, 6.656 L. and 91.2, 6.658 L., where black signals over-drying. In these passages, blackness recalls an object that is burnt (i.e., exposed to too much fire).

[109] *Vict.* 88.2–3, 6.642–644 L., 89.1, 6.644 L., 93.2, 6.660 L.   [110] *Vict.* 90.5, 6.656 L.

middle circuit) are perceived as moving from east to west, representing a movement from the central fire (= the east; i.e., the rising of the sun) to the extremities (= the west; i.e., the setting of the sun, from which the sun then "turns around" and comes back to its point of origin). "Inbound" souls (i.e., souls that are moving *toward* the middle circuit) are perceived as moving from west to east, since these souls will return to the middle circuit (= the east) after reaching their "western" extremity in either the belly or the flesh.[111] If an inbound soul is "pure" and "shining," then the patient has nothing to worry about. If a soul is "dark" and "obscure" and moving "westward," however, that means the soul is conveying morbid humors to either the belly or the flesh. If the soul appears to move upwards in its westward movement, this means that the morbid humors are gathering in the head.[112] If it falls on the land, this signifies a flux to the flesh, while if it falls into the sea, this signifies a flux to the belly.[113] If the soul comes to a region that is excessively dry, it will not be able to draw sufficient nutriment to itself. As a result, its fire will dim and it will produce images of heavenly bodies in which their fire, too, is weakened.[114] Specific humors will give rise to dream visions that reflect their particular characteristics. Phlegm produces visions of heavenly bodies afflicted with water, ice, the extinction of light, and the halting of movement, all because phlegm is cold and wet and will accordingly slow down or even stop the soul's movement.[115] Bile, meanwhile, produces visions of heavenly bodies afflicted with fire, heat, and rapid movement, the reason being that bile naturally stokes the fire within the soul and makes it move faster.[116] Images of battle literalize the metaphorical battle between the body and peccant humors,[117] while wandering, eating, running, and being afraid reflect the activity of the soul as it moves throughout the body.[118]

In addition to perceiving an excess or deficiency of moisture in the body, the soul can also perceive the *pneuma* that enters via respiration. In these cases, dreamers perceive the effects as happening either to themselves or to their homes. What is most interesting about this particular subset of dreams is that they seem to depict the actual source of the *pneuma* that we breathe. If we dream that we are receiving something from a god, from

---

[111] *Vict.* 89.10, 6.650 L. For previous attempts to explain this tricky passage, see Jouanna (1998: 171) and van der Eijk (2004: 200).

[112] *Vict.* 89.11, 6.650 L.   [113] *Vict.* 89.10–11, 6.650 L.

[114] *Vict.* 89.6, 6.646 L. See note 55 in this chapter.   [115] *Vict.* 89.2, 6.644–646 L.

[116] *Vict.* 89.7, 6.648 L.

[117] *Vict.* 88.2, 6.642–644 L., 93.4–5, 6.660–662 L. For a direct reference to this battle, see 6.3, 6.480 L.

[118] On the violence of running, see pp. 239–240. If one dreams that the soul is running, this presumably means that some external force is driving it to move at a quickened pace.

a dead person, from the *aither*, or from the *aer*, that is because we are *actually* receiving substances from these entities.[119] The dead sometimes wear clothes and they sometimes do not; their clothes are sometimes clean and white and sometimes they are dirty and black. What this represents is our inhalation of *pneuma* that is sometimes moist and sometimes dry, sometimes healthy and sometimes laden with morbid humors. Likewise, the dead can take items out of our homes, just as *pneuma* can take substances out of our bodies.[120] As for the gods, they can give us items that are clean or dirty, just as our bodies receive either good or bad substances whenever we inhale fire-driven *pneuma*.[121]

In all of these dreams, the soul sees the cosmic analogies that a waking person might otherwise miss. Even if we do not consciously recognize the connection between the body and the cosmos, our souls inherently know that the body is a "resemblance of the whole," and it activates this set of analogies during sleep; that is, when the soul is unencumbered by the sensory information that comes in from the phenomenal world. In our dreams, we see that the flesh is equivalent to the earth, while the belly is equivalent to the sea. We see that the entire cosmos is a "home" (οἶκος) for the soul, and that this soul is connected to the heavenly bodies that occupy the *aither*. We see that these heavenly bodies require nourishment to prevent their fires from dimming, and that they are specifically fed by moisture that is "clean" and "bright." We also see that the *aer* is pervaded by both the dead and the gods, fiery beings who are sometimes clothed in moisture, but who can also fly around without any clothing at all. Both the dead and the gods enter our bodies in the form of inhaled *pneuma*. These beings can either help or harm our bodies, and they do so by either adding material or taking it away.

Another important set of analogies for *On Regimen* can be found in chapters 11–24. In this section, the author chides his fellow humans for failing to ascertain a divinely inspired analogy between the arts (τέχναι) and nature (φύσις), according to which everything that we do in our daily

---

[119] The author is very clear about this point in chapter 92: "To see the dead in a clean state and in white cloaks is a good sign, and to receive something clean from them signals the health of both the body and the things that enter it. For it is from the dead that nourishment, growth, and seeds arise, and for these things to enter the body in a clean state signals health." By the "dead," the author means the small, invisible souls that had previously been exhaled by another person as their own life was dissipating, the "seeds" that will be confined to the realm of "Hades" (i.e., the air) until they are inhaled by another, "large" animal (p. 224). See also 89.12–13, 6.650–652 L., where the author notes that visions of the heavenly bodies signal the entrance of some substance from the *aither*, while visions of rain and other forms of precipitation signal the entrance of some substance from the *aer*.
[120] *Vict.* 92.2, 6.658 L.   [121] *Vict.* 89.13, 6.652 L.

occupations has some parallel in human physiology. In some of these
analogies, the activities of the craftsmen mirror what the doctor himself
should do when treating a patient. Seers, for example, model the same
approach to knowledge that the doctor should employ: they relate the
visible to the invisible, the past to the future, the dead to the living, and the
intelligent to the unintelligent (12, 6.488 L.). In other analogies, the activity
of the craftsman mirrors the activity of the body, or even the universe as
a whole.

These craft analogies fit into a broader approach to the attainment of
knowledge that the author invokes throughout *On Regimen*. When tend-
ing to the body and its various functions, our intelligence is weaker than
the intelligence of the gods.[122] The gods assist our inquiries, but the
majority (οἱ πολλοί) fail to recognize the true nature of things,[123] since
they hold to opinion rather than knowledge, and they do not even know
the correct method by which insights are to be achieved.[124] It is possible to
"chance upon" (ἐπιτυγχάνειν) a correct statement here or there,[125] but
anyone who truly seeks understanding must sift through many particulars
in order to find the hidden truth. We must "investigate the things that are
invisible from the things that are visible" (11.1, 6.486 L.), and we must
recognize that "the things here [in the realm of the visible] perform the
actions of the things there [in the realm of the invisible]" (5.1, 6.476 L.).
The problem with humans is that they do not even recognize the invisible
truths that they mimic with their own actions. They "recognize what they
do, but they do not recognize what they reflect" (γινώσκοντας ἃ ποιέουσι,
καὶ οὐ γινώσκοντας ἃ μιμέονται, 11.1, 6.486 L.), and they "do not have
knowledge about what they do, whereas they think they have knowledge
[δοκέουσιν εἰδέναι] about what they actually do not do" (5.2, 6.476 L.).
The greatest irony, of course, is that the truth lies hidden in plain sight.
"The eyes are not sufficient," however, "to judge even about the things that
are seen," for what we see must further be considered by the mind
(γνώμη).[126] Even though humans do not use their intelligence correctly,
failing to recognize (γιγνώσκειν) the cosmic principles that they reflect in
their everyday actions, a divine necessity forces them to perform these
actions "whether they intend to or not" (ἃ βούλονται καὶ ἃ μὴ βούλονται,
5.2, 6.478 L.).

---

[122] *Vict.* 1.1, 6.466 L., 11, 6.486 L., 93.6, 6.662 L.
[123] *Vict.* 1, 6.466–468 L., 4.2–3, 6.474–476 L. Note, however, 68.2, 6.594 L.: "I divide the year into four
parts, a thing that the majority recognize most of all."
[124] *Vict.* 1.1, 6.466 L., 11.1, 6.486 L.   [125] *Vict.* 1.1, 6.466 L., 87, 6.640–642 L.
[126] *Vict.* 4.2, 6.474–476 L.

There is a clear parallel between the soul that "tends its own household" while the body is asleep and the enlightened humans who move beyond the senses to catch a glimpse of the hidden truth. When the body is asleep, our souls perceive the analogies between the body and the cosmos, associating the flesh with land, the belly with the sea, and the three circuits of the vascular system with the three circuits of the sun, moon, and stars. Our souls also identify the *pneuma* that we inhale as the real manifestation of what we conventionally call both the "dead" and the "gods," who are simply invisible emanations of a single cosmic fire. The author's goal is to make our souls perform while we are awake what they already tend to do when the body is asleep. Since we cannot shut off our senses while we are awake, we need to find another way to rise above them, and the author's solution is to make us look for analogies that conceal the high-level commonalities that transcend particular differences.

6.8   The Mind of Gods

In chapter 11, the author says that a "mind of gods" (θεῶν νοῦς) teaches human beings to mimic the things that occur within their bodies (11.1, 6.486 L.). This "mind of gods" makes humans perform certain actions even when they are not aware of what they are imitating, "recognizing what they do, but not recognizing what they reflect" (11.1, 6.486 L.). "Humans establish a *nomos*," the author writes, "setting it down for themselves, but they do not recognize [οὐ γινώσκοντες] the things concerning which they establish it" (11.2, 6.486 L.). In this passage, the author stresses that humans possess only a partial "recognition" of the universe. They are guided by some external principle that dictates everything that they do, and yet they are unaware of the extent to which this "mind of gods" governs their actions. In chapter 10, the author refers to another sort of "mind," defining it as the "hottest and strongest fire" that occupies the body's middle circuit. This fire contains "soul, mind [νοῦς], thought, movement, growth, decrease, change, sleep, and waking. It steers all things in all circumstances, both these things here and those things there, never staying still" (10.3, 6.486 L.). Since this fire ultimately controls everything in the body, every *movement* that we make, one presumes that the only way in which a "mind of gods" could conceivably control the body is to do so by way of the fiery intelligence within our chests. The author is also eager to stress that the "mind" within our bodies occupies a circuit that is itself analogous to the circuit of the sun, and that it steers "both these things here and those things there" in an apparent analogy between our central soul and some overarching, cosmic fire. The upshot of these observations is that the author of *On Regimen* seems to believe that the "mind" of human beings and the "mind" of gods are actually two forms of the same thing. The mind of human beings is weaker than the mind of gods, but both minds arise from the same source. We have already seen a microcosmic echo of this macrocosmic process in the author's discussion of the human body. When the soul in the middle circuit secretes a portion of itself to distribute moisture to the flesh, that portion of the soul is weaker than the "hottest and strongest" fire that is located in the middle circuit. These weaker divisions of the soul are loaded with more moisture than the fire in the middle circuit, with the result that they have far less intelligence (γνώμη) than the purer fire in the heart and its adjacent vessels. Given this author's deep commitment to his analogy between the body and the cosmos, this all suggests that the author associates the "mind of gods" with the sun/*aither*, and that he further believes that all other forms of intelligence – and, indeed, all other *divinities*, including the undying soul within our bodies – have been "separated off" from this central source, sent off in various directions to give soul, mind, thinking, movement, growth, and diminution to all things.

As the author stresses on multiple occasions, there is only one soul, only one fire that steers the universe as a whole. This fire is what constructed and now governs the cosmos in its various cycles, while its weaker exhalations construct and govern individual things, including the bodies of human beings. We should not be surprised, therefore, if the body turns out to be a reflection of the whole, nor should we be surprised that we mimic human physiology in our daily occupations. Since everything can ultimately be traced back to the cosmic fire, it is by necessity that everything else that depends on this fire will perform the same actions. An obvious benefit of this insight is that we can use observations about the phenomenal world to learn about the universe as a whole. We can move from the microcosm to the macrocosm, from "parts" to the "whole," from the visible to the invisible. This is the method of inquiry that the author of *On Regimen* advocates very forcefully, and it is inextricably linked to his theory about a single intelligence that governs all things.

So how do the traditional gods of Greek myth fit into this system? As we have already noted, the author seems to believe that there is a central fire, concentrated in the sun, that is the source of all divinity. Our souls are likewise divine because they spring from this central intelligence. As for the traditional gods, they are presumably offshoots of the same cosmic fire. Sophocles writes that certain "wise men" call Helios (i.e., the sun) "the begetter of the gods and the father of all" (fr. 752 Radt). Although his divine principle is air rather than fire, Anaximenes is similarly said to have asserted that all gods are merely offspring of the air (DK 13 A10) and to have linked the soul within our bodies to the air that governs the universe as a whole (DK 13 B2). Like Anaximenes, Xenophanes reduced all divinity to a single, nonanthropomorphic being, referring to this being as "one god, greatest among both gods and humans, similar to mortals neither in body nor in thought" (DK 21 B23). In other fragments, Xenophanes speaks of a god who "without toil shakes all things with the thought of his mind" (DK 21 B25) and who "sees as a whole, apprehends as a whole, and hears as a whole" (DK 21 B23), appropriating descriptions of Helios as a divinity who "sees all things and hears all things" (*Od.* 12.323) and of Zeus as a god who "knows all things well" (*Od.* 20.75), possessing an eye that "sees all things and apprehends all things" in the same manner as the sun (Hes. *Op.* 267). In *On Flesh*, the author appropriates the same descriptions of Helios and Zeus when he claims that the "hot" is immortal, that it "apprehends, sees, and hears all things," and that it "knows all things, both what is and what is going to be" (2.1, 8.584 L.). Similar repetitions of this formula can be found in Epicharmus's assertion that "mind sees and mind hears, while everything else is deaf and blind" (DK 23 B12; cf. Iamb. *VP* 228) and in the description of an all-seeing, all-hearing "intelligence" (φρόνησις) that mirrors our "mind" (νοῦς) and permeates the universe at X. *Mem.* 1.4.17–18.[127] Parmenides, Heraclitus, and Empedocles also advance reinterpretations of the gods in terms strongly reminiscent of *On Regimen*. Parmenides begins his poem by driving a blazing chariot along the path of a "divinity" (δαίμων). Parmenides's escorts on this journey are the Heliades (i.e., the daughters of the sun), and he attributes his insights to a female divinity who "steers all things" (πάντα κυβερνᾷ, DK 28 B12.3) from the middle of the heavenly circuits, not unlike *On Regimen*'s soul that "steers all things in all circumstances" (πάντα διὰ παντὸς κυβερνᾷ, 10.3, 6.486 L.) from the center of the vascular system. Heraclitus similarly refers to a fiery "intelligence" (γνώμη) that "steers all things in all circumstances" (ἐκυβέρνησε πάντα διὰ πάντων, DK 22 B41).[128] Like Xenophanes, Heraclitus seems to have reduced all divinity to a single essence, claiming that the one wise

---

[127] In Ennius's *Epicharmus* (a Roman imitation of Epicharmus), it is claimed that our souls are fiery emanations from the sun (fr. 8 Warmington) and that the sun is entirely made of "soul" (fr. 9 Warmington). Compare further Critias DK 88 B25.10–24 and Pl. *Lg.* 10.901d.

[128] For other divine forces that "steer" the cosmos, see Philol. DK 44 B21, Diog. Apoll. DK 64 B5, Epich. DK 23 B57, Pl. *Phlb.* 28d, *Plt.* 272e–273e, *Smp.* 186e, 197b–e, *Phdr.* 247c–e, Arist. *Ph.* 203b7–15 (= Anaximand. DK 12 A15), *Mete.* 339a23, [*Mu.*] 400b6–8, and Men. fr. 372 K–A.

thing is fiery in nature and "both willing and not willing to be called by the name of 'Zeus' alone" (DK 22 B32). Empedocles also reinterprets the traditional gods as cosmological principles, asserting that the sun-god Apollo is "a sacred and ineffable thought organ [φρήν] darting through the entire cosmos with swift thoughts" (DK 31 B134, trans. Inwood). Similar reinterpretations of the gods as "mind" (νοῦς), fire, or *aither* were advanced by other thinkers from this era, including Pherecydes of Syros, Hippasus of Metapontum, Ecphantus of Syracuse, and the author of the Derveni papyrus. These ideas were so widespread that they even found reflection in drama. In Euripides's *Trojan Women*, Hecuba asks whether Zeus should be called "necessity of nature" (ἀνάγκη φύσεος) or "mind of mortals" (νοῦς βροτῶν, 886). In his comedies, Aristophanes parodies such acts of theological reinterpretation. In the *Clouds*, the chorus prays to *aither* as the "most august nourisher of all living things" and to Helios as a "great divinity among gods and mortals" (570–574). Elevated above the stage, the comic Socrates "contemplates the sun" and seeks to gain insights into "the gods" and "the things on high" by mixing his mind with its kindred air (225–230). Plato also reinterprets the gods in a manner reminiscent of *On Regimen*. In his discussion of how the circular movement of the soul is reflected in the heavenly bodies, Plato writes that "this soul – whether it is by riding in the car of the sun, or from outside, or otherwise, that it brings light to us all – every man is bound to regard as a god" (*Lg.* 10.899a, trans. Bury). Within this cultural context, it would hardly be surprising for the author of *On Regimen* to engage in similar acts of theological reinterpretation. With so many of his contemporaries reframing traditional divinities as cosmic principles, it would in fact be strange if *On Regimen*'s author did *not* think about the gods along similar lines.

To test this hypothesis, I would like to consider the author's discussion of dreams, in which he describes the prayers one should perform in response to various visions. In this section, the author lists a number of dream visions and offers prescriptions for each, but there are only three conditions for which he supplements his prescriptions with prayer. The first is a case in which an *apokrisis* of moisture falls upon the soul and "disturbs" it (88.2–3, 6.642–644 L.). In this case, the author simply notes that one should "pray to the gods," without specifying any gods by name. In this instance, the generalized call to pray to the gods seems to be a request to join forces with these fiery beings, since the uniting of their fire with the patient's own soul would help the patient's fiery soul overcome the invading moisture. The second time that prayer is prescribed is for a series of "heavenly" signs that are caused by the inhalation of foreign substances into the body (89.12–14, 6.650–652 L.). For these conditions, the author says that if the signs are *good*, the patient should pray to Helios, Heavenly Zeus, Zeus the Protector of Property, Athena the Protector of Property, Hermes, and Apollo, while if the signs are *bad*, the patient should pray to the apotropaic gods, Ge (i.e., the earth), and the heroes. The third reference to prayer relates to a particularly dangerous drying of the flesh (90.6–7, 6.656–658 L.). In this case, the patient is instructed to moisten the flesh, to avoid both the sun and cold, and to pray to Ge, Hermes, and the heroes.

The author's choice of these specific divinities has never been definitively explained.[129] As van der Eijk (2004: 205n69) observes, "The selection of these particular deities (as against others, e.g. Asclepius) is a question which deserves to be further pursued, perhaps in relation to the doctrine of the soul." Now that we have come to a better understanding of what this author thinks about the soul, we can hazard a few guesses about his selection of these divinities. First, we have already noted that the gods in *On Regimen* are best interpreted as particularized manifestations of a single cosmic fire. The sun contains the highest concentration of fire in the universe, and so we should hardly be surprised that Helios comes first in the list of gods in chapter 89. As for the other gods in this list, the author had reinterpreted Zeus already in chapter 5, where he used "Zeus" to denote the visible realm, illuminated by the fiery *aither*. "Heavenly Zeus" might therefore represent the *aither* that contains the "heavenly" bodies (i.e., the sun, the moon, and the stars). In a fragment from Euripides, one character asks, "Do you see this *aither* on high, unlimited and holding the earth all around in its moist arms? Think that this is Zeus, consider this to be a god" (fr. 941 K.). In another fragment, a character says, "the *aither* gives birth to you, maiden, which is called Zeus by humans" (fr. 877 K.).

A similar interpretation can be applied to the next two gods: "Zeus the Protector of Property" and "Athena the Protector of Property." The adjective *ktesios* ("protector of property") was a cult epithet of Zeus, but it is otherwise unattested for Athena. When applied to Zeus, the epithet indicates his role as the protector of the home and its storeroom.[130] We have already seen several references to "homes" and "storerooms" in *On Regimen*. In particular, we have seen the body described as the "house" of

---

[129] For earlier discussions, see Fredrich (1899: 216n1), Hey (1908: 38–39), Palm (1933: 77–79), Hoessly (2001: 304n278), van der Eijk (2004: 203–205), Gorrini (2005: 143n59), and Craik (2015: 275).

[130] Compare especially A. *Supp.* 443–445 and Men. fr. 410 K–A.

the soul (86.2, 6.640 L., 90.5, 6.656 L., 92.2, 6.658 L.) and the belly described as the "storeroom" of the body (10.1, 6.484 L.). At one point, the author even refers to dreams in which souls take items from one's home (92.2, 6.658 L.) – the very type of theft that Zeus Ktesios was deemed effective at preventing.[131] Thus, Zeus the Protector of Property and his daughter, Athena the Protector of Property, could potentially be invoked as protectors of the various "homes" within the universe, especially the house that represents our bodies.[132] In chapter 10, the author suggests that the belly's analogue (i.e., the sea) is the "storeroom" (ταμιεῖον) for the universe as a whole. At the macrocosmic level, the author might have therefore believed that the intelligent fire (= Zeus) acts as a "steward" (ταμίας) of the universe, distributing water throughout the cosmos by directing a cycle of evaporation and precipitation.[133] The epithet *ktesios* could even invoke the idea that human souls are the "property" (κτήματα) of the gods – an idea that Plato attributes to mystic thinkers.[134] Along this reading, Zeus and Athena would be the "Protectors of Property" insofar as they oversee the various divisions of the cosmic soul.

It may also be significant that Athena, Hermes, and Apollo – the last three gods in this list – are all traditionally identified as the children of Zeus. Thus, they could represent the "children" of *aither*; that is, the offshoots of the cosmic soul that the *aither* sends down to earth. In the *Timaeus*, Plato describes "young gods" (νέοι θεοί) who are also called "children" (παῖδες) in relation to the central intelligence, and who are specifically given the task of "steering the mortal creature in the fairest and best way possible" (42d–e, trans. Bury, modified). We have already quoted a fragment from Euripides in which an unknown character is called a "child of the *aither*" (fr. 877 K.). In another fragment, the *aither* itself is said to be the creator of both gods and men (fr. 839.1–2 K.), while

---

[131] For Zeus Ktesios's role as a protector from theft, see Faraone (1992: 6–7).

[132] In early Greek thought, both the *aither* and the body are frequently called a "home" for the soul. There is also an interesting reference to two "homes" in Plato's *Protagoras* (321d–322a), one belonging to Zeus and the other shared by Hephaestus and Athena, paralleling the twin references to a Zeus Ktesios and an Athena Ktesia in *On Regimen*. In this passage, Prometheus is said to have stolen fire and craft-knowledge from the home of Hephaestus and Athena in order to give humans a "divine portion" (θεία μοῖρα), recalling *On Regimen*'s assumption that the human *technai* are guided by a divine intelligence that is fiery in nature and emanates from the sun.

[133] In Isocrates's *Busiris*, Zeus is called the "dispenser" (ταμίας) of rains and droughts (11.13). Greek poetry is also replete with references to Zeus as the "dispenser" of all things. For the comparison of *On Regimen*'s soul to a "steward" who distributes moisture from the belly's "storeroom," see note 56 on p. 234.

[134] Pl. *Phd.* 62b–c, *Criti.* 109b, and *Lg.* 10.902b–c, 906a–b. According to Plato, what makes humans the "property" of the gods is the fact that they have a share of the divine soul within themselves (τῆς ἐμψύχου μετέχει φύσεως, *Lg.* 10.902b).

Aristophanes describes how the *aither* "gave birth" to living creatures through an act of separation (*Th.* 14–15), using language strongly reminiscent of the soul-divisions that we find in *On Regimen*. In the so-called Orphic gold tablets, initiates are instructed to refer to themselves as "children" of the starry heaven (*OF* 474–484, 488–490). Parmenides also claims that his journey to the central intelligence was guided by the "daughters of the sun," while Cleanthes opens his *Hymn to Zeus* with the assertion that all living creatures are "born from Zeus," who possesses many names, "steers" the universe with his intelligence, and imparts to everything that lives a "likeness of a god" (fr. 537 von Arnim).

This identification of the "children" of Zeus with the offspring of the cosmic soul would work especially well for Athena, who is said to have arisen fully grown from the head of Zeus, and who is also sometimes said to have access to Zeus's thunderbolt. Democritus and Plato both allegorize Athena as a form of "mind" (νοῦς), "thought" (διάνοια), or "thinking" (φρόνησις).[135] In Aeschylus's *Eumenides*, Athena asserts that she received her "understanding" (φρονεῖν, 850) from Zeus, a mythological precedent that could very well have suggested that Athena is nothing more than an offshoot of the intelligent *aither*. In his astronomical system, Philolaus is said to have associated the "motherless" number seven with both Athena and the sun (DK 44 B20), while he called the central fire the "house of Zeus" (DK 44 A16). If the author of *On Regimen* similarly gave his gods specific domains, one hypothetical arrangement could include a "Heavenly Zeus" embracing all things, a "Zeus the Protector of Property" governing the two "homes" for divine souls (i.e., the *aither* and the earth), and an "Athena the Protector of Property" governing the lower one of these "homes" (i.e., the earth) by steering the sun through its revolutions. In this way, Athena would recall the Dike ("Justice") of Heraclitus (DK 22 B94), who ensures that the sun does not overstep its limits. She would also recall Hesiod's description of Dike, the "offspring of Zeus" (Διὸς ἐκγεγαυῖα), who sits at her father's side and reports to her father the "unjust mind" of wicked men (*Op.* 256–262).[136]

As for Hermes, he is traditionally identified as the messenger of the gods and as the escort of souls to the afterlife. In the context of *On Regimen*, both of these functions would have been relevant to the author's system. The

---

[135] Democr. DK 68 B2 and Pl. *Cra.* 407b.

[136] In Homer, the only divinity who is Διὸς ἐκγεγαυῖα is Athena (*Od.* 6.229). Note also Parmenides's reference to a goddess who "steers all things" from the middle of the heavenly circuits (DK 28 B12.3) – presumably the same goddess who gives Parmenides his insights into the universe as a whole.

author may have speculated, for example, that Hermes is simply another name for the fiery *pneuma* that transmits substances between the *aither* and the earth, sometimes bringing substances down to the earth (i.e., serving as the "messenger" of heavenly Zeus) and sometimes bringing substances up to the *aither* (i.e., escorting souls to the afterlife by helping them rejoin the cosmic fire). Hermes is included in the list of heavenly gods at 89.14, 6.652 L., but he is paired with Ge and the heroes at 90.7, 6.656–658 L. This implies that *On Regimen*'s Hermes moves between two realms, just as he does in Greek myth. As for Apollo, he carries an obvious connection with the sun. In some ancient allegories, Apollo is specifically said to represent the *rays* of the sun (e.g., Macr. *Sat.* 1.17), and it is possible that he holds a similar association here. At Heraclit. DK 22 B118, the sun's rays are called a "dry soul, wisest and best." We may also recall Empedocles's description of Apollo as "a sacred and ineffable thought organ [φρήν] darting through the entire cosmos with swift thoughts" (DK 31 B134, trans. Inwood).[137] In a fragment from Scythinus, the universe is compared to a golden lyre "which well-shaped Apollo, son of Zeus, tunes as a whole, taking together beginning and end, and as his shining plectrum he holds the light of the sun" (fr. 1 West). Like Scythinus, the author of *On Regimen* compares the universe to a lyre (18, 6.492 L.; cf. 8.2, 6.482 L.). He also associates the "circuit" (περίοδος) of the sun with the establishment of harmonious cycles in both the body and the cosmos. Thus, *On Regimen*'s pairing of Apollo with Hermes (the inventor of the lyre) may suggest that Apollo regulates these cycles by using his "plectrum" (= the sun's rays) to play the "lyre of Hermes" (= the cycle of evaporation and precipitation), whereby the "up" and "down" movements of water reflect the "up" and "down" movements of notes upon a lyre (cf. 18.3, 6.492 L.). This macrocosmic harmony, in turn, would reflect the microcosmic process whereby the body's "sun" (= the central circuit) uses its "rays" (= the inner and outer circuits) to establish a harmonious *summetria* between drying and mois-tening, moving back and forth from a central circuit that, like the middle string on a lyre, is also called the *mese* (89.2, 6.644 L.).

All of these "heavenly" gods receive prayers in response to positive signs, most likely because the author views the dry *aither* as healthier than the earth and its surrounding *aer*.[138] When something unhealthy has entered the body, the author recommends prayer to a different set of deities: the apotropaic gods, Ge, and the heroes. Because all divinity is derived from

---

[137] For the use of similar language to describe the "darting" of the sun's rays, see *Il.* 18.210–212.
[138] On the relative healthiness of *aither* versus *aer*, see p. 226.

a single, cosmic fire that steers the universe as a whole, we can start by observing that this second set of divinities will also be fiery in nature. The main difference is that instead of inhabiting the heavens, these gods inhabit the earth. As we have already observed, the author of *On Regimen* appears to have believed that the earth, like the flesh, is simply a concretion of cold water. He may have also believed that the earth contains passageways for "hot and cold *pneuma*" just as the flesh contains passageways for *pneuma* to enter and exit the body. Other thinkers from this period talk about winds that circulate through the earth, creating earthquakes and providing humans with both sickness and divine inspiration.[139] In the body, the soul that runs through the outermost circuit is a secretion of the "hottest and strongest" fire in the middle circuit. By referring to a goddess called Earth (= Ge), the author may be suggesting that a similar fire is also embedded in the earth. In *On Flesh*, the author observes that the earth, being cold and dry, also contains a large quantity of the hot (2.2, 8.584 L.). Aristotle similarly observes that the earth contains "a large quantity of fire and heat" (*Mete.* 360a6), while Empedocles observes that "many fires burn under the earth" (DK 31 B52). A reservoir of subterranean fire would explain such phenomena as volcanoes and hot springs, and it would also explain why the winds that blow across the earth's surface originate in the frozen poles. When discussing the "death" of human beings, the "death" of coals, and the cooling of freshly cooked foods, the author of *On Regimen* envisions a process whereby fiery *pneuma* is ejected from a larger object wherever water has "gained the upper hand" over fire. Since the frozen poles manifest the extreme ascendancy of water over fire, it is possible that the author would have applied this same model to the earth, postulating that the fiery soul of the earth is ejected and sent into the *aer* wherever water has "gained the upper hand" over fire.[140] As this *pneuma* blows across the earth, some of it becomes sickly, while some of it becomes healthy. The healthy variety could well be what the author associates with the apotropaic gods, as this *pneuma* would literally "turn away" unhealthy substances from the body.[141] The author's use

---

[139] Compare Arist. [*Mu.*] 395b26–30: "Many vent-holes for wind open in every part of the earth; some of them cause those who draw near to them to become inspired, others make them to waste away, others make them utter oracles, as at Delphi and Lebadia, others utterly destroy them, as the one in Phrygia" (trans. Forster *apud* Barnes, modified).

[140] For the violent ejection of a substance by its opposite, compare 6.2, 6.478 L. and 78.1, 6.622 L. Since water dominates fire in the frozen poles, the *pneuma* that arises from the poles will start off with the qualities of being cold and wet, eventually losing this moisture when it passes through drier regions.

[141] For the medical use of the verb ἀποτρέπειν, compare *Hum.* 4, 5.482 L., where the doctor is instructed to "turn away" (ἀποτρέπειν) and "combat" (μάχεσθαι) adverse symptoms, and *Epid. II* 3.8b, 5.112 L. (= *Epid. VI* 2.7, 5.282 L.), where the doctor is told to "turn away" (ἀποτρέπειν)

of the term "apotropaic" might even be related to the "turning points" (τροπαί) in which fire and water give way to one another (for which cf. the use of the verb ἀποτρέπεσθαι at 3.2, 6.472 L., quoted on p. 217), which would imply that the "fiery" nature of these divinities is combating the "watery" nature of the humors. The "heroes," meanwhile, might have some connection with the free-floating souls of human beings, which are breathed out of living bodies during the transition from "life" to "death."[142] Commentators on this passage have often pointed to the association of heroes with both healing cults and, more specifically, incubation rites. In the Classical period, there were numerous cults of "healing heroes" across the Greek-speaking world. Some noteworthy examples include Asclepius and his sons Machaon and Podalirius, Amphiaraus, Heracles, Protesilaus, Pancrates and Palaemon, Amynus, and the anonymous *heros iatros*. It is unclear whether the author of *On Regimen* would have viewed the heroes as always benevolent, or whether he would have also considered them potential sources of harm. The pathogenic nature of heroes is famously parodied in a fragment from Aristophanes's *Heroes* (fr. 322 K–A, trans. Henderson, modified):

> Wherefore, gentlemen, stand
> guard and worship the heroes, as
> we are the dispensers [ταμίαι]
> of what's bad and what's good,
> and keeping a lookout for the unjust
> and for thieves and robbers
> we give them diseases:
> distended spleens, coughs, dropsy,
> catarrh, mange, podagra,
> madness, canker-sores,
> buboes, shivers, fever.[143]

---

inappropriate movements of the humors. Similar uses of this verb can be found at *Hum.* 5, 5.482 L., *Coac.* 513, 5.702 L., *Aff.* 25, 6.236 L., *Loc. Hom.* 11, 6.296 L., 13.4, 6.300 L., 18, 6.310 L., 21, 6.312–314 L., 23, 6.314 L., 40.2, 6.330 L., and *Ulc.* 1.3, 6.400 L. Given the common use of this term in medical contexts, it seems likely that the author of *On Regimen* envisioned the "apotropaic" gods as performing a similar function of "turning away" harmful moisture.

[142] Compare D.L. 8.32 (on the views of Pythagoras): "All the air is full of souls, and these are called both *daimones* and heroes."

[143] On this fragment, see Gelzer (1969) and Henrichs (1991: 192–193). For other references to heroes as potential sources of harm who need to be turned away, see *Morb. Sacr.* 1.11, 6.362 L., Ar. *Av.* 1485–1493, Men. fr. 348 K–A, Ath. 11.4 (= Chamael. fr. 9 Wehrli), Aët. 1.8.2, Babr. 63, Paus. 9.38.5, Philostr. *Her.* 18.1–6, Hsch. s.v. κρείττονας, Phot. s.v. κρείττονες, and perhaps also Ar. fr. 712 K–A. Note also the reference to "vengeful souls" who are also called *daimones* at *P. Derv.* col. VI.1–4.

As suggested by Lanata (1967: 33n69), the author of *On Regimen* may invoke a notion of harmful heroes in chapter 92. In this passage, the author refers to souls of the dead who bring substances into the body, some of which are healthy and others that are not. If these dead souls are the equivalent of what the author calls "heroes," then this passage would explain the ambiguous nature of these divinities in Greek culture. It should be stressed, however, that the term "heroes" does not appear in this passage. It is therefore possible that the author distinguishes the heroes from a separate class of spirits, blaming the latter for conveying unhealthy substances into the body, while viewing the former as always helpful, perhaps even giving them the job of regulating other beings.[144] Heraclitus famously claimed that people who pray to empty statues and try to purify themselves with blood "do not at all recognize what gods and heroes really are" (DK 22 B5). In another fragment, he presents the heroes as "guardians" of all things, both living and nonliving (DK 22 B63), suggesting that the author of *On Regimen* may have similarly viewed the heroes as the guardians of matters here on earth. Also worth noting in this context are the references to heroes in the so-called Orphic gold tablets. In these documents, initiates identify themselves as children of the *aither* who hope to break the cycle of life and death and thereby enter the ranks of the "heroes." If the author of *On Regimen* is working within a similar intellectual framework, then he, too, would have associated the heroes with both the soul and the *aither*, perhaps identifying them as a subset of human souls who, in contrast to the majority of free-floating souls who "wander without intelligence" (πλανᾶται … ἀγνώμονα, 6.3, 6.478–480 L.), have maintained their intelligence even after being reduced to the realm of the invisible.

The last instruction for prayer in *On Regimen* advises that we pray to Ge, Hermes, and the heroes in cases of overdried flesh (90.6–7, 6.656–658 L.). The purpose of this prayer seems to be to ensure the proper rehydration of the flesh, which our souls can either assist or hinder as they make their way through the outermost circuit.[145] The author presumably targets the

---

[144] Compare the distinction between malevolent souls who wander the earth and just souls who rejoin the gods at Pl. *Phd.* 81c–e. Aët. 1.8.2, by contrast, attributes to Thales, Pythagoras, Plato, and the Stoics the belief that the heroes are souls that have been separated from their bodies, with "good souls" becoming "good" heroes and "evil souls" becoming "harmful" heroes. For *On Regimen*'s description of "clean" and "dirty" souls, compare Pl. *R.* 10.614d–e, where bad souls, inhabiting the earth, are said to be "full of squalor and dust," while good souls, inhabiting the heavens, are said to be "clean."

[145] For the soul's role in both delivering and removing moisture as it travels through the outermost circuit, see p. 234.

"earthly" gods in this instance not only because the *aer* near the earth is less healthy than the *aither* up above but also because the *aer* is loaded with moisture, which these deities can help our souls deliver to the flesh. There might even be a connection with *On Regimen*'s association of the flesh with the earth, implying that just as the chthonic deities tend to the macrocosmic earth, so too will they care for the microcosmic "earth" that represents the flesh. As for the inclusion of Hermes in this list, I would suggest that this god again has something to do with the cycle of evaporation and precipitation.[146] One might imagine, for example, that Hermes, as the agent of evaporation and precipitation, is called upon in this passage to assist the body's soul in "evaporating" the nutriment from our bellies (= the sea). After evaporating this moisture, Hermes would then assist our souls in redistributing this water to the overdried flesh by way of the outermost circuit (= the sky).[147] In this prayer, Hermes replaces an earlier reference to the apotropaic gods in chapter 89. The main difference between these two prayers is that the one in this chapter asks the gods to *add* moisture, while the one in chapter 89 asks the gods to *remove* moisture from the body. This might explain why Hermes and the apotropaic gods trade places between these two prayers, since the messenger Hermes is an agent for transmitting moisture-laden *pneuma*, while the apotropaic gods literally "turn away" that same *pneuma*. Ge and the heroes seem to be more versatile in nature, not unlike how the souls within our bodies can both add nutritive moisture and remove excess moisture as they move through the outermost circuit.

In all of these prayers, the gods are only asked to intervene for affections pertaining to the soul. The first prayer involves an *apokrisis* of moisture that falls upon the soul and "disturbs" it (88.2, 6.644 L.). The second involves the inhalation of foreign substances – an action that again involves the soul inasmuch as inhaled air pours directly into the soul (89.12–14, 6.650–652 L.; cf. pp. 228–229). The third prayer involves a severe case of over-drying, which, as we have noted, would require the involvement of the soul inasmuch as it is the soul that needs to distribute moisture to the flesh during its rounds through the outermost circuit (90.6–7, 6.656–658 L.). In all three cases, the gods would interact with the soul by way of respiration, essentially "steering"

---

[146] Compare Empedocles's claim that Iris, another divine messenger, "brings wind or great rain from the sea" (DK 31 B50).

[147] For *On Regimen*'s use of a water-cycle metaphor to describe the soul's distribution of nutriment from the belly to the flesh, see p. 232.

our souls just as our souls "steer" everything within the body.[148] This observation supports the interpretation of divinity that I have advanced in this chapter. For the author of *On Regimen*, human souls and "gods" are two forms of the same substance. The "mind of gods" is able to exercise more power than the souls within our bodies, but both emanations of the cosmic fire/soul/intelligence regulate their respective "homes." Whereas the author of *On Regimen* believes that doctors can leverage the healing power of the microcosmic soul through the administration of foods, drinks, and exercise, there are some situations in which additional guidance is needed. In these cases, the doctor should call on something higher, leveraging an even more powerful form of "soul" that governs the world in which we live.

There is certainly more that can be said about this system, but the preceding survey should suffice to illustrate both its breathtaking range and the interconnectedness of its ideas. What is most remarkable about this system is the sheer extent to which both the macrocosm and the microcosm are shaped by similar processes. They are governed by divine hierarchies derived from the splitting of one soul into parts, and they are primarily driven by the "hottest and strongest fire" that inhabits the middle circuit and is associated with the sun. It should come as little surprise, therefore, that a problem within the body can be assisted by the gods: the gods perform the same actions wherever they are found, no matter the scale. The sun within the *aither* is analogous to the sun within the body, and so a prayer to the gods will activate them both.

---

[148] The involvement of the soul in all three prayers speaks against Gregory's (2015: 92–94) proposal that the prayers in *On Regimen* are not meant to be intercessory. For general discussions of divine inspiration through the agency of breath, see Murray (1981, 2015), Sissa (1990: 9–70), Padel (1992: 88–98), Katz and Volk (2000), and Holmes (2010: 64–69).

Conclusion

In Chapter 1, we encountered the following testimony for Alcmaeon of Croton, a nebulous figure who seems to have been active at some point in the fifth century BCE (DK 24 B4):

> Alcmaeon says that the containing cause of health is equality among the powers [τὴν ἰσονομίαν τῶν δυνάμεων] – wet, dry, cold, hot, bitter, sweet, and the rest – while the single rule among these [τὴν ἐν αὐτοῖς μοναρχίαν] is productive of disease.

In this study, I have shown that such a theory of opposites does not require the extreme form of therapeutic reductionism that is attacked in *On Ancient Medicine*, whereby diseases can only be treated by balancing the hot with the cold, the cold with the hot, the dry with the wet, and the wet with the dry. Instead, the treatment of "opposites with opposites" was primarily directed toward the remote cause of a disease, while the proximate cause could still be treated by identifying and then purging harmful humors from the body. The doxographer understands this distinction between remote and proximate causes when he calls Alcmaeon's principle of *isonomia* the "containing cause" of health (τῆς μὲν ὑγιείας ... συνεκτικήν). In ancient discussions of causation, a "containing cause" was understood to be a cause that *maintains* a state of being. It does not restore that state after it is lost, but simply keeps it where it is. For Alcmaeon, the balance of the hot, the cold, the dry, and the wet is like the nail that holds a picture on a wall. Once the nail is removed, the picture falls to the ground, but the restoration of the nail will not magically make the picture jump back into place.[1]

This two-tiered model of pathogenesis is vital to understanding the systems of the cosmological doctors. These doctors did not replace humors

---

[1] Compare Aristotle's likening of falling ill to the irreversible act of throwing a stone (*EN* 1114a16–18).

262

with *hupotheseis*, but they combined their first principles with more traditional views of health and disease. This observation is important for the larger question of whether we can say that the cosmological doctors belonged to an intellectual "movement" in any restrictive sense of the term. On the one hand, these doctors certainly share many points in common. We have noted, for example, that they often use arguments from induction to establish the existence of universal principles, that they believe that the microcosm of the body can shed light on the macrocosm of the universe, and that they seek to overcome individual differences by identifying high-level commonalities that transcend all particulars. At the same time that we recognize these similarities, it must be admitted that the systems of the cosmological doctors are hardly parallel in form. For some, the first principles of the universe are the material stuffs from which all things are composed; for others, their first principles resemble what an Aristotelian would call an "efficient cause." Some are happy to speculate about what is invisible, while others, such as Polybus, specifically renounce any interest in substances that cannot be confirmed through the senses. Such variations suggest that the cosmological doctors were not primarily in dialogue with each other. Instead, they seem to have responded to more general trends in early Greek medicine, sometimes focusing on the "powers" (δυνάμεις) that bring about health and disease, and sometimes considering the shared "nature" (φύσις) of both the human body and the universe as a whole.

Instead of separating themselves from the rest of the medical tradition, the cosmological doctors fell along a continuum with other doctors from this period. There is no clear distinction between these doctors and other medical writers who sought out high-level commonalities. The author of *On the Seed-Nature of the Child*, for example, makes many claims that may be labeled "cosmological." He never explicitly defines the first principles of the universe, but he is nevertheless engaging in essentially the same mode of inquiry that we see in *On the Nature of the Human Being*, *On Breaths*, *On Flesh*, and *On Regimen*. What makes the category of "cosmological doctor" so amorphous is that these doctors did not see themselves as significantly departing from their peers. They maintained the same general understanding of *pneuma*, humors, and the "powers" of food and drink that we find in other texts, and they built on preexisting approaches to medical inquiry, especially as regards the comparison of dissimilar phenomena in the hope of finding "one similarity" that unites and governs them all. Some contemporaries of these doctors would certainly have criticized them for investigating "the things on high," but what actually qualified as medically relevant in this period was still up for debate. The cosmological doctors saw themselves primarily as doctors and only secondarily as cosmologists. It is with this in mind that I have approached them in this study, and I hope that future research will further integrate these doctors into our broader understanding of early Greek thought.

References

Adams, F. 1886. *The Genuine Works of Hippocrates*. Wood.

Agge, K. 2004. *Die pseudo-hippokratische Schrift von der Siebenzahl*. Tectum.

Allen, J. 2000. "Galen as (Mis)informant about the Views of His Predecessors." *Archiv für Geschichte der Philosophie* 83: 81–89.

Althoff, J. 1992. *Warm, kalt, flüssig und fest bei Aristoteles*. Steiner.

Arbøll, T. P. 2021. *Medicine in Ancient Assur: A Microhistorical Study of the Neo-Assyrian Healer Kiṣir-Aššur*. Brill.

Baader, G., and Winau, R. (eds.). 1989. *Die hippokratischen Epidemien: Theorie, Praxis, Tradition*. Steiner.

Bardinet, T. 1995. *Les papyrus médicaux de l'Égypte pharaonique*. Fayard.

Barnes, J. 1983. "Aphorism and Argument." In K. Robb (ed.), *Language and Thought in Early Greek Philosophy*. Hegeler Institute. 91–109.

(ed.). 1984. *The Complete Works of Aristotle*. Princeton University Press.

Barton, J. 2005. "Hippocratic Explanations." In van der Eijk (2005b), 29–47.

Bartoš, H. 2015. *Philosophy and Dietetics in the Hippocratic On Regimen*. Brill.

2020. "Heat, Pneuma, and Soul in the Medical Tradition." In Bartoš and King (2020), 21–31.

Bartoš, H., and King, C. G. (eds.). 2020. *Heat, Pneuma, and Soul in Ancient Philosophy and Science*. Cambridge University Press.

Bergsträsser, G. 1914. *Pseudogaleni in Hippocratis de septimanis*. Teubner.

Bertier, J. 1972. *Mnésithée et Dieuchès*. Brill.

Betegh, G. 2016. "Archelaus on Cosmogony and the Origins of Social Institutions." *Oxford Studies in Ancient Philosophy* 51: 1–40.

2020. "Fire, Heat, and Motive Force in Early Greek Philosophy and Medicine." In Bartoš and King (2020), 35–60.

Bidez, J., and Leboucq, G. 1944. "Une anatomie antique du cœur humain: Philistion de Locres et le *Timée* de Platon." *REG* 57: 7–40.

Blass, F. 1901. "Die pseudippokratische Schrift περὶ φυσῶν und der *Anonymus Londinensis*." *Hermes* 36: 405–410.

Böck, B. 2009. "On Medical Technology in Ancient Mesopotamia." In A. Attia and G. Buisson (eds.), *Advances in Mesopotamian Medicine from Hammurabi to Hippocrates*. Brill. 105–128.

2014. *The Healing Goddess Gula: Towards an Understanding of Ancient Babylonian Medicine*. Brill.

Bonnet-Cadilhac, C. 1993. "Traduction et commentaire du traité hippocratique *Des maladies des jeunes filles.*" *History and Philosophy of the Life Sciences* 15: 147–163.

Bourbon, F. 2017. *Hippocrate: Femmes stériles, Maladies des jeunes filles, Superfétation, Excision du fœtus.* Les Belles Lettres.

Bourgey, L. 1953. *Observation et expérience chez les médecins de la collection hippocratique.* Vrin.

Brătescu, G. 1980. "Les éléments vitaux dans la pensée médico-biologique orientale et dans la Collection hippocratique." In Grmek (1980), 65–72.

Brisson, L. 2013. "Le *Timée* de Platon et le traité hippocratique *Du régime*, sur le mécanisme de la sensation." *Études Platoniciennes* 10.

Brock, A. J. 1916. *Galen: On the Natural Faculties.* Harvard University Press.

Burgess, T. C. 1902. "Epideictic Literature." *The University of Chicago Studies in Classical Philology* 3: 89–261.

Burkert, W. et al. (eds.). 1998. *Fragmentsammlungen philosophischer Texte der Antike.* Vandenhoeck & Ruprecht.

Burnet, J. 1930. *Early Greek Philosophy.* Fourth edition. Black.

Bury, R. G. 1926. *Plato: Laws, Volume II, Books 7–12.* Harvard University Press.

   1929. *Plato: Timaeus, Critias, Cleitophon, Menexenus, Epistles.* Harvard University Press.

   1932. *The Symposium of Plato.* Second edition. Heffer.

Calvus, F. M. 1525. *Hippocratis Coi ... octoginta volumina.* Minutius.

Capelle, W. 1912. "Μετέωρος – μετεωρολογία." *Philologus* 71: 414–448.

Carrick, P. 2001. *Medical Ethics in the Ancient World.* Georgetown University Press.

Chang, H.-H. 2008. "Rationalizing Medicine and the Social Ambitions of Physicians in Classical Greece." *Journal of the History of Medicine and Allied Sciences* 63: 217–244.

Clifford, R. J. (ed.). 2007. *Wisdom Literature in Mesopotamia and Israel.* Society of Biblical Literature.

Cohn-Haft, L. 1956. *The Public Physicians of Ancient Greece.* Smith College.

Cooper, G. L., and Krüger, K. W. 1998. *Attic Greek Prose Syntax.* University of Michigan Press.

Cooper, J. M. 1997. *Plato: Complete Works.* Hackett.

   2004. *Knowledge, Nature, and the Good: Essays on Ancient Philosophy.* Princeton University Press.

Cornarius, J. 1538. *Hippocratis Coi medici ... libri omnes.* Froben.

Craik, E. M. 1998. *Hippocrates: Places in Man.* Oxford University Press.

   2001a. "Thucydides on the Plague: Physiology of Flux and Fixation." *CQ* 51: 102–108.

   2001b. "Plato and Medical Texts: *Symposium* 185c–193d." *CQ* 51: 109–114.

   2009. *The Hippocratic Treatise On Glands.* Brill.

   2015. *The "Hippocratic" Corpus: Content and Context.* Routledge.

   2018. "Hippocrates and Early Greek Medicine." In P. T. Keyser and J. Scarborough (eds.), *The Oxford Handbook of Science and Medicine in the Classical World.* Oxford University Press. 215–232.

Cross, J. 2018. *Hippocratic Oratory: The Poetics of Early Greek Medical Prose.* Routledge.

Cruse, A. 2004. *Roman Medicine.* Tempus.

Curd, P., and Graham, D. W. (eds.). 2008. *The Oxford Handbook of Presocratic Philosophy.* Oxford University Press.

de la Villa Polo, J. et al. 2003. *Tratados hipocráticos,* vol. 8. Editorial Gredos.

Dean-Jones, L. 1994. *Women's Bodies in Classical Greek Science.* Oxford University Press.

2003. "Literacy and the Charlatan in Ancient Greek Medicine." In Yunis (2003), 97–121.

Dean-Jones, L., and Rosen, R. M. (eds.). 2016. *Ancient Concepts of the Hippocratic.* Brill.

Deichgräber, K. 1933. "Πρόφασις: eine terminologische Studie." *Quellen und Studien zur Geschichte der Naturwissenschaften und der Medizin* 3: 209–225.

1935. *Über Entstehung und Aufbau des menschlichen Körpers (Περὶ σαρκῶν).* Teubner.

1937. "Petronas." *RE* 19.1: 1191–1192.

1971. *Die Epidemien und das Corpus Hippocraticum.* Second edition. De Gruyter.

Demont, P. 1993. "Die epideixis über die techne im V. und IV. Jh." In Kullmann and Althoff (1993), 181–209.

Denyer, N. 2008. *Plato: Protagoras.* Cambridge University Press.

di Benedetto, V. 1966. "Tendenza e probabilità nell'antica medicina greca." *Critica Storica* 5: 315–368.

1986. *Il medico e la malattia.* Einaudi.

Diels, H. 1893a. *Supplementum Aristotelicum, vol. 3, pars 1. Anonymi Londinensis Iatrica.* Reimer.

1893b. "Über die Excerpte von Menons *Iatrika* in dem Londoner Papyrus 137." *Hermes* 28: 407–434.

1911. "Hippokratische Forschungen II. III." *Hermes* 46: 261–285.

Diller, H. 1932. "Ὄψις τῶν ἀδήλων τὰ φαινόμενα." *Hermes* 67: 14–42.

1936. Review of Deichgräber (1935). *Gnomon* 12: 367–377.

1938. "Philistion (4)." *RE* 19.2: 2405–2408.

1959. "Der innere Zusammenhang der hippokratischen Schrift *De victu.*" *Hermes* 87: 39–56.

1964. "Ausdrucksformen des methodischen Bewusstseins in den hippokratischen *Epidemien.*" *Archiv für Begriffsgeschichte* 9: 133–150.

1971. "Zum Gebrauch von εἶδος und ἰδέα in vorplatonischer Zeit." In G. Mann et al. (eds.), *Medizingeschichte in unserer Zeit.* Enke. 23–30.

Dodds, E. R. 1973. *The Ancient Concept of Progress and Other Essays on Greek Literature and Belief.* Oxford University Press.

Dover, K. 1980. *Plato: Symposium.* Cambridge University Press.

Ducatillon, J. 1977. *Polémiques dans la collection hippocratique.* Champion.

1983. "Le traité des *Vents* et la question hippocratique." In Lasserre and Mudry (1983), 263–276.

Duchesne-Guillemin, J. 1956. "Persische Weisheit in griechischem Gewande?" *Harvard Theological Review* 49: 115–122.

Duminil, M.-P. 1998. *Hippocrate: Plaies, Nature des os, Cœur, Anatomie.* Les Belles Lettres.

Dümmler, F. 1889. *Akademika.* Ricker.

Edelstein, L. 1931. Περὶ ἀέρων *und die Sammlung der hippokratischen Schriften.* Weidmann.

1953. "Hippokrates." *RE Supplement* 6: 1290–1345.

1967. *The Idea of Progress in Classical Antiquity.* Johns Hopkins University Press.

Elman, Y. 1975. "Authoritative Oral Traditions in Neo-Assyrian Scribal Circles." *Journal of the Ancient Near Eastern Society* 7: 19–32.

Enache, C. 2015. "The Intelligence Typology in Hippocrates' *De victu* I 35." *Wiener Studien* 128: 37–48.

Ermerins, F. Z. 1859–64. *Hippocratis et aliorum medicorum veterum reliquiae.* Kemink.

Faraone, C. A. 1992. *Talismans and Trojan Horses: Guardian Statues in Ancient Greek Myth and Ritual.* Oxford University Press.

Farrington, B. 1953. *Greek Science.* Second edition. Penguin.

Ferguson, J. 1969. "The Opposites." *Apeiron* 3: 1–17.

Festugière, A. 1948. *Hippocrate: L'ancienne médecine.* Klincksieck.

Flemming, R., and Hanson, A. E. 1988. "Hippocrates' *Peri partheniôn* ('Diseases of Young Girls'): Text and Translation." *Early Science and Medicine* 3: 241–252.

Ford, A. 2009. *The Origins of Criticism: Literary Culture and Poetic Theory in Classical Greece.* Princeton University Press.

Fredrich, C. J. 1899. *Hippokratische Untersuchungen.* Weidmann.

Furley, D. J., and Wilkie, J. S. 1984. *Galen on Respiration and the Arteries.* Princeton University Press.

Garofalo, I. 1988. *Erasistrati fragmenta.* Giardini.

Geller, M. J. 2004. "West Meets East: Early Greek and Babylonian Diagnosis." In Horstmanshoff and Stol (2004), 11–61.

2007. "Phlegm and Breath: Babylonian Contributions to Hippocratic Medicine." In I. L. Finkel and M. J. Geller (eds.), *Disease in Babylonia.* Brill. 187–199.

2010. *Ancient Babylonian Medicine: Theory and Practice.* Wiley-Blackwell.

2018. "Babylonian Medicine as a Discipline." In Jones and Taub (2018), 29–57.

Gelzer, T. 1969. "Zur Versreihe der 'Heroes' aus der Alten Komödie (Pap. Mich. inv. 3690)." *Zeitschrift für Papyrologie und Epigraphik* 4: 123–133.

Gillespie, C. M. 1912. "The Use of εἶδος and ἰδέα in Hippocrates." *CQ* 6: 179–203.

Gomperz, T. 1901. *Greek Thinkers.* Scribner's.

Gorrini, M. E. 2005. "The Hippocratic Impact on Healing Cults: The Archaeological Evidence in Attica." In van der Eijk (2005b), 135–156.

Götze, A. 1923. "Persische Weisheit in griechischem Gewande: eine Beitrag zur Geschichte der Mikrokosmos-Idee." *Zeitschrift für Indologie und Iranistik* 2: 61–98, 167–177.

Gourevitch, D. 1989. "L'Anonyme de Londres et la médecine d'Italie du Sud." *History and Philosophy of the Life Sciences* 11: 237–251.

Grapow, H. (ed.). 1954–73. *Grundriss der Medizin der alten Ägypten.* Akademie-Verlag.

Gregory, A. 2015. *The Presocratics and the Supernatural.* Bloomsbury.

Grensemann, H. 1968. "Der Arzt Polybos als Verfasser hippokratischer Schriften." *AbhMainz* 2: 53–95.

    1974. "Polybos (8)." *RE Supplement* 14: 428–436.

    1975. *Knidische Medizin,* vol. 1. De Gruyter.

    1987. *Knidische Medizin,* vol. 2. Steiner.

Grmek, M. (ed.). 1980. *Hippocratica.* Centre national de la recherche scientifique.

Gundert, B. 1992. "Parts and Their Roles in Hippocratic Medicine." *Isis* 83: 453–465.

Guthrie, W. K. C. 1962. *A History of Greek Philosophy,* vol. 1. Cambridge University Press.

Hadot, P. 1998. *The Inner Citadel: The Meditations of Marcus Aurelius.* Harvard University Press.

Hahm, D. E. 1977. *The Origins of Stoic Cosmology.* Ohio State University Press.

Hankinson, R. J. 1991. "Greek Medical Models of Mind." In S. Everson (ed.), *Psychology.* Cambridge University Press. 194–217.

    2001. *Cause and Explanation in Ancient Greek Thought.* Oxford University Press.

    2018. "Aetiology." In Pormann (2018), 89–118.

Hanson, A. E. 1975. "Hippocrates: *Diseases of Women 1.*" *Signs* 1: 567–584.

Hardie, W. F. R. 1976. "Concepts of Consciousness in Aristotle." *Mind* 85: 388–411.

    1980. *Aristotle's Ethical Theory.* Second edition. Oxford University Press.

Harris, C. R. S. 1973. *The Heart and the Vascular System in Ancient Greek Medicine.* Oxford University Press.

Heeßel, N. P. 2004. "Diagnosis, Divination and Disease: Towards an Understanding of the *rationale* behind the Babylonian *Diagnostic Handbook.*" In Horstmanshoff and Stol (2004), 97–116.

    2010. "Einleitung zu Struktur und Entwicklung des Corpus der therapeutischen Texte." In B. Janowski and D. Schwemer (eds.), *Texte aus der Umwelt des Alten Testaments,* vol. 5. Gütersloher Verlagshaus. 31–35.

Heidel, W. A. 1912. "On Anaximander." *CP* 7: 212–234.

    1914. "Hippocratea, I." *HSCP* 25: 139–203.

    1941. *Hippocratic Medicine: Its Spirit and Method.* Columbia University Press.

Henrichs, A. 1991. "Namenlosigkeit und Euphemismus: Zur Ambivalenz der chthonischen Machte im attischen Drama." In H. Hoffman (ed.), *Fragmenta dramatica.* Vandenhoeck & Ruprecht. 161–201.

Herter, H. 1976. "The Problematic Mention of Hippocrates in Plato's *Phaedrus.*" *Illinois Classical Studies* 1: 22–42.

Hey, O. 1908. *Der Traumglaube der Antike.* Staub.

Hoessly, F. 2001. *Katharsis: Reinigung als Heilverfahren.* Vandenhoeck & Ruprecht.

Holmes, B. 2010. *The Symptom and the Subject: The Emergence of the Physical Body in Ancient Greece.* Princeton University Press.

Horky, P. S. 2019. "When Did *Kosmos* Become the *Kosmos*?" In P. S. Horky (ed.), *Cosmos in the Ancient World.* Cambridge University Press. 22–41.

Horstmanshoff, H. F. J., and Stol, M. (eds.). 2004. *Magic and Rationality in Ancient Near Eastern and Graeco-Roman Medicine.* Brill.

Hort, A. 1916. *Theophrastus: Enquiry into Plants,* vol. 1. Harvard University Press.

Huffman, C. A. 1993. *Philolaus of Croton: Pythagorean and Presocratic.* Cambridge University Press.

    2021. "Alcmaeon." In E. N. Zalta (ed.), *The Stanford Encyclopedia of Philosophy* (summer 2021 edition). https://plato.stanford.edu/archives/sum2021/entries/alcmaeon.

Hüffmeier, F. 1961. "Phronesis in den Schriften des *Corpus Hippocraticum.*" *Hermes* 89: 51–84.

Hulskamp, M. A. A. 2012. "Space and the Body: Uses of Astronomy in Hippocratic Medicine." In P. Baker, H. Nijdam, and K. van 't Land (eds.), *Medicine and Space.* Brill. 149–167.

    2013. "The Value of Dream Diagnosis to the Hippocratics and Galen." In S. Oberhelman (ed.), *Dreams, Healing, and Medicine in Greece.* Routledge. 33–68.

    2016. "*On Regimen* and the Question of Medical Dreams in the Hippocratic Corpus." In Dean-Jones and Rosen (2016), 258–270.

Hunter, R. 2004. *Plato's Symposium.* Oxford University Press.

Ilberg, J. 1894. "Die medizinische Schrift *Über die Siebenzahl* und die Schule von Knidos." In *Griechische Studien.* Teubner. 22–39.

    1925. *Die Ärzteschule von Knidos.* Hirzel.

Inwood, B. 2001. *The Poem of Empedocles.* Revised edition. University of Toronto Press.

Jacques, J.-M. 2008. "Aristōn (I)." In Keyser and Irby-Massie (2008), 139.

Jaeger, W. 1938. *Diokles von Karystos.* De Gruyter.

    1944. *Paideia: The Ideals of Greek Culture,* vol. 3. Oxford University Press.

Joly, R. 1960. *Recherches sur le traité pseudo-hippocratique Du régime.* Les Belles Lettres.

    1961. "La question hippocratique et le témoignage du *Phèdre.*" *REG* 74: 69–92.

    1967. *Hippocrate: Du régime.* Les Belles Lettres.

    1970. *Hippocrate: De la génération, De la nature de l'enfant, Des maladies IV, Du fœtus de huit mois.* Les Belles Lettres.

    1972. *Hippocrate: Du régime des maladies aiguës, Appendice, De l'aliment, De l'usage des liquides.* Les Belles Lettres.

    1978. *Hippocrate: Des lieux dans l'homme, Du système des glandes, Des fistules, Des hémorroïdes, De la vision, Des chairs, De la dentition.* Les Belles Lettres.

    1983. "Platon, *Phèdre* et Hippocrate: vingt ans après." In Lasserre and Mudry (1983), 407–422.

1984. *Hippocrate: Du régime*. Akademie-Verlag.

Jones, A., and Taub, L. (eds.). 2018. *The Cambridge History of Science*, vol. 1. Cambridge University Press.

Jones, W. H. S. 1923a. *Hippocrates*, vol. 1. Harvard University Press.

1923b. *Hippocrates*, vol. 2. Harvard University Press.

1931. *Hippocrates*, vol. 4. Harvard University Press.

1946. *Philosophy and Medicine*. Johns Hopkins University Press.

1947. *The Medical Writings of Anonymus Londinensis*. Cambridge University Press.

Jouanna, J. 1961. "Présence d'Empédocle dans la *Collection Hippocratique*." *Bulletin de l'Association G. Budé* 20: 452–463.

1965. "Rapports entre Mélissos de Samos et Diogène d'Apollonie à la lumière du traité hippocratique *De natura hominis*." *Revue des Études Anciennes* 67: 306–323.

1966. "La théorie de l'intelligence et de l'âme dans le traité hippocratique *Du Régime*: ses rapports avec Empédocle et le *Timée* de Platon." *REG* 79: xv–xviii.

1969. "Le médecin Polybe est-il l'auteur de plusieurs ouvrages de la *Collection hippocratique*?" *REG* 82: 552–558.

1974. *Hippocrate: pour une archéologie de l'école de Cnide*. Les Belles Lettres.

1977. "La *Collection hippocratique* et Platon (*Phèdre* 269c–272a)." *REG* 90: 15–28.

1983. *Hippocrate: Maladies II*. Les Belles Lettres.

1984. "Rhétorique et médecine dans la *Collection hippocratique*." *REG* 97: 26–44.

1988. *Hippocrate: Des vents, De l'art*. Les Belles Lettres.

1989. "Note sur l'histoire de la subdivision du traité hippocratique *Du régime* en livres et sur le problème de l'existence de l'ΥΓΙΕΙΝΟΝ dans la *Collection hippocratique*." *Studi Classici e Orientali* 29: 13–19.

1992. "La naissance de la science de l'homme chez les médecins et les savants à l'époque d'Hippocrate: problèmes de méthode." In López Férez (1992), 91–111.

1998. "L'interpétation des rêves et la théorie micro-macrocosmique dans le traité hippocratique du *Régime*: sémiotique et mimésis." In K.-D. Fischer, D. Nickel, and P. Potter (eds.), *Text and Tradition: Studies in Ancient Medicine and Its Transmission*. Brill. 161–174.

1999. *Hippocrates*. Translated by M. B. DeBevoise. Johns Hopkins University Press.

2000. *Hippocrate: Épidémies V et VII*. Les Belles Lettres.

2002. *Hippocrate: La nature de l'homme*. Second edition. Akademie-Verlag.

2003a. *Hippocrate: La maladie sacrée*. Les Belles Lettres.

2003b. "Sur la dénomination et le nombre des sens d'Hippocrate à la médecine impériale: réflexions à partir de l'énumération des sens dans le traité hippocratique du *Régime*, c. 23." In I. Boehm and P. Luccioni (eds.), *Les cinq sens dans la médecine de l'époque impériale: sources et développements*. de Boccard. 9–20.

2007. "La théorie de la sensation, de la pensée et de l'âme dans le traité hippocratique du *Régime*: ses rapports avec Empédocle et le *Timée* de Platon." *Annali dell'Università degli Studi di Napoli "L'Orientale"* 29: 9–39.

2012. *Greek Medicine from Hippocrates to Galen*. Brill.

2016. *Hippocrate: Épidémies I et III*. Les Belles Lettres.

Jüthner, J. 1909. *Philostratos: Über Gymnastik*. Teubner.

Kahn, C. H. 1960. *Anaximander and the Origins of Greek Cosmology*. Columbia University Press.

1979. *The Art and Thought of Heraclitus*. Cambridge University Press.

Katz, J., and Volk, K. 2000. "'Mere Bellies'? A New Look at *Theogony* 26–8." *JHS* 120: 122–131.

Kerferd, G. B. 1981. *The Sophistic Movement*. Cambridge University Press.

Keyser, P. T., and Irby-Massie, G. L. (eds.). 2008. *The Encyclopedia of Ancient Natural Scientists*. Routledge.

Kind, F. E. 1936. Review of Deichgräber (1935). *Philologische Wochenschrift* 56: 625–639, 676–684.

King, H. 1998. *Hippocrates' Woman: Reading the Female Body in Ancient Greece*. Routledge.

Kirk, G. S. 1954. *Heraclitus: The Cosmic Fragments*. Cambridge University Press.

Kleingünther, A. 1933. Πρῶτος εὑρετής: *Untersuchungen zur Geschichte einer Fragestellung*. Dieterich.

Konstan, D., and Young-Bruehl, E. 1982. "Eryximachus' Speech in the *Symposium*." *Apeiron* 16: 40–46.

Kranz, W. 1938. "Kosmos und Mensch in der Vorstellung frühen Griechentums." *Nachrichten von der Gesellschaft der Wissenschaften zu Göttingen, Philologisch-historische Klasse* 2: 121–161.

Kudlien, F. 1967. *Der Beginn des medizinischen Denkens bei den Griechen*. Artemis.

1970. "Medical Education in Classical Antiquity." In C. D. O'Malley (ed.), *The History of Medical Education*. University of California Press. 3–37.

Kühn, C. G. 1821–33. *Claudii Galeni opera omnia*. Cnobloch.

Kühn, J.-H. 1956. *System- und Methodenprobleme im Corpus Hippocraticum*. Steiner.

Kullmann, W., and Althoff, J. (eds.). 1993. *Vermittlung und Tradierung von Wissen in der griechischen Kultur*. Narr.

Kuriyama, S. 2002. *The Expressiveness of the Body and the Divergence of Greek and Chinese Medicine*. Zone Books.

Kurz, D. 1970. Ἀκρίβεια: *Das Ideal der Exaktheit bei den Griechen bis Aristoteles*. Kümmerle.

Laks, A. 1998. "Éditer l'influence? Remarques sur la section C du chapitre Diogène d'Apollonie dans les *Fragmente der Vorsokratiker* de Diels-Kranz." In Burkert et al. (1998), 89–105.

2006. *Introduction à la "philosophie présocratique."* Presses Universitaires de France.

2008. *Diogène d'Apollonie*. Academia Verlag.

Laks, A., and Most, G. W. 2016a. *Early Greek Philosophy*, vol. 5. Harvard University Press.

2016b. *Early Greek Philosophy*, vol. 6. Harvard University Press.

Lami, A. 2007. "[Ippocrate], *Sui disturbi virginali*: testo, traduzione e commento." *Galenos* 1: 15–59.

Lanata, G. 1967. *Medicina magica e religione popolare in Grecia fino all'età di Ippocrate*. Edizioni dell'Ateneo.

Langholf, V. 1986. "Kallimachos, Komödie und hippokratische Frage." *Medizinhistorisches Journal* 21: 3–30.

1989. "Generalisationen und Aphorismen in den Epidemienbüchern." In Baader and Winau (1989), 131–143.

1990a. *Medical Theories in Hippocrates: Early Texts and the Epidemics*. De Gruyter.

1990b. "L'air (*pneuma*) et les maladies." In Potter, Maloney, and Desautels (1990), 339–359.

2004. "Structure and Genesis of Some Hippocratic Treatises." In Horstmanshoff and Stol (2004), 219–275.

Laskaris, J. 2002. *The Art Is Long: On the Sacred Disease and the Scientific Tradition*. Brill.

Lasserre, F., and Mudry, P. (eds.). 1983. *Formes de pensée dans la Collection hippocratique*. Droz.

Le Blay, F. 2005. "Microcosm and Macrocosm: The Dual Direction of Analogy in Hippocratic Thought and the Meteorological Tradition." In van der Eijk (2005b), 251–269.

Lebedev, A. V. 2014. *Логос Гераклита: реконструкция мысли и слова* [= *The Logos of Heraclitus: A Reconstruction of His Thought and Word*]. Nauka.

Leichty, E. 1988. "Guaranteed to Cure." In E. Leichty and M. Ellis (eds.), *A Scientific Humanist*. University Museum. 261–264.

Lesher, J. H. 2008. "The Humanizing of Knowledge in Presocratic Thought." In Curd and Graham (2008), 458–484.

Levin, S. B. 2014. *Plato's Rivalry with Medicine: A Struggle and Its Dissolution*. Oxford University Press.

Lewis, O. 2017. *Praxagoras of Cos on Arteries, Pulse and Pneuma*. Brill.

Licciardi, C. 1989. "Tendance et probabilité dans les *Epidémies II. IV. VI*." In Baader and Winau (1989), 117–130.

Lichtenthaeler, C. 1991. *Le traité des Vents est typiquement pseudo-hippocratique*. Droz.

Littré, É. 1839–61. *Oeuvres complètes d'Hippocrate*. Ballière.

Lloyd, G. E. R. 1963. "Who Is Attacked in *On Ancient Medicine*?" *Phronesis* 8: 108–126.

1964. "The Hot and the Cold, the Dry and the Wet in Greek Philosophy." *JHS* 84: 92–106.

1966. *Polarity and Analogy: Two Types of Argumentation in Early Greek Thought*. Cambridge University Press.

1968. "Plato as a Natural Scientist." *JHS* 88: 78–92.

1975. "The Hippocratic Question." *CQ* 25: 171–192.

1979. *Magic, Reason, and Experience: Studies in the Origin and Development of Greek Science.* Cambridge University Press.

1987. *The Revolutions of Wisdom: Studies in the Claims and Practices of Ancient Greek Science.* University of California Press.

1991a. *Methods and Problems in Greek Science: Selected Papers.* Cambridge University Press.

1991b. "The Definition, Status, and Methods of the Medical τέχνη in the Fifth and Fourth Centuries." In A. C. Bowen (ed.), *Science and Philosophy in Classical Greece.* Garland. 249–260.

2002. "Le pluralisme de la vie intellectuelle avant Platon." In A. Laks and C. Louguet (eds.), *Qu'est-ce que la philosophie présocratique?* Septentrion. 39–53.

2003. *In the Grip of Disease: Studies in the Greek Imagination.* Oxford University Press.

2007. "The Wife of Philinus, or the Doctors' Dilemma: Medical Signs and Cases and Non-Deductive Inference." In D. Scott (ed.), *Maieusis: Essays on Ancient Philosophy in Honour of Myles Burnyeat.* Oxford University Press. 335–350.

Lo Presti, R. 2016. "Perceiving the Coherence of the Perceiving Body: Is There Such a Thing as a 'Hippocratic' View on Sense Perception and Cognition?" In Dean-Jones and Rosen (2016), 163–194.

Long, A. A. 1999. "The Scope of Early Greek Philosophy." In A. A. Long (ed.), *The Cambridge Companion to Early Greek Philosophy.* Cambridge University Press. 1–21.

Longrigg, J. 1963. "Philosophy and Medicine: Some Early Interactions." *HSCP* 67: 147–175.

1983. "[Hippocrates'] *Ancient Medicine* and Its Intellectual Context." In Lasserre and Mudry (1983), 249–256.

1993. *Greek Rational Medicine: Philosophy and Medicine from Alcmaeon to the Alexandrians.* Routledge.

2001. "Medicine in the Classical World." In I. Loudon (ed.), *Western Medicine: An Illustrated History.* Oxford University Press. 25–39.

Lonie, I. M. 1977. "A Structural Pattern in Greek Dietetics and the Early History of Greek Medicine." *Medical History* 21: 235–260.

1981. *The Hippocratic Treatises On Generation, On the Nature of the Child, Diseases IV.* De Gruyter.

López Férez, J. A. (ed.). 1992. *Tratados hipocráticos.* Universidad Nacional de Educación a Distancia.

López Férez, J. A., and García Novo, E. 1997. *Tratados hipocráticos*, vol. 2. Editorial Gredos.

López Morales, D. 2001. *Hipòcrates, tractats mèdics, vol. IV: El règim de vida.* Fundació Bernat Metge.

Magdelaine, C. 1997. "Microcosme et macrocosme dans le *Corpus hippocratique*: réflexions sur l'homme et la maladie." In J.-L. Cabanès (ed.), *Littérature et médecine.* Université Michel de Montaigne Bordeaux III. 11–39.

Manetti, D. 1990. "Doxographical Deformation of Medical Tradition in the Report of the *Anonymus Londinensis* on Philolaus." *Zeitschrift für Papyrologie und Epigraphik* 83: 219–233.

1992. "Hippo Crotoniates." *Corpus dei papiri filosofici greci e latini* I.1**: 455–461.

1999a. "'Aristotle' and the Role of Doxography in the *Anonymus Londinensis* (PBrLibr inv. 137)." In P. J. van der Eijk (ed.), *Ancient Histories of Medicine: Essays in Medical Doxography and Historiography in Classical Antiquity*. Brill. 95–141.

1999b. "Philolaus 1 T." *Corpus dei papiri filosofici greci e latini* I.1***: 16–31.

1999c. "Plato 129 T." *Corpus dei papiri filosofici greci e latini* I.1***: 528–578.

2005. "Medici contemporanei a Ippocrate: problemi di identificazione dei medici di nome Erodico." In van der Eijk (2005b), 295–313.

2008a. "Euruphōn of Knidos." In Keyser and Irby-Massie (2008), 321–322.

2008b. "Petrōn(as) of Aigina." In Keyser and Irby-Massie (2008), 638–639.

2008c. "Philistiōn of Lokroi." In Keyser and Irby-Massie (2008), 649–650.

2008d. "Polubos." In Keyser and Irby-Massie (2008), 681–682.

2011. *Anonymus Londiniensis: De medicina*. De Gruyter.

Manetti, D., and Roselli, A. 1982. *Ippocrate: Epidemie, libro sesto*. La Nuova Italia.

Mansfeld, J. 1971. *The Pseudo-Hippocratic Tract Περὶ ἑβδομάδων Ch. 1–11 and Greek Philosophy*. Van Gorcum.

1975. "Alcmaeon: 'Physikos' or Physician? With Some Remarks on Calcidius' 'On Vision' Compared to Galen, *Plac. Hipp. Plat.* VII." In J. Mansfeld and L. M. de Rijk (eds.), *Kephalaion*. Van Gorcum. 26–38.

1980a. "Plato and the Method of Hippocrates." *Greek, Roman, and Byzantine Studies* 21: 341–362.

1980b. "Theoretical and Empirical Attitudes in Early Greek Scientific Medicine." In Grmek (1980), 371–390.

2018. *Studies in Early Greek Philosophy*. Brill.

Mansfeld, J., and Runia, D. T. 2010. *Aëtiana: The Method and Intellectual Context of a Doxographer*, vol. 3. Brill.

Matsui, S., and Cornelli, G. 2017. "O tratado pseudo-hipocrático *Sobre as carnes* e o testemunho do *Fédon*." *Humanitas* 70: 25–36.

Maucolin, B. 2009. *Untersuchungen zur hippokratischen Schrift Über die alte Heilkunst*. De Gruyter.

Meyerhof, M., and Schacht, J. 1931. *Galen: Über die medizinischen Namen*. Akademie der Wissenschaften.

Michler, M. 2003. *Westgriechische Heilkunde: eine Skizze*. Königshausen & Neumann.

Miller, H. W. 1949. "*On Ancient Medicine* and the Origin of Medicine." *Transactions and Proceedings of the American Philological Association* 80: 187–202.

Mudry, P. 1980. "Sur l'étiologie des maladies attribuée à Hippocrate par Celse, *De medicina*, préf. 15." In Grmek (1980), 409–415.

1982. *La préface du De medicina de Celse*. Institut suisse de Rome.

Müller, C. W. 1965a. *Gleiches zu Gleichem*. Harrassowitz.

1965b. "Schreibkunst oder Malerei?" *Sudhoffs Archiv* 49: 307–311.

Müri, W. 1936. *Arzt und Patient bei Hippokrates*. Jahresbericht des Städtischen Gymnasiums Bern.

Murray, P. 1981. "Poetic Inspiration in Early Greece." *JHS* 101: 87–100.

2015. "Poetic Inspiration." In P. Destrée and P. Murray (eds.), *A Companion to Ancient Aesthetics*. Wiley-Blackwell. 158–174.

Naddaf, G. 2005. *The Greek Concept of Nature*. State University of New York Press.

Nails, D. 2002. *The People of Plato: A Prosopography of Plato and Other Socratics*. Hackett.

Nelson, A. 1909. *Die hippokratische Schrift περὶ φυσῶν: Text und Studien*. Almqvist & Wiksell.

Nightingale, A. W. 1995. *Genres in Dialogue: Plato and the Construct of Philosophy*. Cambridge University Press.

2004. *Spectacles of Truth in Classical Greek Philosophy: Theoria in Its Cultural Context*. Cambridge University Press.

Nikitas, A. 1968. Untersuchungen zu den Epidemienbüchern II, IV, VI des Corpus Hippocraticum. Dissertation. Hamburg.

Nunn, J. F. 1996. *Ancient Egyptian Medicine*. University of Oklahoma Press.

Nutton, V. 2004. *Ancient Medicine*. Routledge.

2007a. "Philistion (1)." *BNP* 11: 46–47.

2007b. "Polybus (6)." *BNP* 11: 504–505.

2020. *Galen: A Thinking Doctor in Imperial Rome*. Routledge.

O'Brien, D. 1970. "The Effect of a Simile: Empedocles' Theories of Seeing and Breathing." *JHS* 90: 140–179.

Oldfather, C. H. 1933. *Diodorus Siculus: Library of History*, vol. 1. Harvard University Press.

Olerud, A. 1951. *L'idée de macrocosmos et de microcosmos dans le Timée de Platon: étude de mythologie comparée*. Almqvist & Wiksell.

Olson, S. D. 2007. *Athenaeus: The Learned Banqueters, Books 3.106e–5*. Harvard University Press.

Orelli, L. 1998. "Vorsokratiker und hippokratische Medizin." In Burkert et al. (1998), 128–145.

Oser-Grote, C. M. 1997. "Das Auge und der Sehvorgang nach Aristoteles und der hippokratischen Schrift De carnibus." In W. Kullmann und S. Föllinger (eds.), *Aristotelische Biologie: Intentionen, Methoden, Ergebnisse*. Steiner. 333–349.

2004. *Aristoteles und das Corpus Hippocraticum: die Anatomie und Physiologie des Menschen*. Steiner.

Padel, R. 1992. *In and Out of the Mind: Greek Images of the Tragic Self*. Princeton University Press.

Palm, A. 1933. *Studien zur hippokratischen Schrift Περὶ διαίτης*. Tübinger Chronik.

Parker, R. 1983. *Miasma: Pollution and Purification in Early Greek Religion*. Oxford University Press.

Pease, A. S. 1926. "Things without Honor." *CP* 21: 27–42.

Peck, A. L. 1928. Pseudo-Hippocrates Philosophus. Dissertation. Cambridge.

1936. "The Hippocratic Treatise *On Flesh*." *The Classical Review* 50: 62–63.

Pelling, C. 2000. *Literary Texts and the Greek Historian*. Routledge.

Pelosi, F. 2016. "Music for Life: Embryology, Cookery and *Harmonia* in the Hippocratic *On Regimen*." *Greek and Roman Musical Studies* 4: 191–208.

Pendrick, G. J. 2002. *Antiphon the Sophist*. Cambridge University Press.

Perilli, L. 2001. "Alcmeone di Crotone tra filosofia e scienza." *Quaderni Urbinati di Cultura Classica* 69: 55–79.

Pfleiderer, E. 1896. *Sokrates und Plato*. Laupp.

Pigeaud, J. 1990. "La maladie a-t-elle un sens chez Hippocrate?" In Potter, Maloney, and Desautels (1990), 17–38.

Plambӧck, G. 1964. "*Dynamis* im *Corpus Hippocraticum*." *AbhMainz* 2: 58–110.

Pohlenz, M. 1938. *Hippokrates und die Begründung der wissenschaftlichen Medizin*. De Gruyter.

Pormann, P. E. (ed.). 2018. *The Cambridge Companion to Hippocrates*. Cambridge University Press.

Potter, P. 1988a. *Hippocrates*, vol. 5. Harvard University Press.

1988b. *Hippocrates*, vol. 6. Harvard University Press.

1995. *Hippocrates*, vol. 8. Harvard University Press.

2010. *Hippocrates*, vol. 9. Harvard University Press.

2018. *Hippocrates*, vol. 11. Harvard University Press.

Potter, P., Maloney, G., and Desautels, J. (eds.). 1990. *La maladie et les maladies dans la Collection hippocratique*. Éditions du Sphinx.

Primavesi, O. 2009. "Medicine between Natural Philosophy and Physician's Practice: A Debate around 400 BC." In S. Elm and S. N. Willich (eds.), *Quo Vadis Medical Healing: Past Conceptions and New Approaches*. Springer. 29–40.

Prince, S. 2016. "The Peripatetic Hippocrates and Other Monists in the *Anonymus Londiniensis*." In Dean-Jones and Rosen (2016), 99–116.

Rawlings, H. R. 1975. *A Semantic Study of Prophasis to 400 B.C.* Steiner.

Regenbogen, O. 1931. "Eine Forschungsmethode antiker Naturwissenschaft." *Quellen und Studien zur Geschichte der Mathematik, Astronomie und Physik* 1: 131–182.

Reinhardt, K. 1916. *Parmenides und die Geschichte der griechischen Philosophie*. Cohen.

Rey, A. 1946. *La science dans l'antiquité*, vol. 4. Albin Michel.

Rochberg, F. 2004. *The Heavenly Writing: Divination, Horoscopy, and Astronomy in Mesopotamian Culture*. Cambridge University Press.

Roselli, A. 2016. "The Gynaecological and Nosological Treatises of the *Corpus Hippocraticum*: The Tip of an Iceberg." In G. Colesanti and L. Lulli (eds.), *Submerged Literature in Ancient Greek Culture*, vol. 2. De Gruyter. 187–203.

2018. "Nosology." In Pormann (2018), 180–199.

Rowe, C. 1999. "The Speech of Eryximachus in Plato's *Symposium*." In J. J. Cleary (ed.), *Traditions of Platonism*. Ashgate. 53–64.

Salles, R. (ed.). 2021. *Cosmology and Biology in Ancient Philosophy: From Thales to Avicenna*. Cambridge University Press.

Schibli, H. S. 1990. *Pherekydes of Syros*. Oxford University Press.

Schiefsky, M. J. 2005. *Hippocrates: On Ancient Medicine*. Brill.

Schluderer, L. R. 2018. "Imitating the Cosmos: The Role of Microcosm-Macrocosm Relationships in the Hippocratic Treatise *On Regimen*." *CQ* 68: 31–52.

Schöne, H. 1900. Review of Fredrich (1899). *Göttingische Gelehrte Anzeigen* 162: 654–662.

Schöner, E. 1964. *Das Viererschema in der antiken Humoralpathologie*. Steiner.

Scurlock, J. 1999. "Physician, Conjurer, Magician: A Tale of Two Healing Professionals." In T. Abusch and K. van der Toorn (eds.), *Mesopotamian Magic*. Styx. 69–79.

2014. *Sourcebook for Ancient Mesopotamian Medicine*. SBL Press.

Scurlock, J., and Andersen, B. R. 2005. *Diagnoses in Assyrian and Babylonian Medicine*. University of Illinois Press.

Shcherbakova, E. 2018. "The Paths of the Soul in the Pseudo-Hippocratic *De victu*." In C. Ferella and C. Breytenbach (eds.), *Paths of Knowledge: Interconnection(s) between Knowledge and Journey in the Greco-Roman World*. Edition Topoi. 75–91.

Sisko, J. E. 2006. "Cognitive Circuitry in the Pseudo-Hippocratic *Peri Diaites* and Plato's *Timaeus*." *Hermathena* 180: 5–17.

Sissa, G. 1990. *Greek Virginity*. Translated by A. Goldhammer. Harvard University Press.

Smith, W. 1867. *A Dictionary of Greek and Roman Biography and Mythology*, vol. 3. Little, Brown, and Co.

Smith, W. D. 1979. *The Hippocratic Tradition*. Cornell University Press.

1983. "Analytical and Catalogue Structure in the *Corpus Hippocraticum*." In Lasserre and Mudry (1983), 277–284.

1989. "Generic Form in *Epidemics* I to VII." In Baader and Winau (1989), 117–130.

1994. *Hippocrates*, vol. 7. Harvard University Press.

1999. "The Genuine Hippocrates and His Theory of Therapy." In I. Garofalo et al. (eds.), *Aspetti della terapia nel Corpus Hippocraticum*. Olschki. 107–118.

Spät, F. 1897. *Die geschichtliche Entwickelung der sogenannten Hippokratischen Medicin im Lichte der neuesten Forschung*. Karger.

Spoerri, W. 1983. "L'anthropogonie du Περὶ σαρκῶν (et Diodore 1,7,3s.)." In Lasserre and Mudry (1983), 57–70.

Squillace, G. 2012. *Menecrate di Siracusa*. Olms.

2015. "Menecrates of Syracuse: Reality and Fiction." In J. Althoff, S. Föllinger, and G. Wöhrle (eds.), *Antike Naturwissenschaften und ihre Rezeption*, vol. 25. Wissenschaftlicher Verlag Trier. 79–92.

2017. *Filistione di Locri*. Olms.

Steckerl, F. 1945. "Plato, Hippocrates, and the Menon Papyrus." *CP* 40: 166–180.

1958. *The Fragments of Praxagoras of Cos and His School*. Brill.

Stol, M. 1991–2. "Diagnosis and Therapy in Babylonian Medicine." *Jaarbericht Ex Oriente Lux* 32: 42–65.

Taylor, A. E. 1911. *Varia Socratica*. Parker.

Taylor, C. C. W. 1999. *The Atomists: Leucippus and Democritus*. University of Toronto Press.

Temkin, O. 1953. "Greek Medicine as Science and Craft." *Isis* 44: 213–225.

Thivel, A. 1981. *Cnide et Cos? Essai sur les doctrines médicales dans la Collection hippocratique*. Les Belles Lettres.

1983. "Médecine hippocratique et pensée ionienne, réponse aux objections et essai de synthèse." In Lasserre and Mudry (1983), 211–232.

1992. "¿Quienes son los adversarios de Pólibo en los dos primeros capítulos del tratado *De la Naturaleza del hombre*?" In López Férez (1992), 145–155.

Thomas, R. 1993. "Performance and Written Publication in Herodotus and the Sophistic Generation." In Kullmann and Althoff (1993), 225–244.

2000. *Herodotus in Context*. Cambridge University Press.

2003. "Prose Performance Texts: *Epideixis* and Written Publication in the Late Fifth and Early Fourth Centuries." In Yunis (2003), 162–188.

Touwaide, A. 2007. "Petron(as)." *BNP* 10: 874–875.

Trédé, M. 1992. *Kairos: l'à-propos et l'occasion. Le mot et la notion, d'Homère à la fin du IVe siècle avant J.-C.* Klincksieck.

van der Eijk, P. J. 1990. "Aristoteles über die Melancholie." *Mnemosyne* 43: 33–72.

1995. "Aristotle on 'Distinguished Physicians' and on the Medical Significance of Dreams." In P. J. van der Eijk, H. F. J. Horstmanshoff, and P. H. Schrijvers (eds.), *Ancient Medicine in Its Socio-Cultural Context*, vol. 2. Rodopi. 447–459.

2000–1. *Diocles of Carystus*. Brill.

2004. "Divination, Prognosis, Prophylaxis: The Hippocratic Work 'On Dreams' (*De victu* 4) and Its Near Eastern Background." In Horstmanshoff and Stol (2004), 187–218.

2005a. *Medicine and Philosophy in Classical Antiquity: Doctors and Philosophers on Nature, Soul, Health and Disease*. Cambridge University Press.

(ed.). 2005b. *Hippocrates in Context*. Brill.

2008. "The Role of Medicine in the Formation of Early Greek Philosophical Thought." In Curd and Graham (2008), 385–412.

2012. "Hippocrate aristotélicien." *Comptes rendus des séances de l'Académie des Inscriptions et Belles-Lettres* 4: 1501–1522.

2018. "Medicine in Early and Classical Greece." In Jones and Taub (2018), 293–315.

Vegetti, M. 1976. *Opere di Ippocrate*. Unione Tipografico Editrice Torinese.

1999. "Culpability, Responsibility, Cause: Philosophy, Historiography, and Medicine in the Fifth Century." In A. A. Long (ed.), *The Cambridge Companion to Early Greek Philosophy*. Cambridge University Press. 271–289.

Vlastos, G. 1947. "Equality and Justice in Early Greek Cosmologies." *CP* 42: 156–178.

von Staden, H. 1989. *Herophilus: The Art of Medicine in Early Alexandria.* Cambridge University Press.

1990. "Incurability and Hopelessness: The Hippocratic Corpus." In Potter, Maloney, and Desautels (1990), 75–112.

1998. "*Dynamis*: The Hippocratics and Plato." In K. J. Boudouris (ed.), *Philosophy and Medicine*, vol. 2. International Centre for Greek Philosophy and Culture. 262–277.

2002. "ὡς ἐπὶ τὸ πολύ: 'Hippocrates' between Generalization and Individualization." In A. Thivel and A. Zucker (eds.), *Le normal et le pathologique dans la Collection hippocratique*, vol. 1. Publications de la Faculté des Lettres, Arts et Sciences Humaines de Nice-Sophia Antipolis. 23–44.

Walshe, T. M. 2016. *Neurological Concepts in Ancient Greek Medicine.* Oxford University Press.

Wee, J. Z. (ed.). 2017. *The Comparable Body: Analogy and Metaphor in Ancient Mesopotamian, Egyptian, and Greco-Roman Medicine.* Brill.

Wellmann, M. 1901. *Die Fragmente der sikelischen Ärzte Akron, Philistion und des Diokles von Karystos.* Weidmann.

1926. "Hippokrates, des Thessalos Sohn." *Hermes* 61: 329–334.

1929. "Alkmaion von Kroton." *Archeion* 11: 156–169.

1930. "Die ps. hippokratische Schrift περὶ ἀρχαίης ἰητρικῆς." *Sudhoffs Archiv* 23: 299–305.

1933. "Die pseudo-hippokratische Schrift περὶ ἑβδομάδων." *Quellen und Studien zur Geschichte der Naturwissenschaft und Medizin* 4: 6–10.

Wenskus, O. 1983. "Vergleich und Beweis im *Hippokratischen Corpus*." In Lasserre and Mudry (1983), 393–406.

1995. "Ist die gegliederte Rede für *De carnibus* eine Form der sinnlichen Wahrnehmung?" *Rheinisches Museum für Philologie* 138: 129–133.

West, M. L. 1971. "The Cosmology of 'Hippocrates,' *De hebdomadibus*." *CQ* 21: 365–388.

2003a. *Greek Epic Fragments.* Harvard University Press.

2003b. *Homeric Hymns, Homeric Apocrypha, Lives of Homer.* Harvard University Press.

Westendorf, W. 1999. *Handbuch der altägyptischen Medizin.* Brill.

Weygoldt, G. P. 1882. "Die pseudo-hippokratische Schrift περὶ διαίτης." *Neue Jahrbücher für Philologie und Paedagogik* 125: 161–175.

Wilamowitz-Möllendorff, U. von. 1901. "Die hippokratische Schrift περὶ ἱρῆς νούσου." *Sitzungsberichte der Königlich Preußischen Akademie der Wissenschaften zu Berlin*: 2–23.

Willerding, F. 1914. *Studia hippocratica.* Officina Academica Dieterichiana.

Withington, E. T. 1928. *Hippocrates*, vol. 3. Harvard University Press.

Witt, M. 2018. "Fabio Calvo: Übersetzer, Herausgeber und Fälscher hippokratischer Schriften." *Sudhoffs Archiv* 102: 33–88.

Wittern, R. 1974. *Die hippokratische Schrift De morbis I.* Olms.

Yunis, H. (ed.). 2003. *Written Texts and the Rise of Literate Culture in Ancient Greece.* Cambridge University Press.

Zatta, C. 2019. *Interconnectedness: The Living World of the Early Greek Philosophers.* Second edition. Academia Verlag.

Zeller, E. 1862. *Die Philosophie der Griechen in ihrer geschichtlichen Entwicklung, II.2: Aristoteles und die alten Peripatetiker.* Second edition. Fues.

1892. *Die Philosophie der Griechen in ihrer geschichtlichen Entwicklung, I.2: Allgemeine Einleitung, Vorsokratische Philosophie.* Fifth edition. Reisland.

Zwinger, T. 1579. *Hippocratis ... viginti duo commentarii tabulis illustrati.* Episcopiorum opera atque impensa.

Index of Passages Discussed

General Index

Abas/Aias, 202
Acumenus, 38
acute diseases, 119, 149, 171
aer. See also *aither* versus *aer*
    material composition, 178–180, 184, 232, 257
    unhealthiness, 226, 247, 256, 260
aither
    and soul, 101, 226–227, 247–261
    divided into zones, 231, 233–234, 245
    divinity of, 178, 226, 247–261
    healthiness, 226, 256, 260
    material composition, 178–180, 184, 222
    versus *aer*, 178–181, 184, 226, 247, 256, 260
    versus earth, 178–181, 184, 222, 231, 255
akribeia, 90–91, 123–128, 131–134, 138, 143, 171, 216, 240–244
Alcidamas, 91
Alcmaeon, 7, 33, 35–36, 44, 46, 78, 262
allopathy, 76–79, 107, 120–121
analogy, 48, 101–102, 164–166, 247–249
    between patients, 140–147
    with coals, 227, 229
    with cooking, 105, 190
    with macrocosm, 11, 16, 184–189, 211–217, 230–235, 245–261
    with music, 46, 161, 256
    with plants, 94, 99–102
    with rivers, 26, 100
    with seasons, 31, 46–47, 71–72, 164
    with *technai*, 39, 86, 160–163, 172, 247
    with weather, 195
    with wine, 195
Anaxagoras, 28, 171
Anaximander, 28
Anaximenes, 85, 115, 251
animals versus humans, 61, 62, 166, 223–225, 230
anomalia, 30
Anonymus Londiniensis, 2, 18–37, 69, 92–104, 163, 207
anthropogony, 2, 150, 171, 176–205
Antiphon, 116, 172

antispasis, 236
aphorism, 142–144
apokrisis, 28, 35, 45–47, 51, 55, 70–71, 74, 76–77, 78–79, 113–115, 120, 145, 194–197, 210, 218, 226, 234, 243, 252, 260
Apollo, 171, 252, 253, 256
apoplexy, 20, 39, 113, 146
apotropaic gods, 253, 257, 260
arche
    of disease, 3, 23–24, 59, 76, 82, 106, 107, 118–120, 147–160, 193–197, 243
    of medicine, 9, 61
    of the body, 154
Archelaus, 172, 202, 208
Ariston, 18, 206
Aristophanes, 37, 91, 252, 255, 258
Aristotle
    and *Diseases of Unwed Girls*, 159
    and doxography, 18, 25, 26, 27, 99, 102, 218
    and *On Regimen*, 207, 210, 218
    on bile, 29
    on drying, 183
    on elements, 27, 178–179, 257
    on *epideixeis*, 88, 91
    on hot and cold, 26
    on medicine, 5, 87, 125, 142, 169, 171, 262
    on movement, 239
    on *perittomata*, 21
    on plants, 101–102
    on *pneuma*, 39, 224
    on Polybus, 69
    on the glutinous, 191
    similarity to cosmological doctors, 103
Asclepiades, 12
Asclepius, 131, 253, 258
āšipu versus *asû*, 130
astronomy, 46, 168, 231
Athenaeus of Attalia, 28
Athenaeus of Naucratis, 27, 57
autarkeia, 125, 212–217
Ayurveda, 8, 209

292

For EU product safety concerns, contact us at Calle de José Abascal, 56–1°,
28003 Madrid, Spain or eugpsr@cambridge.org.

www.ingramcontent.com/pod-product-compliance
Ingram Content Group UK Ltd.
Pitfield, Milton Keynes, MK11 3LW, UK
UKHW020307140625
459647UK00006B/76